QUALITATIVE METHODS IN PUBLIC HEALTH

QUALITATIVE METHODS IN PUBLIC HEALTH

A Field Guide for Applied Research

Second Edition

ELIZABETH E. TOLLEY
PRISCILLA R. ULIN
NATASHA MACK
ELIZABETH T. ROBINSON
STACEY M. SUCCOP

WILEY

First edition *Qualitative Methods in Public Health: A Field Guide for Applied Research* by Priscilla R. Ulin, Elizabeth T. Robinson, and Elizabeth E. Tolley © 2005

Published by Jossey-Bass A Wiley Brand One Montgomery Street, Suite 1000, San Francisco, CA 94104-4594—www.josseybass.com

Library of Congress Cataloging-in-Publication Data

Names: Tolley, Elizabeth E., author.

Title: Qualitative methods in public health : a field guide for applied research / Elizabeth E. Tolley [and four others].

Description: Second edition. | San Francisco, CA : Jossey-Bass & Pfeiffer Imprints, Wiley, [2016] | Series: Jossey-Bass public health | Revision of: Qualitative methods in public health / Priscilla R. Ulin, Elizabeth T. Robinson, Elizabeth E. Tolley. c2005. 1st. ed. | Includes bibliographical references and index.

Identifiers: LCCN 2015042723 (print) | LCCN 2015042794 (ebook) | ISBN 9781118834503 (paperback) | ISBN 9781118834671 (pdf) | ISBN 9781118834657 (epub)

Subjects: LCSH: Public health–Research–Methodology. | Qualitative research. | BISAC: MEDICAL / Public Health.

Classification: LCC RA440.85 .U43 2016 (print) | LCC RA440.85 (ebook) | DDC 362.1072/1–dc23

LC record available at http://lccn.loc.gov/2015042723

Cover Design: Wiley

Cover Image: ©Click Bestsellers/Shutterstock

Printed in the United States of America

SECOND EDITION

PB Printing SKY10048143_051823

Dedicated to Andy Pasternack—our Jossey-Bass editor whose vision and encouragement inspired the first edition of this book.

CONTENTS

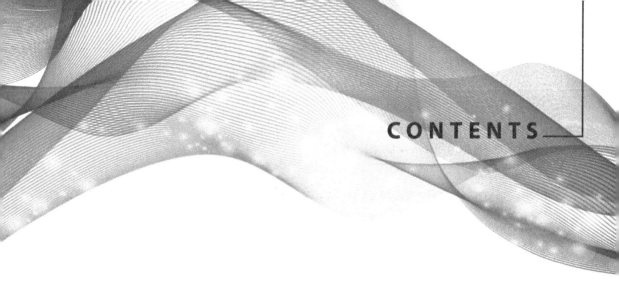

LIST OF FIGURES, TABLES, AND BOXES

Figures

Tables

Boxes

LIST OF CASE STUDIES

FOREWORD

For the past 10 years, I have taught an introductory course to master of public health (MPH) students using the first edition of *Qualitative Methods in Public Health: A Field Guide for Applied Research* (Ulin, Robinson, and Tolley, 2005). It has been an invaluable guide for students eager to understand how and why things work the way they do. The new edition continues that approach. It gives students a solid grounding in the methods of inquiry into the anatomy of a public health problem, teaching them to explore beneath the surface and discover why a problem exists as well as what the practitioner can do to address the problem.

Now in this new edition, examples have been updated and broadened to speak to greater diversity in the public health field. We see in the new material how the field is growing and how research methods have kept pace with new concepts and challenges. Qualitative research methods have found a footing in applied public health, with funding agencies now expecting to see many proposals incorporate a qualitative component in the development, implementation, or evaluation of public health interventions. The second edition takes the reader beyond evaluation of public health interventions and goes directly to research for change. Inequities in power and privilege must be addressed by actively seeking participation of neglected voices, such as women and minorities. Vivid illustrations show how research participants become potential change agents if they have been included in the conduct of the research. This is a bold new approach accompanied by research techniques for making it happen, including more emphasis on the value of mixed methods and on participatory design in which community members actually become partners in the research process.

Readers inexperienced in qualitative research will welcome the clear steps outlined in the chapter on methods, expanded in this edition. They will also discover the utility of mobile devices such as tablets for data collection and consider greater linkages between individual, organizational, and institutional behavior as well as more ambitious goals related to health systems strengthening, health security, human rights, and health equity. The new edition also places more emphasis on qualitative analysis software and on writing for journals, a discussion that seasoned researchers as well as students will find useful.

Given greater recognition today of what qualitative research methods can do to help us understand and solve public health challenges, this book will have a wide audience. Examples in the text cut across problems encountered in public health, community medicine, and social science practice in many parts of the world. Common to all of these is the need for practical, down-to-earth advice on how to apply the methods of qualitative research to real-world settings. Numerous case studies and examples throughout the text and in the appendices provide practical guidance on many aspects of research that conventional text books often neglect, such as developing consent forms, managing budgets, designing interview guides, working with field assistants, and training data collectors.

Taken as a whole, the book represents an accumulation of experience and guidance from researchers who have been using these methods in applied public health work in global and domestic settings for many years. They share their wisdom and insight with readers, helping both to raise excitement about the possibilities these methods offer, and to reassure new researchers who may be considering qualitative methods for the first time.

Suzanne Maman, MHS, PhD
University of North Carolina at Chapel Hill

Reference

Ulin, P. R., Robinson, E. T., & Tolley, E. E. (2005). Qualitative Methods in Public Health: A Field Guide for Applied Research. 1st ed. San Francisco, CA: Jossey-Bass.

ACKNOWLEDGMENTS

Many individuals had a hand in bringing this second edition of *Qualitative Methods in Public Health* from plan to press.

There is also history to acknowledge, for a second edition cannot happen without a first edition. We reiterate our thanks to those who helped make that first edition a reality: those at the U.S. Agency for International Development (USAID), who provided both financial support and substantive guidance on the content of the guide, especially Sarah Harbison and the late Erin T. McNeill. We also thank other individuals at FHI 360 (then Family Health International)—particularly Cynthia Woodsong, as well as colleagues at the World Health Organization, the Population Council, and organizations beyond who contributed their assistance, insight, materials, and support. FHI 360 senior management and Cynthia Geary, formerly of FHI 360, saw us through both editions of this book; to them we are further indebted.

We also acknowledge the many program and research staff members at FHI 360 who have shared research materials and stories about what has worked well and not so well when conducting qualitative research in the field. In particular, we offer special thanks to Kathleen MacQueen for contributing the content on qualitative data analysis software. We also thank the contributors of the case studies, a new feature of this second edition: Jean Baker, Aurelie Brunie, Christine Demmelmaier, Natalie Eley, Emily Evens, Cindy Geary, Nemat Hajeebhoy, Michele Lanham, Kathleen MacQueen, Dominick Shattuck, Rose Wilcher, Christina Wong, and Susan Zimicki. Many thanks also to Paul Feldblum, Michele Lanham, Marguerite Marlow, Emily Namey, the Palladium Group, Sonke Gender Justice, and Christina Wong for their contributions to the appendices. We also thank Denise Todloski at the MEASURE

Evaluation project at the University of North Carolina at Chapel Hill for designing many of the graphics in this edition.

We owe a debt of gratitude to Allison Pack, Frances McVay, Seth Zisette, and Amy Mills for assisting us with the complex task of attending to the completeness, accuracy, and organization of the references. As for reviewers both known to us (e.g., Marga Eichleay and Allison Pack for Chapter 6) and anonymous, their feedback has helped us to rethink, reword, and reorganize each of the chapters for the betterment of the entire book. And of course, without the support and excellence of Seth Schwartz, Melinda Noack, and Maria Sunny of Wiley, our collective efforts would never have made it to print.

Last, we thank our families for serving as sounding boards and comic relief throughout the process: Mark, Elise, and Kyle Healy; Don and Marjorie Ulin; Solana Mack and Zorro; and Alan Dehmer.

ABOUT THE AUTHORS

Elizabeth (Betsy) E. Tolley is a senior scientist and Director of the Social and Behavioral Health Sciences division of FHI 360. Since joining Family Health International (now FHI 360) in 1994, Betsy has used qualitative and mixed-methods research to examine acceptability and use of various sexual health, contraceptive, and reproductive behaviors, including new technologies such as microbicides or development of a longer-acting injectable contraceptive, and existing technologies like implants and intra-uterine devices (IUD). An important focus of recent research has been on microbicide acceptability, including identification and measurement of factors that contribute to initiation and sustained use of microbicides in various populations, from Tanzanian adolescents to married women in India or female sex workers in Benin. For example, she conducted mixed-method research in parallel to a phase two microbicide safety trial to first develop scales (e.g., HIV risk perception, couple sexual communication, acceptability of product attributes) and then longitudinally assess their influence on consistent use. More recently, she applied her understanding of how social and sexual contexts shape acceptability in order to develop and test messages and materials for potential microbicide introduction initiatives in Kenya. Other research topics have included assessment of infant feeding practices, as well as adolescent abortion. Betsy brings to FHI experience in the training and use of qualitative research methods, and she is especially interested in exploring ways to make qualitative analysis more systematic and rigorous and to make qualitative and quantitative approaches more compatible. She has a PhD in health behavior from the Gillings School of Public Health, University of North Carolina at Chapel Hill, and an MA in international development from the Nitze School of International Studies, The Johns Hopkins University. Betsy has over 25 years of experience living and working in developing countries, including various countries in West and North Africa, eastern Africa, and India.

Priscilla R. Ulin is retired from Family Health International (now FHI 360), where she was senior research scientist in the Social and Behavioral Sciences division and, through her work in the early days of the AIDS epidemic, she helped establish the organization's qualitative research program. Trained in quantitative social research, she discovered the power of qualitative methods while studying maternal and child health decision making in Botswana in the early 1970s. From then on in her professional career, she combined quantitative and qualitative techniques in research, teaching, and technical assistance in sexual, reproductive, and maternal and child heath in the United States and developing countries. As a medical sociologist, she focused primarily on social change and utilization of health care systems, with an emphasis on the influence of family and community in sexual and reproductive health decision making, and on community participation in research. Dr. Ulin worked in Haiti under the auspices of FHI's USAID-funded AIDSTECH Project, where she pioneered the use of qualitative methods to explore women's sense of vulnerability in the AIDS epidemic. She was deputy director of FHI's Women's Studies Project, a five-year, multinational program of social and behavioral science research, both qualitative and quantitative, on the consequences of family planning for women's lives. She has directed research in sub-Saharan Africa on women's strategies to control their fertility, on the impact of family planning on women's participation in economic development, and on the influence of family on contraceptive decisions. Dr. Ulin received a master's degree in nursing from Yale University and a PhD in sociology from the University of Massachusetts-Amherst.

Natasha Mack is a researcher in the Social and Behavioral Health Sciences division at FHI 360. Originally trained as a linguistic and cultural anthropologist, she has 15 years of experience in qualitative research, as well as scientific writing and editing. Since joining Family Health International (now FHI 360) in 2004, she has conducted qualitative studies in HIV prevention and other public health areas, including studies on the female condom, pre-exposure prophylaxis for HIV prevention, translation issues in informed consent documents, and most recently infant and young child feeding practices. Her work has included sociobehavioral research components of clinical trials as well as standalone qualitative studies in sub-Saharan Africa and Latin America. Writing has been the mainstay of her tenure at FHI 360. This has included a field manual of qualitative methods, funding proposals, research protocols, FAQs and informational briefs, standard operating procedures, executive summaries, presentations, book chapters, and write-up of study results in final reports and peer-reviewed publications. She has also mentored staff in writing peer-reviewed articles. Dr. Mack speaks French and Spanish and has experience in French- and Spanish-to-English translation. She holds a BA (1993) in comparative area studies and Spanish from Duke University. She earned her MA (1997) and PhD (2004) in linguistic and cultural anthropology from the University of Arizona in Tucson.

Elizabeth T. Robinson is the senior advisor for communications at the University of North Carolina at Chapel Hill's $180 million MEASURE Evaluation project, funded by USAID and PEPFAR. She is a communications professional with more than 25 years of experience managing strategic communication, research dissemination, and knowledge management programs for international public health organizations. Prior to joining UNC, Ms. Robinson served as director for knowledge management for the Health Policy Project at Futures Group in Washington, DC, and she previously held several senior-level communication positions at Family Health International (now FHI 360), including director of information programs. Her work experience includes management of large editorial departments, multilingual web development, and writing on topics ranging from Ebola and health systems strengthening to HIV and gender. She has taught scientific paper writing to researchers at the National Institutes of Health, the Pasteur Institute, medical schools, and nongovernmental organizations, and she has worked as a consultant for the Johns Hopkins Bloomberg School of Public Health, the World Health Organization, the University of the Witwatersrand, and elsewhere. She is lead author of the *Communications Handbook for Clinical Trials: Strategies, Tips, and Tools to Manage Controversy, Convey Your Message, and Disseminate Results;* she was the principal communications advisor to the CAPRISA 004 microbicide trial; and she is the author of several qualitative studies on health communications. Ms. Robinson has devoted much of her professional life to providing technical assistance in communications to health organizations, research institutions, and sectoral ministries in Africa, Asia, and Latin America. Early in her career, she worked as a journalist in metropolitan New York; Washington, DC; North Africa; and Francophone West Africa. Ms. Robinson received a master's degree from the Columbia University Graduate School of Journalism and held a fellowship in the Columbia University School of International and Public Affairs.

Stacey M. Succop is a research associate in the Scientific Affairs department at FHI 360. Ms. Succop has been working in global health and development since 2003, and she joined FHI 360 in 2007. While at FHI 360, Ms. Succop spent more than six years working in the social and behavioral health sciences division, building her experience in study management and logistics, quantitative and qualitative data analysis, research proposal and protocol development, study team training, and scientific writing. She also facilitated relationships and communications for large, multicountry teams and was responsible for developing, coordinating, and monitoring work plans, timelines, and budgets for several simultaneous studies and projects. She worked on research studies and projects covering a wide variety of topics such as HIV prevention, mobile health interventions, family planning, and reproductive health, all in global settings. Currently, Ms. Succop serves as a scientific and technical reviewer for health, population, and nutrition-related protocols developed by staff across the organization. She provides guidance and technical support to research teams related to study design, analysis, and implementation. Ms. Succop holds a BA from Duke University; a master's degree in public health (MPH) in health behavior and health education from the University of North Carolina at Chapel Hill, Gillings School of Public Health, with a certificate in global health and a project management professional (PMP) certification.

QUALITATIVE METHODS IN PUBLIC HEALTH

CHAPTER 1

INVITATION TO EXPLORE

OBJECTIVES:

- To introduce researchers to qualitative methods in public health research, including those whose training and experience may be predominantly in quantitative methods
- To describe the basic characteristics of a qualitative research approach
- To show how qualitative methods can shed new light on complex questions in public health
- To highlight the aspects of qualitative research methodology presented in this book, including content new to this second edition

WHY DO SOME PROGRAMS succeed and others fail? Why are screening programs underused? Why does chronic disease go untreated? Why do countless couples know how to protect themselves from sexually transmitted infection but do not do so? How does a community mobilize itself to solve a persistent health problem? Questions like these may be all too familiar to readers of this field guide—public health practitioners, researchers, and program planners, many of whom have worked for years to protect health and prevent disease in highly vulnerable populations.

Advances in the biomedical and population sciences have brought the means to better health within reach of people around the world. Yet, evidence of escalating disease and inadequate health systems and resources in many countries tell us that there is still much we do not know. How do women and men understand and actually use the technical information they receive to make critical decisions that affect their lives and their children's lives? By opening windows on cultural understandings of health and disease, methods of qualitative research can help us comprehend some of these old problems in new ways.

Our Purpose

The purpose of this book is to make the methods of **qualitative** science more accessible to researchers and practitioners challenged by problems that affect the public's health. Qualitative design can help us understand the underlying behaviors, attitudes, and perceptions that determine health outcomes; it can identify the social, programmatic, and structural impediments to use of existing services; and it can shed light on how to design new development interventions so they align with the socioeconomic realities of their intended beneficiaries and therefore have a greater potential for success.

We write not only for the qualitative researcher but also for applied social scientists, epidemiologists, health providers, health educators, program managers, and others whose training and experience may be predominantly in **quantitative** methods. Our readers will be students as well as professionals looking for ways to probe more deeply the whys and hows of questions they may partially have answered in terms of how much and how many. They will want to know what qualitative methods can offer to improve their practice or strengthen their research findings. And many of our readers will be training others to ask the same kinds of questions, to listen, and to observe.

Numerous disciplines have contributed to the phenomenal growth of public health research and practice. Sociology, anthropology, psychology, economics, demography, environmental science, medical geography, medicine, and nursing, among others, have brought their unique perspectives and methods to a multidisciplinary understanding of health and wellness. Parallel advances in these disciplines have resulted in different ways of conceptualizing and addressing issues as diverse as health decision making, health promotion, health systems strengthening, child survival, compliance, substance abuse, adolescent sexuality, domestic violence, and gender relations. Similar progress in service delivery research and evaluation has given us a broader understanding of providers' knowledge and values, client–provider communication, and issues related to the accessibility and quality of health care for populations at risk.

Much of this work has focused on objective questions, such as numbers of births, patterns of illegal drug use, trends in disease prevalence, and numerous factors that predict health behavioral outcomes. Research designs traditionally have been quantitative, describing measurable phenomena, projecting trends, and sometimes discovering causal relationships. Psychological research in health behavior has developed primarily from a quantitative perspective, contributing useful rating scales and behavioral indicators, along with case study methods and tools for **observation**. Anthropologists and qualitative sociologists have approached some of the same problems from different perspectives, focusing on cultural norms and relationships that influence how people interact and act on everyday experiences (Bernard, 1995; Knodel, 1997). Their methods rely primarily on techniques of observation, participation, guided discussion, in-depth interviewing, life histories, and secondary analysis of documentary data. Emerging methods increasingly used in qualitative research include network analysis and geo-health mapping, using innovative technologies such as data visualization applications and mobile data collection tools.

To conduct rigorous research, investigators must use an appropriate study design, data collection methods, and analytic procedures. Yet there is much overlap among different disciplinary approaches. Quantitative researchers at times use qualitative methods to guide a sampling design or to develop a sensitive data collection tool. Anthropologists and qualitative sociologists turn to quantitative methods when they want to describe a population or measure some tendency they may have observed qualitatively. Quantitative research with representative samples can produce hard, factual, reliable outcome data that usually are generalizable to wider populations (Steckler, McLeroy, Goodman, Bird, & McCormick, 1992). But most quantitative studies lack contextual detail and reflect a limited range of responses (Carey, 1993). On the other hand, qualitative methods elicit rich, contextual data, but their small samples and flexible design usually are not appropriate if the study objective is to describe larger populations with statistical accuracy (Patton, 2002). As a result, researchers have increasingly adopted creative new ways to combine techniques in a research design (Creswell, Klassen, Plano Clark, & Smith, 2011; Teddlie & Tashakkori, 2009), letting the strengths of one method compensate for the limitations of another to yield a more powerful methodology.

We have written this guide not to promote one methodology over another, but because many quantitatively trained health professionals, policymakers, and researchers are looking for ways to expand their methodological options with new tools for answering difficult questions.

In searching the literature on qualitative research, we found it divided between manuals that summarize specific techniques for designing and conducting health-related studies (Campbell, 1999; Hudelson, 1994; Yoddumnern, Mahidon, & Sangkhom, 1993) and more comprehensive texts for general academic audiences (Denzin & Lincoln, 2005, 2011; Guest, Namey, & Mitchell, 2012; Patton, 2002; Rossman & Rallis, 1998). Missing from most manuals was a theoretical basis for qualitative decisions, and few texts included strategies to address practical health research issues and problems that arise in the field. Nor did we find clear guidelines for dealing with the large volume of transcripts that qualitative data collection on sensitive topics often generates. Another gap in the literature was the lack of direction for writing and disseminating qualitative results. Our intent, therefore, is to show first how qualitative methods can shed new light on perplexing questions and, second, to provide basic skills to design, conduct, and disseminate the research.

This volume presents practical strategies and methods for using qualitative research, along with the basic logic and rationale for qualitative research decisions. The guide makes researchers aware of the complexities, advantages, and limitations of qualitative research. Its eight chapters cover a wide range of topics and guide readers through every phase of research—from defining the language and logic of qualitative research, to study design, to the collection, analysis, interpretation, reporting, and dissemination of data.

What Is Qualitative Research?

A challenge to the author of any book on qualitative research is to answer the common sense question: What is it? Although there is no short, comprehensive definition, the unique organizing framework is a theoretical and methodological focus on complex relations between (1) personal and social meanings, (2) individual and cultural practices, and (3) the material environment or context. Similarly, there is no universal blueprint for doing qualitative research, but some basic concepts and principles, described next and summarized in Box 1.1, are common in most qualitative research approaches.

Qualitative research is systematic discovery. Its purpose is to generate knowledge of social events and processes by understanding what they mean to people, exploring and documenting how people interact with each other and how they interpret and interact with the world around them. It also seeks to elucidate patterns of shared understanding and variability in those patterns.

Qualitative researchers value natural settings where the researcher can better understand people's lived experiences. The natural context of people's lives is a critical component of qualitative design because it influences the perspectives, experiences, and actions of participants in the study. It is the interpersonal and sociocultural fabric that shapes meanings and actions.

Many problems central to public health research and practice are deeply embedded in their cultural contexts. People in communities confront decisions and challenges that are conditioned by membership in multiple social groups: whether to vaccinate children, how to prevent obesity, where to go for help in times of illness, and how to give young people the skills and confidence they will need for healthy adulthood. Contradictions and competing priorities can make many seemingly commonplace decisions difficult: Spend money on prescription drugs, or

BOX 1.1 CHARACTERISTICS OF QUALITATIVE RESEARCH

- Explores and discovers
- Seeks depth of understanding
- Views social phenomena holistically
- Provides insight into the meanings of decisions and actions
- Asks why, how, and under what circumstance things occur
- Uses interpretive and other open-ended methods
- Is iterative rather than fixed
- Is emergent rather than prestructured
- Involves respondents as active participants rather than as subjects
- Defines the investigator as an instrument in the research process

save for retirement? Protect oneself from sexually transmitted infection and risk losing the attention and economic support of a sexual partner, or accept the risk of disease? Running through the fabric of economic, sexual, and reproductive lives are the pervasive influences of gender and power, themes that resonate in the voices of the women and men in our research.

Researchers express qualitative data in participants' words, in images, and sometimes in numbers. Language, both verbal and nonverbal, has symbolic meaning; an expression may mean one thing to the study participant and a different thing to the interviewer. Qualitative researchers listen carefully to language as participants tell about their experiences without the constraints of externally imposed structure. When we refer to raw data as narrative, we mean participants relating their ideas and experiences in ways that can offer insight into important research concepts and questions.

The fact that people differ in the ways they interpret—and consequently act on—ordinary situations has profound implications for health research. If it is true that what people define as real is real in its consequences (Thomas & Thomas, 1928), then applied behavioral research in public health must have the capacity to uncover multiple perspectives and understand their implications for health decision making. Qualitative researchers have taken this charge seriously, with the result that we now have at our disposal powerful techniques for "hearing data" (Rubin & Rubin, 1995, p. 12), that is, listening to what people are saying about their own lives in their own words.

The qualitative research process is flexible, emergent, and iterative. The study design is never wholly fixed, but enables an interplay between data collection and discovery. Qualitative studies usually include an iterative design, meaning that findings emerge continuously. The investigator is always in touch with the research process, observing how participants respond to the topic and examining data for fresh insights that might lead to altering a technique, modifying questions, or changing direction to pursue new leads. Analysis does not wait until all the data are collected; it begins in the field.

Reflexivity—the researcher's critical self-awareness—is a vital process of questioning and observing oneself while at the same time listening to and observing the participant.

With their emphasis on egalitarian relationships, feminist and transformative methodologies have contributed greatly to this point. In contrast to the detachment required in many quantitative studies, the observer is a vital component of the qualitative research process in two ways. First, the researcher is in partnership with the participant, working together to explore themes and find answers. Second, he or she is also a key research instrument, not only recording information but at the same time influencing how it is elicited. Self-examination, documented with other observations in the field notes, is part of the iterative process of interpretation and revision that moves the data collection toward its goal.

Qualitative researchers know that there are always at least two key players: the participant who contributes the information and the researcher who, as learner and co-interpreter, guides the process toward the understanding that both seek to articulate. Together they form a partnership for exploring different social understandings of reality. Creating a qualitative research partnership requires a high level of skill. It also carries with it profound ethical obligations because the relationship is based on trust and mutual understanding of a common goal.

Quantitative or Qualitative?

What is social reality, and how do we explain it? The question has stirred debate and polarized social science research between quantitative and qualitative methods. The issue of whether a given approach is appropriate centers on "the capacity of the data, as collected by one method or the other, to describe, understand, and explain social phenomena" (Pedersen, 1992, p. 43). Depending on their academic training and theoretical orientation, researchers often have strong opinions about the relative merits of qualitative and quantitative approaches (Guest, 2013). Theoretical purists argue that because each methodology reflects a different understanding of research, human behavior, and the nature of social life, the two are incompatible (Greenhalgh, 1997). A purist would choose one or the other approach on the principle that mixing quantitative and qualitative methods violates the assumptions on which either framework is constructed (Carey, 1993; Patton, 1990). The debate between those who espouse use of either particular approach revolves around fundamental questions such as, "what is health and disease, who decides what are important research questions, and whose 'truth' is the 'real truth'?" (Meetoo & Temple 2003, p. 6).

Our position, like that of many quantitative and qualitative researchers today, chooses pragmatism over "one-sided paradigm allegiance" (Patton, 1990, p. 38). Our purpose in presenting more than one theoretical framework is to help readers understand similarities and differences, strengths and limitations, and the contribution that each can make to applied health research. The methods that emerge from these frameworks "offer a distinct set of strengths and limitations that are markedly different but potentially complementary when combined in a mixed-method research design" (Wolff, Knodel, & Sittitrai, 1991, p. 2).

Throughout this book, we advocate methodological appropriateness—using theory and related methods to make reasoned decisions "appropriate to the purpose of the study, the questions being investigated, and the resources available" (Patton, 1990, p. 39).

Application of Research to Action

We have chosen to focus on applied research because it informs action and enhances decision making on practical issues, unlike basic research, which is conducted to generate theory and produces knowledge for its own end. Although applied research can add immeasurably to our understanding of human, institutional, and systems behavior, its outcomes are "judged by their effectiveness in helping policymakers, practitioners, and the participants themselves make decisions and act to improve the human condition" (Rossman & Rallis, 1998, p. 6). Most well-designed qualitative studies have elements of both the basic and the applied, because rigorous applied research has a theoretical base and scholars ground their theory in concrete findings. Unfortunately, however, too many examples of hastily constructed qualitative research attempt to apply faulty findings to policy or program issues. Such studies often have inadequate theoretical bases or use data collection techniques that are inappropriate to the purpose of the research. These misguided efforts do not constitute science and seldom contribute significantly to solutions to problems.

At least three important developments are fueling the demand for qualitative expertise in both domestic and international health arenas:

1. Advances in cross-cultural understanding of health and health-related behavior
2. Global health patterns
3. Increased awareness of issues in human rights and health equity, particularly implications for access to health care services by the underserved, including the poor and ethnic and sexual minorities

Advances in Cross-Cultural Understanding of Health and Health-Related Behavior

Sophisticated quantitative methods have produced an extensive base of knowledge for understanding such phenomena as population growth, disease patterns, and many aspects of human behavior that are determinants of health and sickness. But each new finding leads to more questions and new research problems that often require a different approach to data collection and analysis. For example, knowing the number of tuberculosis cases in a given region leads us to ask why infection is still high in some populations. Or with the wide availability of primary health care services, we must ask why so many potentially serious diseases continue to go undetected in their early stages. Qualitative methods are adding a new dimension to the ongoing search for answers to these and other complex questions.

Designs for quantitative surveys are increasingly incorporating qualitative techniques in an effort to improve the validity of interview tools through better understanding of the language and perspectives of study populations (see Case Study 1 in Appendix 1). Hearing participants' customary language for sexual issues helps the survey researcher compose standardized items in familiar words or prestructured response categories from actual experience. Program planners too are finding that participation of affected groups in collecting qualitative data and analyzing local problems leads to more relevant programs and a greater sense of community ownership. In eastern North Carolina, for example, a study to investigate the potential impact of industrial swine operations on decreased health and quality of life employed trained interviewers in a household survey of three rural communities. A community resident accompanied each interviewer to explain the purpose and importance of the survey, resulting in a participation rate of 86% (Wing & Wolf, 2000).

At the same time, technological innovations, such as analytic tools based on geographic information systems (GIS), are fueling rapid changes in the range of perspectives that qualitative research can explore. Use of new information, communication, and technology tools for data collection, such as mobile phones and tablets, are fueling creative approaches to implementing study designs, such as participatory action research, that "prioritize flexibility and accessibility in the processes and products of our inquiry" (Cope & Elwood, 2009, p. 171).

Global Health Patterns

Demographic and health statistics speak to the urgent need for solutions to public health problems everywhere. Growing health disparities between rich and poor countries, as well as between urban and rural areas of many countries, highlight different research needs. In an Ebola outbreak, for example, the strength or weakness of a country's health system and deeply rooted cultural practices for burial of the dead, if not understood and addressed, can contribute to a pandemic, endangering global health security (West African Health Organization [WAHO], 2015). In the United States, heart disease, cancer, respiratory diseases, and stroke account for more than half of total annual deaths (Hoyert & Xu, 2012), and many instances of these health issues are related to tobacco use, poor diet, physical inactivity, and alcohol consumption. In the poorest areas of the world, preventable and treatable diseases, such as diarrhea, measles, and malaria, take a heavy toll on human life. In Africa alone, more than 2.3 million people die from vaccine-preventable diseases annually (Carr, 2004). Complications of pregnancy, childbirth, and unsafe abortion claim the lives of over 500,000 women every year, 99% of them in developing countries (World Health Organization [WHO], 2014). Globally, 15% of all women living with HIV (aged 15 years and older) are 15 to 24 years old; of these, 80% live in sub-Saharan. (Joint United Nations Programme on HIV/AIDS [UNAIDS], 2014). Moreover, many health experts are only just beginning to acknowledge the full impact of social problems such as gender-based violence, the feminization of poverty, homelessness and mental illness, economic crises, persistent regional conflict, and refugee resettlement—all play out in a climate of increasing globalization and overburdened resources.

This book illustrates the principles of qualitative research in the context of global health, with reference to social and behavioral determinants of many preventable health problems. Qualitative research is not a solution but rather a route to better understanding of the human condition, with the hope of contributing to more rational decision making for improved health program effectiveness and impact. Given the magnitude of the problems we face, we must use all the tools at our disposal, and use them well.

Increased Awareness of Issues in Human Rights

A growing awareness of the impact of social environment on health has focused attention on the interplay among population and development, human rights, and gender. If we hope to address pressing needs for improved health and social development, we urgently need better understanding of the complexities of human and institutional behavior. The desire to probe interrelationships among, for example, health decisions, human rights, gender equity, equality, and empowerment calls for new ways to address old, intractable questions. Investigators from the fields of women's studies and applied disciplines in the social sciences continue to search for better understanding of key developmental processes such as gender socialization and role awareness, raising new questions that invite a more qualitative approach to research.

Concern for the status of women is a critical element in development policy, but human rights and the ethics of inclusion add another dimension. We are seeing a gradual shift of priorities toward new goals for community participation, human rights advocacy, gender equity, and health equity broadly defined (United Nations Human Rights, 2008). These trends have strengthened research outcomes by influencing how research is conceptualized and conducted. Our research questions are more likely now to include attention to gender relations in health decision making and to status and power as significant factors in the study of health service delivery. Qualitative methods enable researchers to explore more fully the nature and consequences of gender identities and relations not only in reproductive health but also, for example, in access to and use of malaria prevention and treatment services (Kenya Ministry of Health, 2015). As they become more aware of the powerful role of status in everyday life, researchers themselves are increasingly adopting participatory, transformative approaches to research that are consistent with qualitative work. This shift is creating new collaborative relationships with study participants and heightened awareness of the researcher's ethical responsibility in the data collection partnership.

Getting Started

Like the first edition, this second edition takes you step-by-step through the qualitative research process from its theoretical base to its application in public health problems, to dissemination of findings for program and policy change. Key elements in the process are interaction and interpretation. By interaction, we mean broadly the art and science of asking, observing, listening, reflecting, and probing—always with the purpose of engaging people in meaningful dialogue. We advocate qualitative techniques, independent of or in association with quantitative methodology, as a way of discovering how people act and interact in the familiar contexts of their lives. Our purpose is to share what we have learned with other researchers who are similarly committed to systematic analysis to inform policy and program development for healthier and more empowered populations.

The chapters that follow build the qualitative process: understanding, designing, implementing, and using methods to answer questions and solve problems that challenge workers in public health.

Chapter 2, The Language and Logic of Qualitative Research, begins with a brief overview of the theoretical basis for qualitative research, emphasizing the practical application of theory to research design and analysis. To help the reader locate qualitative research in the theoretical universe, we review three important paradigms, or theoretical frameworks, that have guided methodological decisions in social and behavioral health research. We emphasize the complementarity of these frameworks and the added value of linking them in well-coordinated designs to solve complex problems. Chapter 2 also presents examples of substantive theories and conceptual models that public health researchers may use to guide their research designs or synthesize study findings. We conclude Chapter 2 with a discussion of standards for judging the scientific rigor of qualitative research. We maintain that different assumptions and purposes make the criteria for evaluating quality in quantitative and qualitative studies analogous but not interchangeable.

In Chapter 3, Designing the Study, we present and discuss important design questions in a sequence that follows a typical research proposal. Basic steps move from defining the area of inquiry and the purpose and problem of the research to analyzing, writing, and disseminating the findings. We also discuss conceptual frameworks that link concepts and relationships to qualitative data collection strategies. We then review aspects of informed consent that are particularly relevant to qualitative studies, including the ethical responsibility of the researcher in an open-ended interview or discussion.

To underscore the point that combining qualitative and quantitative methods can increase the power of the design and result in a more comprehensive understanding of the topic of study, we present practical strategies and resources for mixed-method design.

Chapter 4, Collecting Qualitative Data: The Science and the Art, describes the principal methods of data collection. We identify three fundamental methods—observation, in-depth interviewing, and focus group discussion. Observation is further divided into nonreactive (including documentary research) and participant observation. Techniques of in-depth interviewing and focus group discussion are presented in detail, along with participatory research methods and other selected structured qualitative approaches: freelisting and pile sorts, photo narrative, storytelling, network analysis, and body mapping. We recommend a semi-structured approach to data collection and discuss the construction and use of topic guides.

In Chapter 5, Logistics in the Field, we focus on implementation. This chapter contains practical recommendations for introducing a study; building a research team; working with stakeholders and policymakers; selecting and training data collectors; developing field materials; and recording, transcribing, and translating data.

Chapter 6, Qualitative Data Analysis, is a comprehensive overview in which the reader learns how to process and interpret text by working through five interrelated steps. We draw on a single case study to provide concrete examples of how to read, code, display, reduce, and interpret qualitative data. Included in this discussion are guidelines for analysis of data in mixed-method studies. We then detail the concept of rigor in qualitative studies, showing how qualitative concepts analogous to validity and reliability can be used to judge the trustworthiness of the findings. In this chapter, we also emphasize the importance of selecting appropriate software for computer text analysis, and we summarize some of the distinguishing features of several programs in common use.

Chapter 7, Disseminating Qualitative Research, outlines ways to effectively disseminate and promote the use of results. We suggest some possible outcome indicators for dissemination and use of study findings and challenge researchers to reconsider their roles in planning and implementing dissemination.

Chapter 8, Putting It Into Words: Reporting Qualitative Research Results in Scientific Journals and Reports, discusses the steps in writing up qualitative study findings. These steps incorporate ethical norms that govern how we present results, integrate thematic ideas into a meaningful narrative, determine our audiences, and select a presentation format that is both appropriate to the study methods and relevant to potential readers. The chapter offers practical advice on how to organize qualitative findings in articles for peer-reviewed journals as well as written reports, how to report combined qualitative and quantitative results, and considerations for enhancing the credibility and communicability of qualitative writing. We include criteria that external reviewers commonly use to evaluate journal manuscripts, discuss authorship issues, and provide suggestions for the submission process.

One of our objectives in writing this field guide is simply to share with readers the rewards and frustrations of doing qualitative research. Therefore, we offer numerous examples from our own research and from the practical experiences of others who already have embarked on this journey. In Appendix 1 you will find short case studies, based on qualitative or mixed-methods research. They provide real-life examples of how different researchers have designed studies to address pressing public health problems, including decisions they have made about theory, data collection methods, data sources, and dissemination approaches, and what they have learned in the process.

Comments about this book are invited, and they can be sent to publichealth@wiley.com.

Key Terms

1. **Qualitative:** An approach to research that seeks to understand the complex relationships between personal and social meanings, individual and cultural practices, and the material environment or context. Preference is given to textual or other non-numeric data.
2. **Quantitative:** An approach to research that seeks to predict, describe, and/or explain observable phenomena using mathematical and/or statistical techniques.
3. **Iterative design:** A nonlinear research approach in which data collection and analysis may occur in parallel, or where preliminary findings may lead to modifications in data collection approaches.
4. **Observation:** A range of data collection methods that rely on observing, as well as listening or use of other senses, to describe social interactions within their social and physical contexts.
5. **Reflexivity:** In qualitative research, recognition that the researcher both influences and is influenced by the research process. A researcher's questions, participants' responses, and the meaning that is constructed from these exchanges will be influenced by the background and prior experiences of those engaged in the research process.

Review Questions

1. What are the key characteristics of qualitative research, and how does it differ from quantitative research?
2. Which trends in health are spurring the demand for use of qualitative approaches?
3. Why is reflexivity an essential aspect of qualitative research?

References

Bernard, H. R. (1995). *Research methods in anthropology: Qualitative and quantitative approaches*. Thousand Oaks, CA: Sage.

Campbell, O. M. R. (1999). *Social science methods for research on reproductive health*. Geneva, Switzerland: World Health Organization.

Carey, J. W. (1993). Linking qualitative and quantitative methods: Integrating cultural factors into public health. *Qualitative Health Research, 3*(3), 298–318. doi:10.1177/104973239300300303

Carr, D. (2004). *Improving the health of the world's poorest people*. Health Bulletin 1. Washington, DC: Population Reference Bureau.

Cope, M., & Elwood, S. (2009). Conclusion: For qualitative GIS. In M. Cope & S. Elwood (Eds.), *Qualitative GIS: A mixed methods approach*. London, UK: Sage. doi: http://dx.doi.org/10.4135/9780857024541.d16

Creswell, J. W., Klassen, A. C., Plano Clark, V. L., & Smith, K. C. for the Office of Behavioral and Social Sciences Research. (2011). *Best practices for mixed methods research in the health sciences*. Bethesda, MD: National Institutes of Health. Available at http://obssr.od.nih.gov/mixed_methods_research

Denzin N. K., & Lincoln, Y. S. (2000). *Handbook of qualitative research*. Thousand Oaks, CA: Sage.

Denzin N. K., & Lincoln, Y. S. (2005). *The Sage handbook of qualitative research* (3rd ed.). Thousand Oaks, CA: Sage.

Denzin, N. K., & Lincoln, Y. S. (2011). *The Sage handbook of qualitative research* (4th ed.). Thousand Oaks, CA: Sage.

Greenhalgh, S. (1997). Methods and meanings: Reflections on disciplinary difference. *Population and Development Review, 23*(4), 819–824. doi:10.2307/2137382

Guest, G. (2013). Describing mixed methods research: An alternative to typologies. *Journal of Mixed Methods Research, 7*(2), 141–151. doi:10.1177/1558689812461179

Guest, G., Namey, E. E., & Mitchell, M. L. (2012). *Collecting qualitative data: A field manual for applied research*. Thousand Oaks, CA: Sage.

Hoyert, D. L., & Xu, J. (2012). Deaths: Preliminary data for 2011. *National Vital Statistics Reports, 61*(6), 1–51. Available at http://www.cdc.gov/nchs/data/nvsr/nvsr61/nvsr61_06.pdf

Hudelson, P. M. (1994). *Qualitative research for health programmes.* Geneva, Switzerland: Division of Mental Health World Health Organization. Available at http://whqlibdoc.who.int/hq/1994/WHO_MNH_PSF_94.3.pdf

Joint United Nations Programme on HIV/AIDS. (2014). *The gap report.* Geneva, Switzerland: UNAIDS. Available at http://www.unaids.org/sites/default/files/en/media/unaids/contentassets/documents/unaidspublication/2014/UNAIDS_Gap_report_en.pdf

Kenya Ministry of Health. (2015). *Gender and malaria in Kenya.* Nairobi, Kenya: Ministry of Health, Malaria Control Unit. Available at http://www.cpc.unc.edu/measure/pima/malaria/gender-and-malaria-in-kenya

Knodel, J. (1997). A case for nonanthropological qualitative methods for demographers. *Population and Development Review, 23*(4), 847–853. doi:10.2307/2137386

Meetoo, D., & Temple, B. (2003). Issues in multi-method research: Constructing self-care. *International Journal of Qualitative Methods, 2*(3), 1–12.

Patton, M. Q. (1990). *Qualitative evaluation and research methods.* Newbury Park, CA: Sage.

Patton, M. Q. (2002). *Qualitative evaluation and research methods* (3rd ed.). Thousand Oaks, CA: Sage.

Pedersen, D. (1992). Qualitative and quantitative: Two styles of viewing the world or two categories of reality? In N. S. Scrimshaw & G. R. Gleason (Eds.), *Rapid assessment procedures: Qualitative methodologies for planning and evaluation of health-related programmes.* Boston, MA: International Nutrition Foundation for Developing Countries.

Rossman, G. B., & Rallis, S. F. (1998). *Learning in the field: An introduction to qualitative research.* Thousand Oaks, CA: Sage.

Rubin, H. J., & Rubin, I. S. (1995). *Qualitative interviewing: The art of hearing data.* Thousand Oaks, CA: Sage.

Steckler, A., McLeroy, K. R., Goodman, R. M., Bird, S. T., & McCormick, L. (1992). Toward integrating qualitative and quantitative methods: An introduction. *Health Education Quarterly, 19*(1), 1–8. doi:10.1177/109019819201900101

Teddlie, C., & Tashakkori, A. (2009). *Foundations of mix methods research: Integrating quantitative and qualitative approaches in the social and behavioral sciences.* Los Angeles, CA: Sage.

Thomas, W. I., & Thomas, D. S. (1928). *The child in America: Behavior problems and programs.* New York, NY: A.A. Knopf.

United Nations Human Rights. (2008). *Claiming the millennium development goals: A human rights approach.* New York, NY: United Nations Human Rights Office of the High Commissioner for Human Rights. Available at http://www.refworld.org/docid/49fac1162.html

West African Health Organization. (2015, June). Annual Meeting Among Directors of National Health Information Systems and Disease Surveillance and Response Systems and Technical and Financial Partners in the ECOWAS Region: General Report. Bobo-Diolasso, Burkina Faso.

Wing, S., & Wolf, S. (2000). Intensive livestock operations, health, and quality of life among eastern North Carolina residents. *Environmental Health Perspectives, 108*(3), 233–238. doi:10.2307/3454439

Wolff, B., Knodel, J. E., & Sittitrai, W. (1991). *Focus groups and surveys as complementary research methods: Examples from a study of the consequences of family size in Thailand.* PSC Research Report No. 91-213. Ann Arbor: University of Michigan, Population Studies Center.

World Health Organization. (2014). *Global health observatory (GHO): Maternal and reproductive health.* Geneva, Switzerland.

Yoddumnern, B., Mahidon, M., & Sangkhom, W. P. L. S. (1993). *Qualitative methods for population and health research.* Nakorn Pathom, Thailand: Institute for Population and Social Research, Mahidol University at Salaya.

CHAPTER 2

THE LANGUAGE AND LOGIC OF QUALITATIVE RESEARCH

OBJECTIVES:

- To describe three main research paradigms (positivist, interpretivist, and transformative) and provide examples of how they influence research topics and approaches
- To describe the use of qualitative research methods in generating theory
- To describe how qualitative researchers use substantive theory or develop conceptual models to inform or guide their research

PUBLIC HEALTH RESEARCHERS and practitioners daily confront a myriad of challenging questions. How should a new vaccine be promoted to achieve better uptake? What health messages will young adolescents tempted to try street drugs or alcohol actually hear? What programs or policies will most effectively reduce street crime in inner-city neighborhoods? How can an HIV-negative woman have a safe relationship with her infected partner? It is useful to have an idea of how an innovation will be disseminated, how a group of people will react to a public health message, how policies or programs influence crime levels, or how a woman will negotiate the use of condoms with her infected partner.

Theories help you locate where your problem lies and where to find likely solutions.

(J. B. Smith, personal communication)

Research across disciplines has at its core a common scientific logic. However, the process of applying the basic logic of scientific inquiry to tangible problems in public health differs depending on the problem and the researcher's theoretical perspective. Individual researchers may approach any one of the research topics previously identified in different ways. Consider, for example, several approaches to research on urban street crime. While one researcher has examined how the physical characteristics of different neighborhoods affect bus riders' security, including the frequency and types of crime that occur within different neighborhood environments (Loukaitou-Sideris, 1999), another has examined the role of the media in shaping public perceptions about the roots of and blame for inner-city crime (Maneri & ter Wal, 2005). A third has engaged African-American youth to assess their experiences with community violence and the criminal justice system as a way to advocate for change (Thomas et al., 2012). All three researchers seek to make sense of a shared public health problem: urban street crime. Yet, their initial research questions and the methods they have used reflect different theoretical frameworks and different orientations to and use of substantive theory.

In this chapter, we present three overarching theoretical frameworks, often called **paradigms**, which underpin the research discussed in this book. We also discuss how more specific substantive theory may emerge from qualitative research or may be used to guide qualitative research. The rationale for and application of qualitative methods and the relationship to either the generation or the use of theory differ within these different paradigms.

Frameworks for Research: Paradigms, Theories, and Conceptual Models

Research frameworks range from broad to very specific theoretical approaches that contain their own vocabulary and logical assumptions. **Paradigms** provide researchers with a set of unified principles and rules for conducting research. Paradigms differ in terms of how they express the nature of reality, what methods are considered appropriate for investigating this reality, and why research should be undertaken in the first place (Willis, 2007, p. 21).

More specific frameworks can be found in substantive theories that propose how a set of concepts interact to influence an outcome. **Substantive theory** may first emerge through empirical observations or more formal, often qualitative, research. It is further established through a process of formal testing and application to multiple research topics and/or contexts. For example, the "broken windows" theory—one of the theories that informed the kind of neighborhood characteristics to be examined in the study on bus rider security—was built on earlier research (Newman, 1972) and continues to be tested in multiple settings with evidence for and against its precepts. It proposes that neglect of the physical environment—including broken windows, cracked sidewalks, or piles of refuse—are signs that no one is in charge, attracting potential criminals to prey on the community (Loukaitou-Sideris, 1999).

Like substantive theories, **conceptual models** posit relationships among specific **concepts** or **constructs**. A model may selectively use constructs from one or more existing theories or from empirical data, but it is organized in new ways to define a specific research problem or explain emergent data. For example, a conceptual model proposing how improved health policies lead to health outcomes may examine political will for policy reform, the role of multisectoral actors on the health system, and factors affecting implementation of policies at the service delivery level (Hardee, Irani, & Rodriguez, 2015). To do so, they may selectively use concepts from the field of health behavior as well as from other fields, including political science or economics.

Three Theoretical Paradigms for Public Health Research

In applied research, a paradigm can be an ally—a powerful strategic tool to guide you through the many practical decisions that arise in the design and implementation of your research. But how to choose a paradigm? In this book, we present three ways of conceptualizing a problem. These are major paradigms that have guided scientific study from the earliest days of public health research to the present. They are not substantive theories but rather are ways of investigating, discovering, and describing concrete reality. Over many years, these paradigms have evolved, adding scientific validity and depth to observations of the world around us.

We start with *positivism*, which emerged from the natural sciences in the nineteenth century and is widely regarded as the taproot of Western scientific methodology. Using quantitative models, positivist thinkers introduced principles of objective reasoning, explanation, verification, and prediction. The *interpretive paradigm* opened scientific research to new questions that could only be addressed by studying the subjective meanings of phenomena. The third approach we present, the *transformative paradigm*, is a relatively recent advance in science. It builds on interpretive principles to understand often-neglected points of view, forging new links between research and advocacy. The three paradigms are not mutually exclusive. They call attention to different aspects of reality, ask different questions in different ways, and often complement each other in mixed-method designs.

One viewpoint proposes that all [social scientific] data can in principle be measured or classified; therefore, when we confront non-quantified data, our task is to refine them through analysis so that they are subject to quantification or categorization.

(Selltiz, Wrightsman, Cook, & Society for the Psychological Study of Social Issues, 1976, p. 460)

As you examine your own views of social life, your theoretical perspective, expressed in a paradigmatic framework, is likely to become an increasingly deliberate choice consistent with the problems you study. In the light of trends in the ever-widening field of qualitative research, however, we advocate a pragmatic approach that recognizes theoretical distinctions but is able to incorporate relevant elements from all three in carefully designed studies.

Table 2.1 summarizes the logic and language of the three approaches as they relate to public health research and outlines major points, with a selection of examples from the methodological toolboxes of each. Interested readers are referred to more comprehensive sources such as the *Sage Handbook of Qualitative Research* (Denzin & Lincoln, 2011; Maxwell, 2008).

Quantitative Research From a Positivist Perspective

Much of what is known today about population and reproductive health can be attributed to research that has developed from quantitative principles in the natural sciences. Quantitative methods have become the norm for describing the state of the world's population—demographic models that project trends in fertility, morbidity, and mortality; epidemiological surveillance techniques to describe patterns of disease, including the spread of vector-borne illnesses such as dengue fever and Chagas disease; and standardized household surveys that provide statistical data on knowledge, attitudes, and practices related to health behavior.

A basic assumption of this paradigm is that the goal of science is to develop the most objective methods possible to get the closest approximation of reality. Researchers who work from this perspective use quantitative terms to explain how **variables** interact, shape events, and cause outcomes. They often develop and test these explanations in experimental studies. Multivariate analysis and techniques for statistical prediction are among the classic contributions of positivist research. This framework has evolved largely from a 19th-century philosophical approach. Inspired by philosophers such as August Compte, John Stuart Mill, and Emile Durkheim (Willis, 2007, p. 43), positivists maintain that reliable knowledge is based on direct observation or manipulation of natural phenomena through empirical, often experimental, means.

Quantitative studies in social science use highly standardized tools with precisely worded questions. Working with representative samples, the interviewer interested in adolescent tobacco use might ask questions about young peoples' motivations for tobacco use, temptations to smoke in a range of circumstances, parents' or friends' use of tobacco, and ability to resist smoking. Specific questions might include: "How much do you agree or disagree with the statement 'Smoking helps you fit in with others'? How tempted are you to smoke when your friends offer you a cigarette? Do you have a parent or guardian who currently smokes cigarettes?" (National Cancer Institute, 2012).

Table 2.1 Three Paradigms for Public Health Research

	Positivist	Interpretivist	Transformative
Basic assumptions	The social world is composed of observable facts. Reality is objective, independent of the researcher.	The social world is constructed of meaning observable in symbolic human acts, interactions, and language. Reality is subjective and multiple as seen from different perspectives.	The social world is governed by power relations, a fact that influences research design by identifying and including all relevant subgroups. Reality is negotiated and differs according to status and power.
Sources of evidence	Facts are revealed through standard scientific processes and are context-free.	Meanings are derived from perceptions, experiences, and actions in relation to social contexts.	Power, control, and contextual factors can be heard in personal accounts that reflect different versions of reality.
Methods	Structured data collection, controlled measurement, and clinical trials are the norm. Examples: surveys, clinical trials, rating scales, structured observation.	Semi-structured, open-ended questions, and observation enable participants to express thoughts and actions in natural ways. Examples: in-depth interviews, focus group discussions, participant observations, case histories.	Participatory forms of observation and guided conversation enable both marginal and dominant groups to voice opinions and tell their stories. Examples: participatory action techniques, reflexive listening, challenges to political and personal barriers to entrenched positions.
Research intention	Quantitative studies seek description, explanation, verification, and prediction of human behavior (as well as natural phenomena) through causal relationships.	Qualitative studies seek discovery, understanding, and insight into the circumstances of human behavior.	Transformative studies seek insight into different experiences as reflected, for example, by gender, race, sexual orientation, or living with a disability; they can influence power and control in an agenda for social change.
Level of participation	Research subjects answer specific, predetermined questions in a structured response format.	Research participants are active partners in data collection and respond to semi-structured questions spontaneously and naturally.	Research participants have relative freedom to direct the data collection process and define follow-up.
Impact on study participants	The impact is neutral. Research subjects may gain new information or insight from the results.	Participants are aware of their engagement in the research process and may gain insight into their own perspectives and behaviors, as well as the research topic.	Participation is empowering. Results may lead to a participant-initiated action agenda and empowerment to propose and/or participate in policy change.

Questions are almost always closed-ended or precoded but may include some open-ended questions. In data analysis the answers to open-ended questions are typically classified according to predefined categories that represent the researcher's theoretical understanding of the problem.

Control of extraneous and competing variables is important in quantitative design. The framework applies rules for incorporating factors from the social environment based on assumptions that are different from other frameworks. Using experimental and quasi-experimental designs, quantitative researchers attempt through randomization to distribute evenly the effect of contextual variables, such as size of enrollment in an evaluation of several school health programs; accessibility of clinic services in a study of child immunization in a rural area; and presence or absence of organized labor in a national study of health risks in the workplace. Their rationale is that context contains hidden determinants that may affect measurement of causal or associative relationships and bias the outcomes of the study. Control is thus fundamental to quantitative research assumptions because it provides a means to isolate extraneous variables and focus more clearly on the relationships that were highlighted in the research problem.

Controlling effects also helps researchers identify and explain in quantitative terms the influence of factors in the study environment on key relationships. For example, if your research problem was to identify factors that predict fertility trends in Peru, you would measure the variable relationships among selected possible determinants of fertility and assess the relative strength with which each factor predicts the number of births per Peruvian woman. You would control for sociodemographic and other variables that might explain the observed relationships. You would obtain accurate measurements, but because it is impossible to identify, measure, and control every variable that could influence whether a woman will give birth, you would always have unanswered or partially answered questions. A versatile investigator might at this point turn to qualitative techniques to explore some of the quantitative findings in greater depth.

In quantitative studies, accuracy, reliability, and relative freedom from bias are critical criteria for judging the quality of findings. The inherent difficulty of ensuring accuracy in any social or behavioral inquiry has led quantitative researchers to stress neutrality, uniformity, objectivity, and replicability. Such goals are consistent with the positivist goal to study phenomena objectively and to express findings in terms of measurable outcomes and relationships. A quantitative strategy emphasizes structure: consistent operational definitions throughout the study, precisely worded questions, and statistical analysis. However, this structure limits the scope of the research by requiring the formulation of research problems and questions in measurable terms.

> **Gender is "the roles that men and women play and the relations that arise out of these roles. They are socially constructed, not physically determined."**
>
> ***(Pan American Health Organization, 1997, p. 28)***

Over the years, demographers, epidemiologists, biostatisticians, and other quantitative scientists have met many methodological challenges. Their painstaking efforts to answer difficult questions have resulted in an impressive knowledge base in population studies and public health. But still missing is a deeper understanding of the circumstances that help to explain why and how people make the decisions they do, and why and how health systems evolve along a given path. Even when working in a quantitative framework, therefore, researchers often seek other ways of understanding human and institutional behavior, specifically in the methods of qualitative research (Pedersen, 1992), based on different principles and theoretical assumptions.

Qualitative Research From an Interpretivist Perspective

The theoretical framework for most qualitative research emerges from an interpretivist perspective, a paradigm that sees the world as constructed, interpreted, and experienced by people in their interactions with each other and with wider social systems (Ulin, 1992). A rejection of the positivist insistence on objectivity and thus value-free inquiry, interpretivism can be viewed as a collection of different movements that share some common principles (Willis, 2007, pp. 53–54). First is the notion that all knowledge is socially constructed. The goal of research, therefore, is not to search for universally generalizable truths, but to understand a group's "lived" experiences as they are played out in a particular place and time. A second and related idea is that, in order to develop true understanding, a researcher must examine the research topic holistically. For this reason, interpretivists prefer to conduct their research in natural settings rather than carefully controlled environments.

Furthermore, interpretivists favor an "emic" perspective, which examines the topic of investigation through the eyes of those being studied, rather than through the lens of an external and impartial researcher (Willis, 2007, p. 100). For this reason, some interpretivist researchers reject the use of substantive theory to help guide their choice of research topics and questions. Instead, they believe that researchers should enter into the research with an open mind and use a flexible and open-ended research process. (See section on Using Qualitative Methods to Develop Theory.) At the same time, interpretivists acknowledge that all research is inherently subjective. As the late

18th-century philosopher Immanuel Kant argued, human beings' perceptions of their world are filtered through the mental faculties they are born with (Willis, 2007, p. 51). Like research subjects themselves, researchers are embedded in historical, social, and environmental contexts that shape the questions they ask, as well as the interactions between themselves and those engaged in their research (Willis, 2007, p. 130).

The kinds of research questions that arise in an interpretivist framework are mainly those that address why, how, and under what circumstances rather than what and how many. Why do people who were abused as children tend to be overrepresented among abusive adults? Under what circumstances will parents accept a school's responsibility for sex education? How do economically dependent women protect themselves from HIV transmission when their partners are at risk? Why has immunization for the human papilloma virus (HPV) been widely accepted in some countries and rejected in others? Each of these questions leads deeper into questions of subjective meaning—the meaning that life events and experiences have related to health decisions and health behavior. The same questions can be addressed from a quantitative perspective but in terms of discrete indicators with measurable dimensions. Qualitative methods of participant observation, in-depth interviews, and focus group discussions would elicit data on subjective understandings.

Methods associated with this perspective enable participants to speak freely and help investigators gain insight into a phenomenon that the participant has experienced (Barnett & Stein, 1998). As subsequent chapters will show, interpretivist methodology seeks information in as natural a context as possible, where the researcher can observe activities and events as they occur and encourage people to respond from their own perspectives and experiences and in their own words. In the previous HPV question, researchers would be looking for understanding of parental concerns about immunizations, parent and provider decisions, and circumstances associated with immunization acceptance. They might not include more descriptive questions such as extent, patterns, and prediction of acceptance or measurable indicators of knowledge and attitudes concerning HPV or immunizations, more generally—issues that a quantitative framework would better address. Notably, a combined methodological strategy in this example would make it possible to use the strengths of each approach while compensating for each one's limitations.

Working on the assumption that "research participants construct [their own] accounts of reality" as they experience it, Meetoo and Temple (2003) used an interpretivist framework to investigate self-care among people with diabetes. Their design included methods that would enable them to see how participants built their different accounts: semi-structured interviews, structured fixed-response interviews, and diaries. The seemingly inconsistent results, especially comparing face-to-face interview data with the more private diary entries, demonstrated to the researchers the importance of circumstances, or context, in determining different dimensions of self-help.

> **Feminist work sets the stage for other research, other actions, and policy that transcend and transform.**
>
> *(Olesen, 2000, p. 215)*

Similarly, Schuler and colleagues employed an interpretivist framework when exploring men's and women's subjective understanding of standardized questions on intimate partner violence (IPV). Their mixed-methods research, conducted in rural Bangladesh, revealed that most respondents first visualized a specific scenario in which a wife was either "blameless" or "at fault" before deciding whether an episode of wife beating was justified. The authors point out that standardized questions typical of Demographic and Health Surveys (DHS) (a positivist framework) may inadvertently misrepresent socially held attitudes toward wife beating (Schuler, Lenzi, & Yount, 2011; Schuler, Yount, & Lenzi, 2012).

Qualitative Research From a Transformative Perspective

Like interpretivist scholars, theorists working in the transformative realm believe that understanding how people perceive and experience their day-to-day interactions with others is not only a valid but an essential focus of research. Inclusiveness is a key concept in a transformative perspective, which assumes that knowledge is a product of all human interests and relationships. Transformative research therefore tends to focus on marginalized groups, highlighting voices of populations not always represented in the findings of other scientific inquiry (Mertens, 1999). This focus is not unique but reflects paradigmatic constructions from the Freirian tradition (Freire, 1970) as well as participatory research approaches and—of particular importance in public health—feminist thinking. In their emphasis on inclusiveness, transformative researchers apply qualitative or mixed-method research to address discriminatory practices associated with vulnerabilities and social inequity, for example, those related to race, poverty, gender, sexual orientation, or disability. Transformative researchers have turned attention to many forms of social and structural inequity and the related dynamics of power, a topic advanced in the past by critical theorists such as Antonio Gramsci and Michel Foucault and grounded in the work of Karl Marx and other critical scholars.

Until a feminist paradigm was articulated in the 1960s, neither the positivist nor the interpretivist perspectives had fully taken into account the profound influence of power relations, especially—but not uniquely—in the area of women's health (Ulin, 1992). The transformative research paradigm, which first emerged in the 1980s and 1990s (Mackenzie & Knipe, 2006), not only gives voice to people's lived experiences and concerns, but also listens to all voices with the goal of both revealing and reducing the social, political, economic, and other structural impediments that marginalize and subordinate marginal populations (Brooks & Hesse-Biber, 2007). Through their research, feminist and other transformative scholars highlight the failure of traditional positivist methods to adequately represent the often-neglected experiences of subjugated minorities and other vulnerable groups.

Increasingly, transformative research is focusing attention in the public health community on the role that gender plays in sexual decisions. A recent example of gender-based research is the Male Engagement Project (Dayton, Lanham, & Wilcher, 2014), which sampled a range of policy, research, and community stakeholders in Kenya and South Africa to identify strategies for including men in the introduction of new HIV prevention products. The project demonstrated that listening to men gave researchers new insight into how men experience sexual relationships, family planning, and protection against infection. Engaging men in program development and research, they conclude, leads to more effective programs and health outcomes. (See Case Study 2 in Appendix 1.)

Power relationships that maintain boundaries in people's lives often cast women in subordinate positions relative to men, but they apply equally to other forms of power imbalance, for example, those defined by race, economic status, and access to scarce resources. Researchers working within a "political economy of health" framework incorporate notions of power when they examine how social structures and institutions create and reinforce the conditions that lead to inequities in health and disease (Anonymous, 2005). In another example of research based on transformative principles, an environmental action group partnered with academic researchers to train local youth to map and monitor air pollution. This community-based participatory approach led not only to findings of higher rates of asthma among black and Latino children, but also encouraged local advocacy for change in environmental policy related to cleaner air (Minkler, 2010).

By alerting us to the potential for bias when researchers do not seek out or listen to the voices of certain groups of people, transformative researchers are helping to reformulate the design and conduct of applied research. Transformative research typically makes pragmatic use of both qualitative and quantitative methods to highlight population-level disparities, while keeping lived experience central to the investigation (Barnett & Stein, 1998; Tolman & Szalacha, 1999). Similarly, community-based participatory research (CBPR) methods are often a central feature of transformative research because they engage community members as partners in the research process.

As these studies illustrate, participatory involvement of intended beneficiaries of research increases the likelihood that both research questions and interpretation of findings reflect the needs and experiences of the local community. Engagement in the research process can also empower local residents by increasing knowledge of their own communities and building skills to address community problems. Case Study 3 in Appendix 1 further supports these transformative principles by documenting how a collaborative council representing local researchers, health practitioners, and community members worked with local artists to translate research findings into HIV prevention messages through art.

Ultimately, transformative researchers identify and work to *transform* the economic, social, and political conditions that disadvantage one group over another. Transformative research has grown out of a commitment to equity and increasing equality across gender, racial, economic, and other divisions; it is about power and the recognition that long-standing differences in access to power have had a profound effect on the health of populations. This perspective is expanding how we conduct qualitative studies, adding concepts and tools to answer numerous important questions that scientists have not before had effective means to ask. In the authors' experiences, the world of social science research is witnessing a transformation from strict allegiance to highly objective, "value-free" inquiry, on the one hand, to inclusion of the more participatory and socially relevant models exemplified by the interpretivist and transformative models we present here, on the other hand. (See Case Study 2 in Appendix 1 for an example of a participatory secondary analysis to examine men's roles in women's access to new HIV prevention methods.)

Using Qualitative Methods to Develop Theory

Grounded theory (Glaser & Strauss, 1967) is theory that emerges from concrete data—an inductive approach. Because the emergent theory must be "grounded in the data," researchers developing grounded theory do not typically start by testing hypotheses. Instead, they identify relationships among different findings that shed light on the central problem. Although the approach can be used with either qualitative or quantitative data, grounded theory studies rely on qualitative analytical methods rather than statistical analysis.

Studies based on grounded theory follow several methodological conventions. Researchers first identify a topic of interest and initial data sources. As data accumulate, they engage in a process of coding and reflection, which means going through the text line by line and applying codes that reflect the key *categories* (themes) and their *properties* (subcategories) as these emerge from the data.

The data are then compared to identify links from which core categories—and ultimately tentative theories—are derived. These nascent theories give rise to research questions that help refine the emerging theory with new categories of participants, different data collection methods or data sources, new observation sites, or additional interview questions.

Thus, constant comparison, data to data and data to theory, is a hallmark of the grounded theory approach. In one example, when Australian researchers set out to study preventive dental practice, they first interviewed dentists and their staffs as well as patients who had been exposed to new preventive protocols (Sbaraini, Carter, Evans, & Blinkhorn, 2011). With their discovery of a wide range of perspectives on different treatments, they compared subsets of the sample, which led to additional explanations for differences in preventive dental procedures. Thus emerged a conceptual framework that could grow with successive levels of new information until they reached a point of saturation at which further inquiry no longer contributed new insight. In this case, the researchers were able to conclude with a conceptual model that illustrated the complex process of adopting new preventive protocols and was grounded in the experience of both dentists and their patients. Moreover, their model had the substantive relevance and rigor to become the basis for further research design on related topics.

Substantive Theories and Conceptual Models

While a paradigm is a broad theoretical framework that helps to conceptualize a problem, the application of a substantive theory or development of a conceptual model takes us directly into research design. The labels *theory* and *model* are often used interchangeably. For example, many recognized substantive theories, such as the Health Belief Model, include the word *model* in their titles. Indeed, both theories and models represent clusters of related variables that guide research. In this chapter, we distinguish substantive theory, which has a higher degree of recognition, replication, and standardization, from conceptual models, which are developed for or emerge from specific research studies. More comprehensive discussion of theories, models, and frameworks can be found in the literature (Glanz, Rimer, & Viswanath, 2008; Imenda, 2014; National Cancer Institute, 2012).

Substantive theory, also called operational or working theory, goes hand in hand with applied public health research because it represents conclusions about the social world that have emerged from concrete findings of research studies directed at specific problems. Substantive theory has been conducted in a range of disciplines, including psychology, sociology, economics, and public health. Applied research in public health often uses substantive theory deductively to define and explain specific behavior in relation to program development and policy.

Conceptual models may be developed by applied qualitative researchers to lay out their initial assumptions about the area of inquiry. In such cases, researchers estimate the scope of their research by referring to concepts or constructs from multiple substantive theories, from the literature, or from their own experience. This initial framework can offer insight into concepts and relationships that help them define qualitative research problems more clearly and guide the research design.

Alternatively, conceptual models may also be an outcome of research—an inductive way to synthesize the findings from the research. Such conceptual models may be a step in theory-building. For example, Indian women's interest in, and use of, microbicidal products led to a revised conceptual model that showed more nuanced inter-relationships among several determinants of product acceptability, including product attributes, marital harmony, and risk perception (Tolley et al., 2006). (For further information, see Case Study 4 in Appendix 1.)

Next, we provide several illustrative examples of substantive theories. The recommended readings at the end of the chapter provide additional examples. See Box 2.1 for further guidelines on how to choose between different substantive theories that could guide your own work.

BOX 2.1 CHECKLIST FOR EVALUATING SUBSTANTIVE THEORY

When applying a theory or model, consider the following:

- What dimensions of the problem does the theory or model concern?
- Is it specific to the unit of study (e.g., individual behavior, group influences, or environmental issues)?
- How does the theory or model explain this portion of your research problem?
- What information does the theory or model suggest that you gather?
- How accurately does the theory or model coincide with your understanding of the problem?
- What aspects of the problem does the theory or model fail to consider?
- In your judgment, how helpful is the theory or model in working with the problem and determining how best to study it?
- What are its limitations?
- Are all relevant voices represented?

Source: Adapted from van Ryn and Heany (1992, pp. 315–330).

Social-Ecological Model

Social-ecological models (SEM) grew out of the recognition that the "healthy lifestyles" approaches to health promotion of the 1970s and 1980s were not always improving health. By focusing almost exclusively on individual behavior, such approaches could be interpreted as "victim-blaming" (Tesh, 1981). Instead, the SEM acknowledges that health behavior is influenced by many social and environmental factors outside the individual's control (Bronfenbrenner, 1994; McLeroy, Bibeau, Steckler, & Glanz, 1988; Stokols, 1996). Various conceptualizations of the SEM may divide these social and environmental levels in different ways, with the goal of identifying and examining those levels most appropriate for intervention. Research designed from a social-ecological perspective typically examines relationships between two or more of the following levels:

- Individual: knowledge, attitudes, skills, physiology directly attributable to a single individual. In health fields, the primary research focus often is on the individual but with attention to aggregate levels of influence on individual and group behavior.
- Interpersonal: interactions between health providers and clients or between members of couples, families, and networks of friends.
- Organizational: formal and informal groupings of individuals around particular interests, including workplaces and social institutions.
- Community: relationships among individuals and/or organizations are linked by social ties, share common perspectives, and engage in joint action (MacQueen et al., 2001). They may or may not be bounded by well-defined geographic settings.
- Policy: legislation at local, national, or international level.

The SEM suggests levels of investigation for study design. Specific constructs are more likely to come from other substantive social and behavioral theories, which may themselves be situated on one or more levels of the SEM, as shown in Box 2.2.

Health Belief Model

One of the most commonly used frameworks in health behavior research, the Health Belief Model, offers useful guidance for understanding sexual risk behaviors (Janz & Becker, 1984; Rosenstock, Strecher, & Becker, 1994).

BOX 2.2 SOCIAL ECOLOGICAL MODEL AND THE POSITION OF SUBSTANTIVE THEORIES ALONG CONCENTRIC LEVELS OF AGGREGATION

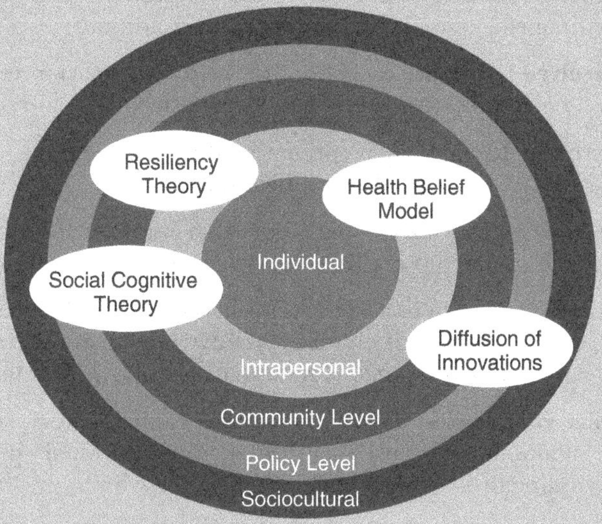

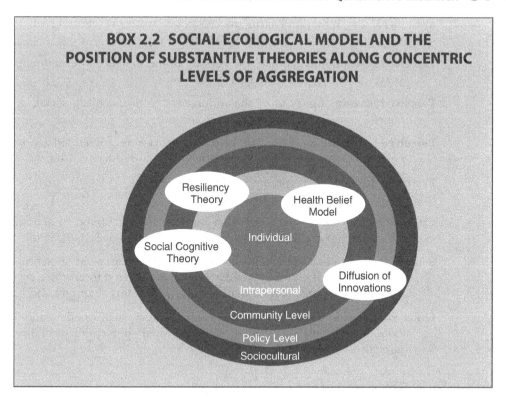

Basic premises of the model are that individuals differ in two ways: (1) how they perceive the personal benefits or value of avoiding illness or getting well, and (2) their expectations that a specific action can prevent illness. People are more likely to take action to prevent or control an ill-health condition if the following apply (Champion & Skinner, 2008):

- They believe it to have potentially serious consequences.
- They believe that a course of action available to them would be beneficial in reducing either their susceptibility to, or the severity of, the condition.
- They believe that the anticipated barriers to (or costs of) taking the action outweigh its benefits.
- This model can address programmatic or practical questions, such as "Why aren't uninsured low-income men accessing government-subsidized health

insurance?" or "Why don't farm workers wear protective clothing when spraying pesticides?" Key concepts are the following:

Perceived susceptibility: people's perception of their chance of developing a preventable condition, such as hypertension

Perceived severity: opinions of the seriousness of the medical, social, or financial consequences of a health condition

Perceived benefits: perceptions of the efficacy of the recommended action (e.g., abstinence, condom use, contraception) to reduce health risks

Perceived barriers: perceptions of the psychological, social, or financial costs of adopting the new health behavior

Cues or triggers to action: events that increase the likelihood of action, including symptoms of infection or exposure to messages on the radio

Self-efficacy: the conviction that one can successfully carry out an action, such as consistent use of preventive measures required to produce certain outcomes (e.g., prevention of obesity or diabetes) (Bandura, 1977)

Other variables: especially sociodemographic factors, such as educational attainment, because they influence an individual's perceptions and thus indirectly influence health-related behavior

Social Cognitive Theory

Bandura's social cognitive theory (SCT) proposes a dynamic and continuous interaction among three components of health behavior—the behavior, the person, and the environment (also known as the situation) (Bandura, 1986). Social cognitive theory begins with the understanding that different behaviors—whether obtaining a recommended immunization, scheduling and attending an annual physical exam, taking daily blood pressure medication, or correctly and consistently using condoms to prevent pregnancy or disease—are associated with different behavioral requirements. Whereas some behaviors require only one-time or intermittent activity, others require long-term and sustained attention. Furthermore, as in more individual-level theories like the Health Belief Model, individual-level constructs—including a person's knowledge, beliefs, skills, and perceived self-efficacy—exert a strong influence on health behavior. However, the social cognitive theory moves beyond the individual level by acknowledging the influence of the situation on behavior. For example, in a study assessing adolescent women's participation in HIV prevention research, the "situation" encompassed the laws or policies regulating adolescent access to health services; the timing and physical location of a study clinic; and the social interactions of peers, sexual partners, or family members relating to trial participation (see Case Study 5 in Appendix 1). Some constructs central to SCT include the following:

- **Reciprocal determinism**—the notion that characteristics of the person, behavior, and environment are constantly interacting and that a change in one component will have an impact on others (Glanz, Rimer, & Viswanath, 2008, p. 273)
- **Psychological determinants**—constructs common to the Health Belief Model and other substantive theories that relate to individuals' beliefs about the behavior, their perceived risk if a behavior were to be enacted (or not enacted), and perceptions about their own or the group's ability to enact a specific behavior
- **Observational learning**—learning to perform a new behavior by watching others perform it, either in person or "virtually" through media
- **Environmental determinants**—characteristics of the environment that exert an influence on the behavior, including policies that reward or punish a behavior, financial costs, and other structures that may make a behavior easier or more difficult to perform

Diffusion of Innovations

The diffusion of innovations theory emerged from a desire to understand and explain why some innovations (ideas, practices, or products) spread rapidly and are widely adopted, while others move slowly or are never adopted, or are quickly abandoned. Similar to the social cognitive theory, this theory identifies characteristics of the innovation, individual adopters (or nonadopters), and the setting as determinants of an innovation's success. For example, the adoption of a new practice (e.g., giving young children foods fortified with micronutrients) will depend on its:

- **Relative advantage:** the degree to which a new idea or practice is better than existing ones
- **Compatibility:** how well the innovation fits the needs of intended users or fits within the delivery system
- **Complexity:** how easy the innovation is to use
- **Trialability:** whether the innovation can be tried before deciding to adopt it
- **Observability:** whether the benefits of the innovation can be easily observed and measured

While some individuals—the innovators or early adopters—will be quick to take up new ideas or practices that exhibit these characteristics, others will wait until the innovation has become more widely accepted or available. Finally, characteristics of the institutional or cultural setting for the innovation influence the degree and pace of adoption (Oldenburg & Glanz, 2008).

Resiliency Theory

Resiliency is a construct that has been applied in research on individuals, families, organizations, societies, health and ecosystems, and cultures using analyses that focus on developmental, demographic, social, and other variables (Southwick, Bonanno, Masten, Panter-Brick, & Yehuda, 2014). From these studies there has emerged a theoretical framework that can be the basis for research in many health-related fields. Determinants of resilience—a mechanism developed in response to intense stress that affects healthy functioning (Johnson et al., 2011)—include "biological, psychological, social, and cultural factors that interact to determine how one responds to stressful experiences." As a theory, it has the potential to offer tentative explanations for individual and societal response to change in many forms, for example, homelessness, natural disasters, global climate change, and epidemics. The theory has been useful in examining issues related to global health security, such as the 2014–2015 Ebola crisis in West Africa, which put enormous strain on health facilities and health systems in affected countries (Kieny, Evans, Schmets, & Kadandale, 2014). Resiliency theory can be useful and aligns well with a transformative perspective, because it:

- Focuses on "positive contextual, social, and individual variables" that "interfere with or disrupt" movement from risk to better health outcomes (Zimmerman, 2013);
- Examines positive deviance, focusing on factors (in individuals, societies, or systems) that can be used to craft change strategies and enhance strengths or healthy functioning;
- Allows health decision makers to shift from a "deficit-based" model of health to "competence-based" models (Southwick et al., 2014) that focus on prevention (e.g., of post-traumatic stress disorder) or disaster preparedness, informing the design of health interventions as well as public health policy.

Standards for Qualitative Research

At the heart of the debate on research standards is the much-used but often misunderstood concept of subjectivity. To a quantitative scientist, data are facts that must be isolated as much as possible from the researcher's personal, or subjective, values; subjectivity can mean distortion. Although the notion of a perfectly objective social science is a widely acknowledged myth, the supposed accuracy of quantitative data often depends on the separation of fact from subjective judgment. In theoretical frameworks that both guide and emerge from qualitative research, on the other hand, subjectivity is an important element in the research process. We believe that we perceive the world only partially and, therefore, as researchers, we must describe as many aspects of reality as we can and be open to many ways of interpreting the social world. Our access to these multiple worldviews is through the subjective experiences and understandings of study participants. The qualitative researcher's use of self as a reflexive (self-aware) partner in collecting and interpreting information further strengthens the position that subjectivity, applied appropriately and systematically, is a positive element in qualitative science.

Judging Quality: The Search for Trustworthy Data

Qualitative and quantitative criteria of excellence are equally important but inherently different (Devers, 1999). All of us who design research or use research findings are concerned with quality, but the criteria of evaluation differ in qualitative and quantitative research practice. They are analogous but not interchangeable. Each has its own appropriate and no less rigorous standards. The most widely adopted criteria, on the one hand, have been those developed from the positivist framework. This framework uses validity, reliability, objectivity, precision, and generalizability to judge the rigor of quantitative studies intended to describe, predict, and verify empirical relationships in relatively controlled settings.

On the other hand, qualitative research aims to explore, discover, and understand; it therefore redefines these criteria for greater relevance in judging quality and outcomes. Several qualitative scientists have articulated standards or criteria for judging qualitative data (Kirk & Miller, 1986; Lincoln & Guba, 1985; Miles & Huberman, 1994). Lincoln and Guba suggest that the fundamental criterion for qualitative reports is trustworthiness. How, they ask, can a researcher be certain that "the findings of an inquiry are worth paying attention to, worth taking account of?" (p. 398). In answer, practitioners and consumers of qualitative science ask a new set of questions: How can we know that the data are credible, dependable, confirmable, and transferable? We introduce these concepts because evaluating the trustworthiness of qualitative data is directly related to the fundamental logic of qualitative theory. In Chapter 6 we discuss standards of quality in greater detail in relation to data analysis.

Credibility. In quantitative science, validity is the extent to which a measurement taps the concept it intends to measure. The outcome is accepted as true within reasonable limits. Credibility, also called truth value, is the corresponding criterion for qualitative research. Validity assumes correct operational measures for the concepts being studied and, in experimental studies, a potential cause–effect relationship (Yin, 1994); credibility focuses on confidence in the truth of the findings, including an accurate understanding of the context and attention to all relevant voices. The credibility of your qualitative findings is increased to the extent that you can answer "yes" to the following questions:

- Do the findings show a logical relationship to each other; that is, are they consistent in terms of the explanations they support?
- Are the findings grounded in, and substantiated by, the narrative data; that is, are the narrative data sufficiently rich to support the specific findings? Do the findings indicate a need for more data?
- Does the original study population consider reports to be accurate? (Miles & Huberman, 1994)

Dependability. An important test of quantitative reliability is the extent to which findings can be replicated. The goal is not only to obtain the same results in a study (which, given intervening time and change, may not be possible) but to be able to replicate the processes used to obtain these results, even though they may be carried out in different cultural contexts (King, Keohane, & Verba, 1994). For qualitative researchers inquiring into unique constellations of multiple phenomena and meanings, this goal would be meaningless. In other words, the same *qualitative* method is not likely to produce the same results because the answers cannot be prestructured to conform to definitions imposed by the research design. Instead, qualitative researchers aim to ensure that their results are dependable. The methodological parallel to reliability, dependability is increased when the research process is consistent and carried out with careful attention to the rules and conventions of qualitative methodology. We ask ourselves:

- Are the research questions clear and logically connected to the research purpose and design?
- Are there parallels across data sources?
- Do multiple field workers have comparable data collection protocols?

Given the contextual nature of qualitative research, we do not expect to produce exactly the same answers. On the other hand, we do anticipate that if the data are dependable, we will find logically consistent patterns of response that remain reasonably stable over time.

Confirmability. Objectivity is a traditional standard of quality in quantitative data. The term generally implies maintaining distance between the observer and the observed and minimizing any possible influence of the researcher's values on the process of inquiry. Either strategy would be counterproductive in most qualitative studies. From a qualitative perspective, the analogous goal is to confirm, by audits and other methods discussed in Chapters 5 and 6, that the data reflect as accurately as possible the participants' perspectives and experiences. Confirmability thus means a way of knowing that, even as a co-participant in the inquiry, the researcher has maintained the distinction between personal values and those of the study participants. Applying the concept of reflexivity, qualitative researchers have an obligation to observe and document their own roles in the research process, including assumptions, biases, or reactions that might influence the collection and interpretation of data. Applying reflexivity contributes to the confirmability of the results.

Transferability. Also called extensibility, transferability is the qualitative analogue to the concept of generalizability. Generalizability of the findings to a wider population is a goal of most quantitative studies. Indeed, if every unit in the study sample has an equal chance of being selected, and the sample is large enough to minimize the probability of error, then this goal can be met within certain specified margins. It is a statistically representative sample. Although generalizability by this definition is not relevant to the goals or the methodology of most interpretive work, it is nevertheless important to know "whether the conclusions of a study … [are] transferable to other contexts" (Miles & Huberman 1994, p. 279). The importance of context in qualitative studies leads some researchers to doubt that results from one context should be transferred to another, while it may lead others to apply conclusions from their data too casually. Our position is on middle ground: Lessons learned from qualitative studies can be applied to other contexts if samples have been carefully selected to represent viewpoints and experiences that reflect key issues in the research problem. Our goal is to produce data that are conceptually, not statistically, representative of people in a specific context. Because context is a key influence in any qualitative research, the researcher must account for contextual factors when transferring data from one situation to another. Repeating the study in another population, with similar conclusions, lends credibility to the results and further specifies the circumstances under which the findings will occur. Thus, well-documented knowledge might be extended to similar populations, but "the burden of proof lies less with the original investigator than with the person seeking to make an application elsewhere. The original inquirer cannot know the sites to which transferability might be sought, but appliers can" (Lincoln & Guba, 1985, p. 404).

Credibility, dependability, confirmability, and transferability are the standards for evaluating the rigor of qualitative studies that are consistent with the worldview, information sources, and methods of the interpretivist paradigm. In subsequent chapters, we will return to these criteria of quality with further discussion of specific techniques for ensuring the rigor of qualitative studies.

Summary

As researchers we each have a fundamental curiosity about our subject of inquiry. But in designing and implementing the research, we must move beyond ordinary curiosity to a disciplined use of the rules and conventions of our theoretical perspective or paradigm. A great deal has been written from the quantitative point of view that will continue to guide much of our work in public health. For this book, we have set our theoretical compass largely, though not entirely, by the interpretivist and transformative paradigms. We believe that, alone or in combination with appropriate quantitative methods, these two theoretical positions can generate qualitative research that addresses many complex issues in public health research and practice. We urge readers to examine their own theoretical perspectives, to ask themselves what perspective their work reflects, where their ideas come from, and whether it might be useful to look at a problem through a different lens. It is important to incorporate self-reflection in the research process to know how one's own worldview influences the questions under investigation. If you understand

and use your theoretical perspective as a guide, you will discover new ways to a better understanding of human thought and individual, institutional, and health systems behavior.

Key Terms

1. **Paradigm:** A broad worldview that presents a definition of the social world linked to related sources of information (data) and appropriate ways (methods) to tap these sources (Guba & Lincoln, 1994). Paradigmatic assumptions establish boundaries for scientific inquiry; that is, researchers draw on paradigmatic concepts and relationships to construct theoretical frameworks for research design.
2. **Substantive theory:** A set of interrelated concepts, definitions, and propositions that systematically explain and/or predict observable phenomena. Theory should be testable and sufficiently abstract to have relevance for a wide range of research topics (see Glanz et al., 2008, p. 26).
3. **Conceptual models**: A set of integrated assumptions that typically draw on one or more substantive theories to define a problem in a specific setting or context. Conceptual models may be developed to guide research domains and questions, or they may emerge from the analysis as a means of synthesizing qualitative data.
4. **Concepts** or **constructs:** The major components of a theory—its building blocks or key elements. The key concepts of the stages of change theory (Prochaska, DiClemente, & Norcross, 1992), for example, describe individual behavior change in the following stages: precontemplation, contemplation, preparation for action, action, and maintenance of the new behavior.
5. **Variables:** Things that can change or differ, quantitatively or qualitatively. Common variables thought to account for differences in health behaviors might include sociodemographic characteristics such as age, sex, or education; measures of, for example, knowledge, attitudes, beliefs, intention, or self-efficacy; and system characteristics that describe communities or institutions in which health care takes place (Fishbein et al. 1991/1997).
6. **Grounded theory**: A systematic approach to social science research that develops theoretical explanations from numerous concrete instances and comparisons of emerging themes.

Recommended Readings

Glanz, K., Rimer, B. K., & Viswanath. K. (Eds.). (2008). *Health behavior and health education: Theory, research, and practice* (4th ed.). San Francisco, CA: Wiley.

National Cancer Institute. (2005). *Theory at a glance: A guide for health promotion practice*. Washington, DC: U.S. Department of Health and Human Services.

Willis J. W. (2007). *Foundations of qualitative research: Interpretive and critical approaches*. Thousand Oaks, CA: Sage.

Review Questions

1. Consider the three main paradigms presented in this chapter. Which paradigm do you feel most closely aligns with your own worldview? Why?
2. Think about a research topic that interests you. What kinds of questions would you ask if you were working from a positivist paradigm?
3. How would your questions differ if you were conducting the same research from a transformative paradigm?
4. Qualitative studies are often guided, either implicitly or explicitly, by the social-ecological model because they examine multiple levels of influence. Thinking again about your topic of interest, what levels would be most relevant to explore?
5. Find a qualitative research publication that makes use of substantive theory or a conceptual model. How was the theory or model used? In your opinion, how helpful was the theory or model in either guiding the study or explaining the findings?
6. Consider this same study. How convincing do you find the results that are presented? Do the authors provide any information in the background or methods sections that affects the trustworthiness of the findings?

References

Anonymous. (2005). Political economy of health. In S. Restivo (Ed.), *Science, technology, and society: An encyclopedia* (pp. 401–405). New York, NY: Oxford University Press.

Bandura, A. (1977). Self-efficacy: Toward a unifying theory of behavioral change. *Psychology Review, 84*(2), 191–215.

Bandura, A. (1986). *Social foundations of thought and action: A social cognitive theory.* Englewood Cliffs, NJ: Prentice-Hall.

Barnett, B., & Stein, J. (1998). *Women's voices, women's lives: The impact of family planning. A synthesis of findings from the Women's Studies Project.* Research Triangle Park, NC: Family Health International.

Bronfenbrenner, U. (1994). Ecological models of human development. In *International encyclopedia of education* (Vol. 3, 2nd ed.). Oxford, England: Elsevier.

Brooks, A. & Hesse-Biber, S. H. (2007). An invitation to feminist research. In S. H. Hesse-Biber (Ed.), *Feminist research practice* (pp. 1–24). Thousand Oaks, CA: Sage.

Champion, V. L., & Skinner C. S. (2008). The health belief model. *Health Behavior and Health Education: Theory, Research, and Practice, 4*, 45–65.

Dayton, R., Lanham, M., & Wilcher, R. (2014). Engaging male partners in women's microbicide use. Available at http://www.fhi360.org

Denzin, N. K., & Lincoln, Y. S. (2011). *The Sage handbook of qualitative research.* Thousand Oaks, CA: Sage.

Devers, K. J. (1999). How will we know "good" qualitative research when we see it? Beginning the dialogue in health services research. *Health Services Research, 34*(5 Pt 2), 1153–1188.

Fishbein, M., Triandis, H. C., Kanfer, F. H., Becker, M., Middlestadt, S. E., & Eichler, A. (1997). *Factors influencing behavior and behavior change: Final report—Theorist's workshop.* Washington, DC: American Cancer Society. [Original work published 1991]

Freire, P. (1970). *Pedagogy of the oppressed.* New York, NY: Herder & Herder.

Glanz, K., Rimer, B. K., & Viswanath, K. (2008). *Health behavior and health education: Theory, research, and practice* (4th ed.). San Francisco, CA: Wiley.

Glaser, B. G., & Strauss, A. L. (1967). *The discovery of grounded theory: Strategies for qualitative research.* Chicago, IL: Aldine.

Guba, E. G., & Lincoln, Y. S. (1994). Competing paradigms in qualitative research. In N. K. Denzin & Y. S. Lincoln (Eds.), *Handbook of qualitative research* (pp. 105–117). Thousand Oaks, CA: Sage.

Hardee, K., Irani, L., & Rodriguez, M. (2015). Linking family planning/reproductive health policies to health programs and outcomes: The importance of the policy implementation space. *International Journal of Gynecology and Obstetrics* (In press).

Imenda, S. (2014). Is there a conceptual difference between theoretical and conceptual frameworks? *Journal of Social Science, 38*(2), 185–195.

Janz, N. K., & Becker, M. H. (1984). The health belief model: A decade later. *Health Education & Behavior, 11*(1): 1–47.

Johnson, D. C., Polusny, M. A., Erbes, C. R., King, D., King, L., Litz, B. T., … & Southwick, S. M. (2011). Development and initial validation of the response to stressful experiences scale. *Military Medicine, 176*(2), 161–169.

Kieny, M.-P., Evans, D. B., Schmets, G., & Kadandale, S. (2014). Health-system resilience: Reflections on the Ebola crisis in western Africa. *Bulletin of the World Health Organization, 92*, 850.

King, G., Keohane, R. O., & Verba, S. (1994). *Designing social inquiry: Scientific inference in qualitative research.* Princeton, NJ: Princeton University Press.

Kirk, J., & Miller, M. L. (1986). *Reliability and validity in qualitative research.* Beverly Hills, CA: Sage.

Lincoln, Y. S., & Guba, E. G. (1985). *Naturalistic inquiry.* Beverly Hills, CA: Sage.

Loukaitou-Sideris, A. (1999). Hot spots of bus stop crime: The importance of environmental attributes. *Journal of the American Planning Association, 65*(4), pp. 395–411.

Mackenzie, N., & Knipe, S. (2006). Research dilemmas: Paradigms, methods and methodology. *Issues in Educational Research, 16*(2), 1–13.

MacQueen, K. M., McLellan, E., Metzger, D. S., Kegeles, S., Strauss, R. P., Scotti, R., ... Trotter, R. T., II. (2001). What is community? An evidence-based definition for participatory public health. *American Journal of Public Health, 91*(12), 1929–1938.

Maneri, M., & ter Wal, J. (2005). The criminalisation of ethnic groups: An issue for media analysis. *Qualitative Social Research, 6*(3), Art. 9.

Maxwell, J. A. (2008). Designing a qualitative study. In L. Bickman & D. Rog (Eds.), *The handbook of applied social research methods* (pp. 214–253). Thousand Oaks, CA: Sage.

McLeroy, K. R., Bibeau, D., Steckler, A., & Glanz, K. (1988). An ecological perspective on health promotion programs. *Health Education Quarterly, 15*(4), 351–377.

Meetoo, D. & Temple, B. (2003). Issues in multi-method research: Constructing self-care. *International Journal of Qualitative Methods, 2*(3), 1–12.

Mertens, D. (1999). Inclusive evaluation: Implications of transformative theory for evaluation. *American Journal of Evaluation, 20*(1), 1–14.

Miles, M. B., & Huberman, A. M. (1994). *Qualitative data analysis: An expanded sourcebook.* Thousand Oaks, CA: Sage.

Minkler, M. (2010). Linking science and policy through community-based participatory research to study and address health disparities. *American Journal of Public Health, 100*(Suppl 1): S81–S87.

National Cancer Institute. (2012). *NCI measures guide for youth tobacco research.* Behavioral Research: Cancer Control and Population Studies. Available at http://cancercontrol.cancer.gov/brp/tcrb/guide_measures.html

Newman, O. (1972). *Defensible space.* New York, NY: Macmillan.

Oldenburg, B., & Glanz, K. (2008). Diffusion of innovations. In. K. Glanz, B. K. Rimer, & K. Viswanath (Eds.), *Health behavior and health education: Theory, research, and practice* (4th ed., pp. 313–333). San Francisco, CA: Wiley.

Olesen, V. L. (2000). Feminisms and qualitative research at and into the millennium. In N. K. Denzin & Y. S. Lincoln (Eds.), *Handbook of qualitative research* (2nd ed., pp. 215–255). Thousand Oaks, CA: Sage.

Pan American Health Organization. (1997). *Workshop on gender, health, and development: Facilitator's guide.* Washington, DC: Regional Program on Women, Health, and Development.

Pedersen, D. (1992), Qualitative and quantitative: Two styles of viewing the world or two categories of reality? In S. Scrimshaw & G. R. Gleason (Eds.), *RAP: Rapid Assessment Procedures. Qualitative methodologies for planning and evaluation of health related programmes* (pp. 39–49). Boston, MA: International Nutrition Foundation for Developing Countries.

Prochaska, J. O., DiClemente, C. C., & Norcross, J. C. (1992). In search of how people change: Applications to addictive behaviors. *American Psychologist, 47*(9), 1102–1114.

Rosenstock, I., Strecher, V.,& Becker, M. (1994). The Health Belief Model and HIV risk behavior change. In R. J. Clemente & J. L. Peterson (Eds.), *Preventing AIDS: Theories and methods of behavioral interventions* (pp. 5–24). New York, NY: Plenum Press.

Sbaraini, A., Carter, S. M., Evans, R. W., & Blinkhorn, A. (2011). How to do a grounded theory study: A worked example of a study of dental practices. *BMC Medical Research Methodology, 11*(1): 128.

Schuler, S. R., Lenzi, R., & Yount, K. M. (2011). Justification of intimate partner violence in rural Bangladesh: What survey questions fail to capture. *Studies in Family Planning, 42*(1), 21–28.

Schuler, S. R., Yount, K. M., & Lenzi, R. (2012). Justification of wife beating in rural Bangladesh: A qualitative analysis of gender differences in responses to survey questions. *Violence Against Women, 18*(10), 1177–1191.

Selltiz, C., Wrightsman, L. S., Cook, S. W., & Society for the Psychological Study of Social Issues. (1976). *Research methods in social relations.* New York, NY: Holt, Rinehart & Winston.

Southwick, S. M., Bonanno, G. A., Masten, A. S., Panter-Brick C., & Yehuda, R. (2014). Resilience definitions, theory, and challenges: Interdisciplinary perspectives. *European Journal of Psychotraumatology, 5.* doi:10.3402/ejpt.v5.25338

Stokols, D. (1996). Translating social ecological theory into guidelines for community health promotion. *American Journal of Health Promotion, 10*(4), 282–298.

Tesh, S. (1981). Disease causality and politics. *Journal of Health Politics, Policy and Law, 6*(3), 369–390.

Thomas, A. J., Carey, D., Prewitt, K., Romero, E., Richards, M., & Velsor-Friedrich, M. (2012). African-American youth and exposure to community violence: Supporting change from the inside. *Journal for Social Action in Counseling and Psychology, 4*(1), 54–68.

Tolley, E. E., Eng, E., Kohli, R., Bentley, M. E., Mehendale, S., Bunce, A., & Severy, L. J. (2006). Examining the context of microbicide acceptability among married women and men in India. *Culture, Health & Sexuality, 8*(4), 351–369.

Tolman, D. L., & Szalacha, L. A. (1999). Dimensions of desire: Bridging qualitative and quantitative methods in a study of female adolescent sexuality. *Psychology of Women Quarterly, 23*(1), 7–39.

Ulin, P. R. (1992). African women and AIDS: Negotiating behavioral change. *Social Science & Medicine, 34*(1), 63–73.

van Ryn, M. & Heany, C. A. (1992). What's the use of theory? *Health Education Quarterly, 19*(3), 315–330.

Willis, J. W. (2007). *Foundations of qualitative research, interpretive and critical approaches.* Thousand Oaks, CA: Sage.

Yin, R. K. (1994). *Case study research: Design and methods.* Thousand Oaks, CA: Sage.

Zimmerman, M. A. (2013). Resiliency theory: A strengths-based approach to research and practice for adolescent health. *Health Education & Behavior, 40*(4), 381–383.

CHAPTER 3

DESIGNING THE STUDY

OBJECTIVES:

- To describe four general purposes for conducting public health research, including formative/exploratory, descriptive, explanatory, and transformative research
- To show how to construct a qualitative research proposal that includes essential elements of study design
- To show how the research purpose affects choice of qualitative, quantitative, or mixed methods
- To show how to link the study purpose to decisions about data sources, sampling approaches, and data collection methods
- To identify other factors that may influence study design, including budgets and timelines
- To describe ethical considerations for research and how to take them into account in choices of study design

A WELL-ARTICULATED DESIGN is the basis for all research proposals. It presents a persuasive argument for why the study is needed, identifies the specific objectives, and provides a logical plan for how those objectives will be met. Design decisions at this stage will demonstrate the value and rigor of your proposed research. They will also clearly show the relationship between your research problem; the conceptual or theoretical framework that will guide your design (see Chapter 2); and the data sources, data collection methods, and analysis procedures through which information will emerge.

As experienced investigators know, the process of designing and implementing qualitative research is rarely linear. In fact, as highlighted in Chapter 1, the flexibility for qualitative researchers to rethink and modify elements of the design even as the data are emerging is an important strength of the qualitative research approach. How can researchers sufficiently demonstrate the value and rigor of their research designs while maintaining the flexibility needed to obtain the in-depth understanding of their topic unique to qualitative research? How can a combination of approaches be structured in a design that will be understood by funders of research?

Health researchers are usually required to develop and submit proposals that will be reviewed and evaluated in order to receive funding. Typically, the elements that make up a study design are described in **research proposals** and include the rationale for the study; its objectives, data sources, and collection methods; a plan for how to analyze study data and disseminate findings to research stakeholders; and an explicit description of how the confidentiality of study participants will be respected. In this chapter, we present and discuss important design questions in a sequence that follows a typical research proposal, as shown in Table 3.1.

Written answers to these questions should provide sufficient detail by which others can judge the relevance and rigor of your proposed research. Such documentation often becomes the basis for proposals submitted to donors for funding or protocols submitted to scientific or ethical review boards prior to research implementation. However, it is important to keep in mind that reviewers often have their own criteria for judging quality and relevance (Creswell, Klassen, Plano Clark, & Smith, 2011). For example, funders often request capacity-building and project management plans to be incorporated with study designs in proposal submissions. Scientific review

Table 3.1 Common Elements of a Research Proposal

Background and rationale	What is the knowledge gap? What is the purpose of the proposed research? What is the larger conceptual framework?
Study objectives	What topics or content areas will be examined, and why? What research questions will be answered?
Data sources	Who should participate? What other information sources should be included?
Data collection methods	What methods, qualitative alone or mixed methods, will best address the research questions? How should the data be collected? How will data collectors be trained and monitored?
Data analysis	How will the data be analyzed?
Dissemination	How will the results be presented, and to whom?
Research ethics	What ethical standards will be implemented to ensure participants' protection?
Other considerations	Timelines and budgets

boards usually have specific requirements about the types of information that must be contained in a protocol for it to be approved.

Background and Rationale

Most applied researchers are drawn to an area of inquiry out of personal interest or experiences or a desire to help solve a problem. In public health, areas of inquiry might be the need for dental care in a community health service, the introduction of a new method of cancer screening, the prevalence of stroke in a low-risk population, or perhaps the high incidence of health-related absenteeism on a factory assembly line. At times, applied researchers engage in a research field that is new to them in response to a request from a stakeholder—whether a Ministry of Health, a nongovernmental organization (NGO), or a foundation. Regardless of how they become engaged in a research topic, most applied researchers will need to secure funding. To do so, they must persuade key stakeholders that the inquiry will benefit society and demonstrate that the proposed research approach will provide useful information and insight into the problem.

The introductory section of a research proposal is where the researcher should make a persuasive case for his or her research. This section should orient the reviewer to the research problem, provide a documented review of what is already known, and identify specific gaps in knowledge that will be addressed by the proposed study. The study objectives should flow logically from this review of the field, and the choice to use a particular qualitative or **mixed-method research** design should be apparent.

For example, a development NGO in Indonesia introduced cleaner, more fuel-efficient cook stoves into one rural area to reduce the negative health impacts of indoor air pollution from traditional stoves, but uptake of the improved cook stoves was lower in some villages than others (see Case Study 6 in Appendix 1). Exploring this issue in the literature, a researcher discovered that most efforts to reduce indoor air pollution caused by traditional cooking methods had focused on individual use; few programs had considered the complex social and cultural factors that influence adoption of this new technology, such as cooking practices, fuel availability, awareness of indoor air pollution, and the structure of work and daily activities. The NGO therefore designed a study that included qualitative components. The rationale given in the study proposal for its selection of methods was that by including focus groups and in-depth interviews in the study design, the development NGO would be better able to address cultural issues relating to adoption of its improved stoves.

Even at this early stage of design, it is important to think ahead to the kinds of information that intended recipients will need. In the cook stoves study, findings led to specific recommendations for development NGOs, policymakers, and health care providers who wanted to increase adoption of environmentally safer cooking methods. The types of questions asked by policymakers and program managers looking for evidence or recommendations on how to make programs more accessible, health care more effective, or services more acceptable are important considerations to address in both your study purpose and your objectives.

Stating the Research Problem

As you narrow your focus to a more manageable field, you begin to define the specific issues that will form the core of the study: the research problem. If the area of inquiry is quality of prenatal care, the research problem might be to explore women's perceptions of the care they receive at a clinic, the nature and consequences of client–provider interaction, or women's decisions about whether to seek prenatal care. If the inquiry focuses on occupational hazards in the workplace, the problem could be to explore the context in which accidents occur and the immediate responses of co-workers in the vicinity.

Study Purpose: Formative, Descriptive, Explanatory, or Transformative Research

One of the first things the reviewer of a proposal or protocol looks for is the purpose of the study. What does it intend to do? Is the proposed study intended to explore a topic that is little understood? Describe in detail a health behavior or its context? Explain whether or how relationships among interacting concepts impact a health outcome? Engage community members in examining a problem of their concern and thus increase their capacity to achieve their own health goals? Once the purpose of the study is established, specific operational objectives should be identified. The study objectives will fine-tune the problem and lead logically into the study design, whether formative, descriptive, explanatory, or transformative.

Formative Research. Formative research is a form of exploratory research that often takes place before a larger program or scientific investigation is initiated. The outcome of a formative study may be to better understand a selected population, create appropriate programs or research procedures, or ensure that the program or study to follow will be culturally relevant and acceptable. A thorough literature or desk review and discussions with stakeholders can help determine the need for a formative stage prior to a larger study and suggest the best methods to use.

Wong and Noriega (2013), for example, conducted formative research in Bangladesh and Papua New Guinea in order to identify potential interventions aimed at reducing gender-based violence (GBV) among sexual minorities, including men who have sex with men, male sex workers, and transgendered women. (See Case Study 7 in Appendix 1.) In addition to conducting small numbers of focus group discussions with these marginalized groups, they involved a range of key informants—including NGO representatives, health care workers, law enforcement officers, and local policymakers—to explore sources and forms of GBV and potential approaches to reducing the violence experienced by those groups.

A different but common application of formative research can be found in some pharmaceutical and biomedical studies. For example, social and behavioral scientists have conducted formative research prior to implementation of several multicountry HIV prevention trials to examine community attitudes toward the clinical research; identify potential barriers to recruitment, retention, and adherence; and to field-test informed consent documents (MacQueen et al., 2012; Tolley & Severy, 2006). Increasingly, such formative research constitutes a first set of activities intended to engage stakeholders in biomedical research (Mack et al., 2013). (See Case Study 8 in Appendix 1 for an example of formative research to prepare for the rollout of new HIV prevention methods internationally.)

Whether paving the way for a health intervention, informing policy, or creating appropriate tools for any research design, formative research can produce valuable information for evidence-based decisions at all levels of practice.

Descriptive Research. Descriptive research describes and documents a health context, whether related to program implementation or to economic or sociocultural structures or practices that are believed to affect health outcomes. When combined with survey methodology, descriptive research can provide a more detailed picture of the issue under study. For example, a mixed-method descriptive study to document and describe attitudes toward voluntary male medical circumcision (VMMC) in Uganda integrated information from household-based surveys, community-level focus group discussions, and provider surveys (Albert et al., 2011). While the household survey provided information about the overall level of support for VMMC, as well as differences by region and among men and women, the focus group discussion data provided more detailed information about community members' reasons for accepting or rejecting VMMC.

Explanatory Research. Explanatory research is most often a quantitative approach that attempts to establish cause-and-effect relationships among variables in a carefully controlled design. The use of qualitative techniques in explanatory research is therefore a departure from its more traditional foundation (Maxwell, 2008, 2013). However, many researchers have discovered that incorporating qualitative methods in mixed-method designs can yield powerful new insights that help to explain patterns and relationships observed in the data. For this reason, for example, in an evaluation of the Malawi Male Motivator project (see Case Study 9 in Appendix 1) (Shattuck et al., 2011), researchers included in-depth interviews with a subsample of program participants. Their study design, which was guided by the information-motivation-behavioral skills (IMB) model (a substantive theory) and included randomization of program participants to either an intervention or a control arm, sought to determine whether men's exposure to the intervention increased contraceptive uptake. The study found that men exposed to the program were more likely to initiate partners' contraceptive use. Adding a qualitative dimension revealed important explanatory information—that improving men's communication skills was a key to the success of the program (Shattuck et al., 2011).

Transformative Research. Research based on a transformative paradigm typically incorporates methods that engage and empower community members (see Chapter 2). These may be qualitative, quantitative, or a mix of both. Action-oriented community diagnosis, for example, a tool developed by Eng and Blanchard (1991), enables researchers to identify group as well as individual health needs. By bringing community residents into the diagnostic process at the level of community assessment, researchers can empower them to find and implement solutions to their own problems. This transformative approach, which employs participatory methods, is particularly useful for linking the health perceptions and needs of individuals to empowerment or conscious behavioral change. In a separate action-oriented study in Darfur, South Sudan, local research partners trained in the use of community mapping techniques were able to engage their communities in identifying needs and resources, and thus take ownership in community development efforts informed by study results (FHI 360, 2011).

Community-Based Participatory Research. Particularly if you are working within a transformative paradigm, you may consider using a participatory approach for your research. Over the last five or more decades, a number of adaptations have existed, including rapid rural appraisal (Chambers, 1981), participatory rural or rapid appraisal (Chambers, 1994), participatory action research (Kemmis & McTaggart, 2008), and community-based participatory research (Wallerstein & Duran, 2006).

More than a set of data collection methods, participatory research is an approach that engages local community members to varying degrees in the process of identifying the research problem and designing, collecting, analyzing, and utilizing the data. In earlier applications of participatory research, ultimate decisions about the research tended to remain with external researchers. For example, while a rural farmer might lead an outside researcher through his fields, naming indigenous plants and describing their uses, outsiders still determined how such information was to be used (Chambers, 1994). Increasingly, participatory research approaches have emphasized the need to share decision-making power and control over research agendas and processes with the local community (Horowitz, Robinson, & Seifer, 2009). In **community-based participatory research** (CBPR), community members play an active role in determining what questions are asked and of whom. They work alongside their research partners to collect and interpret the data and to translate study findings into social action (Wallerstein & Duran, 2006).

While many elements of a participatory research design may resemble other types of research, the process for arriving at design decisions, as well as implementation and dissemination processes, are likely to differ. For example, a CBPR approach may include specific strategies, such as community collaborative councils or joint learning activities, to build community trust and the development of a shared vision of the research (see Case Study 3 in Appendix 1). Bidirectional training may be required, providing community researchers with methods-related knowledge and skills and academic researchers with knowledge and skills related to community norms and processes. During study implementation, regularly scheduled meetings provide opportunities to communicate what is being learned and make adjustments, if needed. Finally, additional and/or alternative approaches to dissemination may be needed to ensure that the community can access, understand, and utilize study findings (Horowitz et al., 2009).

Conceptualizing the Problem in a Larger Framework

One way to keep your design centered on the research problem is to take the time to develop a conceptual model or framework (see Chapter 2). A conceptual framework is a set of related ideas behind the research design. It may be a simple list of concepts and their possible associations or a more elaborate schematic diagram of key influences, presumed relationships, and possible outcomes of the research problem, such as how advocacy influences health policy and in turn health outcomes. (See Box 3.1). Motivated by a compelling

BOX 3.1 CONCEPTUAL FRAMEWORK: SOCIAL DRIVERS OF ADOPTION OF IMPROVED COOK STOVES

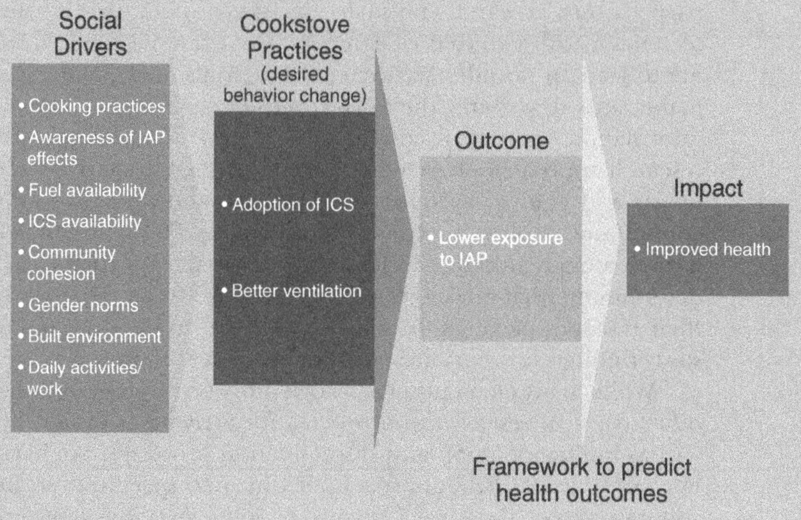

problem or some critical gap in knowledge, most researchers begin a study with at least a tentative notion of what factors may be important and how they might fit together in a logical scheme. Whether a simple list of concepts or a more elaborate schematic diagram, your framework will be the springboard from which you determine important research design decisions, including the specific aims of your study and whether to use a qualitative-only or mixed-method approach. A literature review can identify findings from previous research that will suggest ways of conceptualizing the current problem.

In the cook stove example described in Case Study 6 in Appendix 1 and shown in Box 3.1, by reviewing prior research and substantive theory, the researcher identified a number of factors that might influence people's willingness and ability to adopt new technologies such as improved cook stoves (ICS).

The model included the following potential "drivers" that could be operationalized into interviewer questions or observations:

Cooking practices: type of cook stove and fuel currently used; location of cook stove within/outside of home; frequency, timing, and duration of cook stove use

Awareness of indoor air pollution (IAP) dangers: awareness of linkage between household smoke and respiratory illnesses; perceived susceptibility to and severity of illnesses; barriers to and perceived benefits of improved cook stove technologies among community members, health care providers, and others

Fuel availability: cost of and access to traditional and cleaner fuel sources

Availability of improved cook stoves: cost, procurement, and distribution of improved cook stoves; potential for adaptation of existing cook stove technologies or local manufacturing of improved ones

Community cohesiveness: presence or absence of influential leaders or cohesive organizations to support adoption; mechanisms for social learning and shared decision making; potential for pooling resources for loans or labor

Gender norms: responsibilities for gathering fuel, preparing and cooking food; access to finances to purchase fuel; perceived norms related to women's use of technology

Built environment: type of household structure and external surroundings; ventilation; storage space

Daily activities/work: location, duration, importance, and compatibility of other activities (i.e., childcare, gardening, cleaning, or paid work) relative to cooking activities

Developing Study Objectives

In a proposal, the research problem is generally stated in a set of carefully defined and broadly stated objectives and research questions. Study objectives map the overall purpose of your study and tend to begin with action words, such as *to explore, to describe,* or *to examine.* For example, the specific objectives of a study of caregiver–practitioner interactions related to childhood pneumonia were to:

- Investigate private providers' acute respiratory infection/pneumonia diagnosis and treatment attitudes and practices;
- Explore and document the factors affecting families' care choices for children suspected to have pneumonia;
- Examine the care-seeking and treatment behaviors of caregivers who take children to private providers for suspected pneumonia.

The language included in your objectives will focus attention on the meaning, process, or social contexts underlying your research topic, which can be further articulated in the form of research questions. For example, research questions in a formative study to explore microbicide acceptability among Indian women (see Case Study 4 in Appendix 1) as part of larger global efforts to prevention HIV in vulnerable populations, included the following (Tolley et al., 2006):

- Within what circumstances do married women and men in India perceive a risk of HIV? Does perception differ for women and men?
- How do married couples discuss sexual risk or risk-reduction behaviors? Does discussion differ for couples who are at identified risk versus low or unidentified risk?
- What individual-, couple-, or structural-level factors might affect their willingness or ability to use microbicides?

Research questions should be broad enough to guide qualitative exploration yet concrete and specific enough to support the rationale for the research. Moreover, research questions should not be confused with qualitative interview questions in topic guides, which may be revised or adapted as the study progresses (Maxwell, 2008). (See discussion on topic guides in Chapter 4.) Interview questions, which flow from research questions, yield the data that, in the analysis, will answer broader research questions. Determining the objectives or overarching research questions for your research will, by extension, help you determine which data sources, data collection methods, and data analysis strategies should be included in your protocol. For example, the objectives of the childhood pneumonia study mentioned previously clearly point to the need to include a sample of "private practitioners" and a sample of "caregivers." How such participants are identified and recruited, and whether data collection should include individual interviews, observations of clinic visits, review of clinic records, or group discussions with parents or practitioners remain important choices for research design.

Using Documentary Sources

Documentary sources are often useful when defining and conceptualizing a research problem. From large databases to personal journals and diaries, and even to the lyrics of popular songs, the astute researcher will find clues to a better understanding of the study population. Cultural norms are revealed in radio and TV shows, and blogs and social networking sites contain a wealth of information on people's hopes, fears, and triumphs. Data collected for other purposes, such as the Demographic and Health Survey (DHS) or hospital and clinic records, may shed light on different qualitative questions, for example, what motivates women to seek prenatal care or why there appear to be racial differences in the incidence of workplace injury. Other research problems that might be linked to documentary information include government policy on HIV/AIDS as presented in the press, violence in advertising, gender bias in radio and television dramas, or differences in health information given to different social groups as documented in clinic records. For example, as part of a wider inquiry into AIDS awareness, an AIDS activist in Kenya gathered information on adolescents' concerns about HIV/AIDS from their letters to an AIDS advice column for young people in a local newspaper (L. Kimani, personal communication, November 1990).

All contribute to the cultural context within which a qualitative research problem is formulated, and all are part of the public record. Once data are collected and analysis is in process, the researcher will return again to these sources for insight into the new findings.

Data From Human Subjects

In all research, investigators must decide where and from whom they will gather the data needed to answer their research questions. While documentary sources may offer valuable insight into the context of the research problem, the essence of qualitative research is the human dimension—the people who will help you find your answers.

In decisions about whom to interview, researchers are commonly guided by the paradigm or theoretical framework they have chosen for a study. From an interpretive perspective, the investigator views ordinary people as experts by virtue of the experiences and ideas they can share and their willingness to help explore the research problem. As always in the iterative process of qualitative research, selection criteria may change as the study progresses, allowing the researcher to follow new leads with information from new sources (Rubin & Rubin, 1995).

A typical goal of quantitative research is to generalize findings to larger populations, achieving a high degree of reliability. To minimize sampling error, every case in a sampling frame must have an equal probability of selection. The purpose of most qualitative studies, on the other hand, is to produce information-rich data from a sample chosen for its ability to speak to the research issue (Patton, 1990; Patton 2015, p. 264). Qualitative research emphasizes depth over breadth, insight rather than generalization, illuminating the meaning of human behavior. (See Chapter 1 for a review of the principles of qualitative research.) Although qualitative researchers sometimes use numbers and frequencies to record observations, conceptual rather than numerical considerations determine sample selection. The challenge for the qualitative researcher, therefore, is to select participants who will be able to provide the most meaningful information on the topic. The extent to which results may be relevant to other populations will be enhanced by careful documentation of the conceptual links between research problem, sample selection process, and emerging data.

Selection: Theoretical or *a Priori*?

> **The validity, meaningfulness, and insights generated from qualitative inquiry have more to do with the information-richness of the cases selected and the observational/analytical capabilities of the researcher than with sample size.**
>
> ***(Patton, 1990, p. 185)***

In qualitative design there are two basic approaches to selecting participants; they emphasize experience or insight related to the research problem rather than random selection. One of these approaches, called *theoretical sampling,* is particularly appropriate when the main purpose of data collection is to generate substantive theory (Strauss, 1990). Beginning with a small number of individuals or groups, the researcher asks, "Given what I am learning, what information do I need next and where—or in what groups—will I find it?" (Flick, 1998, p. 65). In other words, theoretical sampling is continuous and gradual, guided by data collection, analysis, and interpretation as theory builds. It is especially consistent with the goals and techniques of grounded theory, which are presented in more detail in Chapter 2.

A priori sampling is the approach most familiar to applied researchers in public health. Based on your research problem and purpose, you define in advance of data collection the sample's characteristics and structure. If your purpose is to understand health attitudes and behaviors of adolescents in a community, you will select participants from this group as well as other individuals whose opinions on adolescent health or whose actual experiences with young people give them special insight into your area of inquiry. If different perspectives and behaviors are known to prevail in the population, then you would choose participants who differ in these respects. At this point you will also decide the numbers of participants in each category and the background characteristics that will help you interpret their responses.

Note that *a priori* selection does not preclude sampling additions and changes as the study progresses. The most important consideration in qualitative sampling is the data's richness or explanatory value. In the adolescent health example, you might discover that young people with conservative religious views perceive sexual norms differently than do their peers with a different religious orientation. The next step could be to invite a sample of religious leaders in the community to help you explore religious influences on adolescent health decisions.

Sample Selection Techniques

Selecting a sample for a qualitative study is not haphazard, nor is it bound by rigid rules of reproducibility. It should be systematic but flexible, guided by clear research questions as articulated in your theoretical framework. Because the purpose of qualitative design is to explore in depth, the investigator carefully selects cases that can typify or shed light on the object of study. Therefore, to identify and gain access to those who can teach you the most about your topic, it follows that sampling methods will generally be based on purpose (*purposive sampling*) rather than on statistical probability of selection (*probabilistic sampling*). In qualitative sampling, purposiveness is a strategic approach, not a single technique, and it means selecting participants for their ability to provide rich information. Purposive sampling should never be confused with sampling for convenience. The latter, motivated primarily by ease of access to respondents, may be economical, but it does not necessarily reflect the study's purpose, and it may significantly weaken the quality of the data (Patton, 2014, p. 300). Although nonprobabilistic sampling is more common than probabilistic sampling for qualitative methods, probabilistic techniques may still be used in qualitative research. See Case Study 10 in Appendix 1 for examples of probabilistic techniques or examples of qualitative research studies that incorporated probabilistic techniques.

There are many purposive strategies, each linked to the purpose of the study as expressed in the initial research question. Following one such typology (Patton, 1990, 2014), we describe several strategies that in our experience have been useful tools for qualitative sampling decisions. Although we present these techniques separately in Table 3.2, readers should be aware that many studies combine more than one.

Sample Size

When a goal of the study is to generalize findings from a sample to a larger population, as in many quantitative designs, the researcher can calculate a representative sample size from a formula. In qualitative studies, optimum size is

Table 3.2 Summary of Sampling Approaches

Sampling Approach	Most Common Use	Benefits	Drawbacks
Probabilistic	Quantitative and mixed methods	Systematic	Typically requires larger sample size
Purposive	Qualitative	Flexible	Selection bias possible
Extreme sampling	Selects extreme or "deviant" cases in order to contrast conditions or characteristics with more typical situations. In using extreme cases, the investigator must take care not to distort reality by making the unusual seem to be the norm. The purpose is not to generalize to all populations or institutions, but to magnify certain characteristics.		
Intensity sampling	Focuses on excellent, but not necessarily extreme, examples of the phenomenon. Samples are small and rich in information but not unusual, such as in the case of people with particular experience in the topic or clinics that provide services relevant to the research problem. In any small exploratory sample, intensive exploration of selected issues with a few well-informed people or groups can add interesting, insightful, and reality-based perspectives and information.		
Homogeneous samples	Whether to emphasize similarities or differences in selecting a sample again depends on the study's purpose. People in homogeneous samples have basically similar characteristics. This type of sample is appropriate if you are studying one or more groups in depth. By limiting sample selection to individuals who meet these criteria, you are better able to focus on a central issue that is relevant to all of them. Focus groups typically use this approach, stimulating people with a common identity to discuss their shared experiences.		
Heterogeneous samples	May be useful for studying issues that cut across individual or program variation. Qualitative investigators sampling from a diverse population may want to highlight variation in some complex phenomenon. Or they may be looking for common themes that emerge even in the presence of other differences. The discovery of similar experiences, behaviors, or perceptions in an otherwise heterogeneous group may warrant further in-depth study in separate homogeneous samples.		
Typical cases	Often in operations research or evaluation, it is useful to describe a typical case, program, or participant that serves as a profile for understanding the principal features of a group of programs or a class of individuals. The researcher may sample a typical case as illustrative or as a unit of analysis. What constitutes typical is a subjective judgment, but key informants who are especially familiar with the general category can likely identify examples that are average—not extreme in any sense related to the study.		

Table 3.2 (*Continued*)

Sampling Approach	Most Common Use	Benefits	Drawbacks
Respondent-driven sampling (RDS)	This is a technique often used for locating hidden or hard-to-reach informants by asking a small number of respondents to recruit others within their networks. These initial "seeds" are often compensated for recruiting a specified number of peers. The second and additional waves of recruited peers may also be compensated for recruiting others in their own networks (Patton 2015, p. 299). Mathematical models may be developed to estimate the degree to which the resulting sample resembles a probabilistic one, although is not a necessary feature of RDS for a qualitative study. Because informants with special expertise can likely identify other knowledgeable people, this technique can be a valuable one when the researcher does not know the field. It is also useful when individuals with the knowledge or experience to provide rich data are difficult to reach, such people whose behavior or lifestyle deviates from social norms, or anyone fearful of public exposure. When such individuals are willing to trust the researcher, it is especially critical to protect their privacy and confidentiality.		
Convenience	Limited budget, short timeline	Rapid	Less rigorous
Opportunistic sampling	Because qualitative strategies can change in response to findings as they emerge in the field, you may need to select additional study participants, making an "on-the-spot decision to take advantage of unforeseen opportunities after fieldwork has begun" (Patton 1990; Patton 2015, p. 300).		

less clear, although there have been attempts to establish minimum criteria (Guest, Bunce, & Johnson, 2006). The investigator is guided by the degree to which incoming data adequately answer the research questions—an ambiguous rule at best. But if sample size depends on completeness of the data (Rubin & Rubin, 1995), how do you know when data are complete?

If the research problem is a simple one, it is possible that one individual could provide the whole answer. In public health, however, most research designs are not that simple. Optimally, you would want to collect data from as many groups or individuals as necessary to answer the research questions. When little new information is coming from your observations, interviews, or focus group discussions, you can be reasonably confident that you have *saturated* that source of information to the point of redundancy (Glaser & Strauss, 1967). For example, in a field experiment aimed at documenting the degree of saturation and variability during thematic coding of 60 in-depth interviews with women from two West African countries, Guest and colleagues found that saturation occurred after analysis of 12 interviews, while most high-level themes were identified after coding the first six in-depth interviews (Guest, Bunce, & Johnson, 2006).

In most funded research, basing participant selection on indeterminate measures such as saturation and redundancy is impractical for determining budgets and timelines. Qualitative researchers might begin with "minimum samples based on expected reasonable coverage... given the purpose of the study and stakeholder interests" (Patton, 1990, p. 186). Once in the field, you will make a decision as to whether you need to expand your sample. Altering the subgroup composition in your design is justified in qualitative research if doing so will enrich your findings. Your research proposal can accommodate alterations to your sampling strategy by describing the types of individuals, groups, or contexts to be sampled and their range, rather than presenting an exact sample size.

The qualitative researcher tries to collect information representative of the range of experiences, perspectives, and behaviors relevant to the research question. In contrast, quantitative approaches are more likely to result in samples that represent the distribution of these variables. The important thing to remember is that "the logic of purposeful sampling is different from the logic of probability sampling" (Patton, 1990, p. 185). Small purposive samples are ideally suited to qualitative inquiry. A large random sample could not accomplish the objectives of an in-depth study any more than a small nonrandom sample could accurately represent a large population. For the qualitative researcher, it is crucial to describe, justify, and explain small sample selection so that others can judge its strengths and weaknesses. "Exercising care not to overgeneralize from purposeful samples, while maximizing to the full the advantages of in-depth, purposeful sampling, will do much to alleviate concerns about small sample size" (Patton, 1990, p. 186).

Recruiting Participants

Study participants are drawn from a community, any of its institutions (e.g., clinics, schools, churches, workplaces, bars), or wherever people are willing to share knowledge and experience related to the research topics. In some studies, researchers visit sites where potential participants gather; they chat informally with people and select an initial sample based on the apparent readiness of individuals to address the research issues. In other studies, clinic records or membership lists serve as a sampling frame, particularly when individuals in the frame share a common characteristic of interest to the research. As in all sampling strategies, decisions must also be made regarding other selection criteria, such as age or marital status. In our study of new contraceptive users in Mali, researchers worked with clinic personnel to identify every married woman who had come to the clinic to begin family planning for the first time (Castle, Konaté, Ulin, & Martin, 1999). But because this study used a longitudinal design, the invitation to participate was extended only to women who were geographically accessible for follow-up interviews.

In community-based studies, you may want to enlist the help of residents to identify and invite eligible individuals to participate. If so, select such recruiters carefully to avoid possible coercion or alienation of important subgroups. As we discuss in Chapter 5, incorporating local people into the field team at this point is especially useful in unfamiliar cultures or in communities with language barriers. It is important to orient helpers to the study's purpose, rehearsing with them how to introduce it, how to invite participation, and how to assure potential participants of confidentiality and freedom to decline.

Data Collection Methods

Because no single research method can tap all dimensions of a complex research problem, it is often valuable to combine two or more methods, drawing conclusions from a synthesis of the results. The use of multiple methods, also called *triangulation,* unquestionably results in a broader perspective on the problem and often more persuasive findings for policymakers. Similar results from two or more methods could increase the credibility of the findings, whereas dissimilar results might raise new questions about alternative interpretations (see Box 3.2). Mixed-method research typically implies the deliberate use of both qualitative and quantitative research—combining the strengths of both—to better understand the research topic.

Note that different results from one method do not necessarily invalidate the results of another. Given that reality is defined in many ways and in many contexts, different data collection tools may reveal a variety of perspectives, different ways that people conceptualize and evaluate the same situation. Like a photographer attempting to capture a perfect likeness, the careful researcher considers the research problem from different angles, using quantitative or qualitative methods or integrating both in various combinations.

Increasingly, researchers are discovering the benefits of using more than one theoretical perspective to study a problem (Obermeyer, 1997; Tashakkori & Teddlie, 1998). Their research reports demonstrate that combining qualitative and quantitative strategies in a single study can result in a more powerful design than either used alone. For example, a study assessing the use of financial incentives to increase adherence to treatment medication might include

BOX 3.2 COMMON WAYS TO MIX METHODOLOGIES

If you understand the following basic principles and techniques of qualitative and quantitative strategies, you will discover useful ways to combine them:

- A formative phase (e.g., focus group discussions) that precedes a quantitative phase (e.g., a household survey) can provide information for generating hypotheses and designing the instrument, as well as identifying language meaningful to the study population.
- Quantitative data can also be used in a formative phase, providing useful background information for designing a qualitative study.
- Quantitative data on study participants (e.g., sociodemographic data and sexual and reproductive histories) can help to interpret qualitative results or highlight important subgroup differences.
- A qualitative phase that occurs at the end of a quantitative study can help to interpret quantitative findings or evaluate an intervention.
- Qualitative and quantitative techniques can be used independently to examine a problem from different perspectives.
- Qualitative (open-ended) questions can be included in a quantitative instrument to collect limited data on issues that cannot be answered in the structured format.
- Qualitative exit interviews can be conducted with a sample of quantitative survey participants to check the external validity or comprehensiveness of the measures.

a structured survey of knowledge, attitudes, and practices among those diagnosed regarding the specific illness and its treatment (a quantitative component) in addition to in-depth interviews with a subset of patients who demonstrate different levels of adherence (a qualitative component) and observation of counseling sessions within clinics (both quantitative and qualitative). Each technique would yield different but complementary results, and together they would give you a more complete picture than one approach alone.

In applied social and behavioral research, few problems do not have the potential for exploration through qualitative and quantitative inquiry. In a study that explored how cultural differences influence minority caretakers' responses to Alzheimer's disease and related dementias (Weitzman & Levkoff, 2000), researchers conducted qualitative interviews with 40 caretakers, followed by 120 structured interviews using several standardized scales. The authors discovered that this combination highlighted the interplay between culture and care more clearly than could any single method alone. They concluded that rigor in research means "not being beholden to a particular research method, but rather letting the questions point to the methods even if it means combining methods" (p. 203).

Similarly, a study of students' use of a school health service might include records of student attendance with age and grade, students' health complaints, the school nurse's observations, and treatment or referral (a quantitative component). In-depth interviews with students, parents, and school personnel (a qualitative component) and observation in the nurse's office (both quantitative and qualitative) would yield three sets of complementary results. Together they could offer a comprehensive understanding of student health care from multiple perspectives.

In a different application of mixed methods, a team of investigators explored hypothetical factors that might influence women's willingness and ability to use an HIV prevention vaginal gel that was still in development. While previous acceptability research had focused mostly on attitudes toward product characteristics, these researchers believed that other factors, including women's perceived risk of HIV and their ability to negotiate sex with partners, would be stronger indicators of predisposition to use a new product. A formative study of high- and low-risk couples in India led the researchers to a better understanding of how women and their partners conceptualized risk, how risk perceptions related to marital relationships, and how men and women negotiated risk—whether for pregnancy, sexually transmitted infections (STIs), or HIV. From these data emerged a conceptual framework that showed relationships among risk perception, couple harmony, and sexual power in relation to sustained use of an HIV prevention gel (Tolley et al., 2006; Tolley, Tsui, Mehendale, Weaver, & Kohli, 2012).

> **Let us be done with the arguments of [qualitative versus quantitative methods]... and get on with the business of attacking our problems with the widest array of conceptual and methodological tools that we possess and they demand.**
>
> *(Trow, 1957, p. 35)*

A Practical Strategy for Mixed-Method Design

Much has been written in support of mixed methodology, but the reader is often left to manage the technical task of combining very different techniques in a coherent design. Once you have established the strategic relevance of two or more methods to the research questions, you will need to decide how to coordinate them. For this purpose we advocate the priority-sequence model (see Box 3.3), an approach that integrates the "complementary strengths of different methods through a division of labor . . . within the same overall project" (Morgan, 1998, p. 366). The division of labor requires two basic decisions, one that assigns priority and one that determines sequence.

The four-cell model represents four basic designs in which "(a) the principal method is either qualitative or quantitative (priority) and (b) the complementary method occurs as a preliminary or a follow-up stage to the primary method (sequence)" (Morgan, 1998, p. 367). In each cell of

BOX 3.3 PRIORITY-SEQUENCE MODEL: DECISIONS FOR INTEGRATING METHODS

Quantitative	Qualitative
1. Qualitative preliminary qual → QUANT* Smaller qualitative study helps guide data collection in a principally quantitative study. Can generate hypotheses, develop content for questionnaires and interventions, and so on. Example: Focus groups shape culturally sensitive versions of a new health promotion campaign.	**2. Quantitative preliminary** quant → QUAL Smaller quantitative study helps guide data collection in a principally qualitative study. Can guide purposive sampling, establish preliminary results to pursue in depth, and so on. Example: A survey of different units in a hospital locates sites for more extensive ethnographic data collection.
3. Qualitative follow-up QUANT → qual Smaller qualitative study helps evaluate and interpret results from a principally quantitative study. Can provide interpretations for poorly understood results, help explain outliers, and so on. Example: In-depth interviews explain why one clinic generates higher levels of patient satisfaction.	**4. Quantitative follow-up** QUAL → quant Smaller quantitative study helps evaluate and interpret results from a principally qualitative study. Can generalize results to different samples, test elements of emergent theories, and so on. Example: A statewide survey of a school-based health program pursues earlier results from a case study.

*In each cell, the primary method is abbreviated in capital letters and the complementary method in lowercase letters.

Source: Morgan (1998, p. 368).

the model, the primary method is abbreviated in capital letters and the complementary method in lowercase letters; arrows indicate their sequence in the design. Thus, the model shows four types of design:

1. A principally quantitative study that begins with a smaller qualitative study.

   The qualitative component might be a formative phase of participant observation or focus group discussions to develop the content of a survey questionnaire. A DHS, for example, might use the results of exploratory work to ensure that the survey instrument covers important topics in language familiar to the respondents. In clinical trials, for example, a preliminary qualitative phase could provide valuable information on the trial population and the likely acceptability of the malaria prevention intervention to be tested.

2. A principally qualitative study that begins with a complementary quantitative study.

   A preliminary survey, for example, might guide selection of study sites and help to define the sample. Qualitative research in public health frequently begins with a review of secondary data from national health, census, and other population surveys in order to relate the research problem to a larger demographic context. Quantitative findings from surveys may highlight important issues that raise questions to explore with qualitative methods.

3. A principally quantitative study with a complementary qualitative study as a follow-up.

   An important purpose of the qualitative phase in this design is to help interpret the results of the quantitative study. The qualitative component may or may not be part of the initial study design. For example, a national survey of HIV/AIDS knowledge, attitudes, and practices might turn up the finding that the majority of respondents understood the basics of prevention but chose not to protect themselves. The researchers could then explore this finding by inviting survey respondents to participate in focus groups to discuss what HIV transmission and protection meant to them and to others in their community. Similarly, quantitative researchers sometimes build into their designs a plan for analysis that includes a small qualitative study at the end, in which individuals from the study population discuss and help interpret selected findings.

4. A principally qualitative study with a complementary quantitative study as a follow-up.

   In this design, the quantitative phase may be a valuable way to test the extent to which qualitative findings are generalizable in a larger population.

> Or one might want to look at qualitative data on attitudes toward STIs from a different perspective by using standardized rating scales in a subsample of the study population. For example, a qualitative study of STI risk among adolescents identified fear of infection, embarrassment, and age as important constructs in attitudes regarding protection. In a follow-up study, the researchers constructed scale items from the adolescent participants' comments; then, having validated the scales and confirmed their reliability, they applied scale analysis techniques to study quantitatively the dimensions—fear and embarrassment—in relation to age.

In some mixed-method studies, qualitative and quantitative components may be equally important. Different methods of data collection may occur simultaneously, guided by complementary objectives. In analysis, the researcher might draw on both at the same time to address the central problem, or analysis of data from one method might serve to illuminate data from the other. Both formative and evaluation research can benefit from the multiple perspectives of a mixed methodology.

Combining different qualitative techniques is also useful, but only if the data collection and methods of analysis are carefully matched to the research questions. For example, a study of adolescent sexuality in Malawi combined in-depth interviews, participant observation, and focus group discussions. The purpose was to examine the social and information networks of adolescent girls: the ways they learn about sexuality, their perception of the risk of HIV infection, their experience with sex, and the skills they learn to avoid infection. The authors reported that "focus group discussion elicited more socially correct answers and produced good data on social norms but not very good data on deviations from those norms. By contrast, in-depth, one-on-one interviews were necessary to elicit good data on actual knowledge and experience." Using more than one qualitative research method, the authors said, "not only broadens the quality of information that can be obtained about sexuality and reproductive health issues in a community, it also opens the way to finding culturally acceptable ways of disseminating information inside your community with the support of and benefit to all its members" (Helitzer-Allen, Makhambera, & Wangel, 1994, p. 81).

When you take your research question to the field, remember that in the iterative process of qualitative inquiry, your design work may not be finished. Qualitative research problems are often deeply stratified, composed of layers of meaning that have not been accessible to other methods in the past. Thus, it may take several iterations before the experienced researcher is satisfied with a set of research questions that will tap the problem's underlying dimensions. The natural evolution of a qualitative research question is a growth process in which a basic question (e.g., Why are people not coming to this clinic?) can continue to generate new and more refined questions.

Selecting Data Collection Methods

Once your research problem has become a set of questions, you are ready to put them to work. Using your conceptual framework as a guide, the challenge now is to match the research questions with the methods and techniques that can yield the richest information. Table 3.3 compares the characteristics, strengths, and weaknesses of four types of data collection, from the least structured, qualitative format to a more structured, typically quantitative design. Although researchers sometimes combine these types to address different dimensions of a research problem, our focus here is mainly on techniques for asking qualitative questions in an open-ended format. Later in this chapter we return to these comparisons in the discussion of collecting data.

Because this book cannot adequately cover all qualitative techniques, we focus on three major methodological strategies: (1) observation, including study of existing documents; (2) in-depth interviews; and (3) focus group discussions (see Chapter 4 for more details). Observing, interviewing, and managing group discussion, aided by careful note-taking and transcription, are basic methods of qualitative science. Once you master the principles and skills of observation and interaction and learn to use documentary materials to understand human behavior, you will have a valuable set of tools that you can adapt to numerous research problems and circumstances, from formative inquiry to program evaluation. Be aware as you design your study that the methods you choose in the beginning may not be the only ones you will use. Even with the study under way, a qualitative researcher must have the flexibility to modify the design, pursue new leads, add new questions, or turn to other subgroups in the population for different perspectives. For example, pilot data from a focus group may reveal that people are reluctant to disclose their views on certain topics in front of others or that they are not accustomed to expressing opinions on controversial issues. You then may decide that individual interviews or one of the techniques discussed in Chapter 4 will be a more comfortable and rewarding approach. If you plan to conduct your data collection activities in phases, and you would like to ensure that you have some flexibility to adjust the methods without having to resubmit an amended protocol for additional review by an institutional review board (see section on Research Ethics), it is important to indicate this in your protocol. You may need to describe each potential method in some detail, including any ethical considerations associated with them.

Table 3.3 Structural Differences in Qualitative Data Collection

Type of Interview	Characteristics	Strengths	Weaknesses
Informal conversational interview	Questions emerge from the immediate context and are asked in the natural course of things; there is no predetermination of question topics or wording.	Increases the salience and relevance of questions; interviews are built on and emerge from observations; interviews can be matched to individuals and circumstances.	Different information collected from different people with different questions; less systematic and comprehensive; certain questions do not arise naturally; data organization and analysis can be quite difficult.
Interview guide approach	Topics and issues to be covered are specified in advance in outline form; interviewer decides sequence and wording of questions in the course of the interview.	The outline increases the comprehensiveness of the data and makes data collection somewhat systematic for each respondent; logical gaps in data can be anticipated and closed; interviews remain fairly conversational and situational.	Important and salient topics may be inadvertently omitted; interviewer flexibility in sequencing and wording questions can result in substantially different responses from different perspectives, thus reducing the comparability of responses.
Standardized open-ended interview	The exact wording and sequence of questions are determined in advance; respondents are asked the same basic questions in the same order; questions are worded in a completely open-ended format.	Respondents answer the same questions, thus increasing comparability of responses; data are complete for each person on the topics addressed in the interview; reduces interviewer effects and bias when several interviewers are used; permits evaluation users to see and review the instrumentation used in the evaluation; facilitates organization and analysis of the data.	Little flexibility in relating the interview to particular individuals and circumstances; standardized wording of questions may constrain and limit naturalness and relevance of questions and answers.
Closed, fixed-response interview	Questions and response categories are determined in advance; responses are fixed; respondent chooses from among these fixed responses.	Data analysis is simple; responses can be directly compared and easily aggregated; many questions can be asked in a short time.	Respondents must fit their experiences and feelings into the researcher's categories; may be perceived as impersonal, irrelevant, and mechanistic; can distort what respondents really mean or experience by so completely limiting their response choices.

Source: Adapted from Patton (1990b, pp. 280–289).

We urge readers to consult the Recommended Readings at the end of this chapter to explore other possibilities for gathering qualitative data. We also encourage you to adapt your data collection methods (such as those presented in Chapter 4) or use of strategic frameworks (such as those presented in Chapter 2) to new research problems and contexts. Many of the innovative techniques reported in qualitative literature today have come from the creative improvisation of researchers seeking better ways to help participants express their perspectives on and experiences with often sensitive topics. These field-driven techniques have included information-generating strategies such as asking young people to photograph significant moments in their lives and training HIV-positive women to interview each other. In both examples, the interpretations of the study participants enhance analysis.

Individual Interviews or Focus Groups?

Whether to interview participants individually or in groups is a common design question that is not always easy to answer. In-depth individual interviews (IDIs) establish a one-to-one relationship between the interviewer and respondent, whereas participants in group interviews—often referred to as focus group discussions (FGDs)—relate to each other as well as to the interviewer (i.e., moderator). The reasons for selecting one or the other method—or using both—can be both theoretical and pragmatic. IDIs are easier to transcribe and analyze, while FGDs can be more efficient, enabling contact with a greater number of people in less time.

In theory, highly sensitive topics, such as injection drug use, sexual behavior, or domestic violence, may argue for an individual interview format with maximum privacy and intimacy. However, if study participants are already accustomed to informal exchange on the topic among themselves—for example, discussion of disease prevention among commercial sex workers—then the investigator might choose a focus group. Ask the question: Sensitive to whom? Questions that would cause embarrassment in a group of middle-class women might be easy for women whose livelihood depends on sexual services at enormous risk to their own health and well-being. In our study of decision making about family planning in Mali, many of the participants were covert users of contraception, often in defiance of the pronatalist wishes of husbands and elders (Castle et al., 1999). Individual interviews were the only option for encouraging these women to share their experiences while protecting their secrets. Researchers encounter similar constraints in studies of injection drug users, women who have broken the law by seeking abortion, or women who engage in commercial sex in places where it is illegal. In such cases, the problem of disclosure can often be resolved in individual interviews with assurance of privacy and confidentiality.

When the research problem focuses on cultural norms, attitudes, or reactions of a group to some aspect of their environment, group discussion can be a rewarding technique. What expectations determine Black or Latino men's use of preventive health care services in the United States? What factors are likely to encourage parents' support of a new program for adolescent health or invite young people's participation? How can local providers create better linkages between their services to ensure that vulnerable women receive protection, treatment, and care from the multiple harmful effects of domestic violence? Questions such as these focus on group norms rather than individual behavior. In each example, a group of people committed to the issue will probably enjoy an opportunity to express their opinions, hear other people's views, challenge one another, and participate in studying a topic of compelling interest. By stimulating interest in a common problem and listening to others' views, participation can also motivate people to initiate change. As they wrestle with questions posed by the moderator (and sometimes by others in the group), participants' comments and debates among themselves will shed light on their community's wider perspectives, revealing clues to the context, or the social environment, in which individuals make decisions that affect their lives. Spontaneous exchange among participants also will show nuances in the language of ideas—the terms people use and the verbal frameworks they commonly construct for understanding their worlds.

IDIs and FGDs may be sequenced in a way that allows for deeper exploration of a given topic. For example, let's consider again the cook stove example at the beginning of this chapter. If you were designing a similar study, you might begin by conducting IDIs with a number of community stakeholders in order to identify the various groups of people within the community who might be more or less likely to adopt the new technology. Were local attitudes most likely to differ by gender, education, or family income? Or perhaps by access to information afforded through participation in community activities or travel opportunities? If so, FGDs with specific groups—for example, among women who volunteered in their communities or tended to travel outside of their local communities and those who stayed at home—could provide more information about facilitators and barriers to new cook stove adoption. A different strategy might be to first conduct FGDs with a range of women representing different ages, marital statuses, or income levels. (See Box 4.7 in Chapter 4 for guidance on deciding how many focus groups to conduct, based on stratification of participant groups and other factors.) Through these discussions, you might identify and invite selected participants to take part in a follow-up individual interview, perhaps to more carefully explore an idea or experience they raised during the FGD.

Collecting Data

Designing the data collection process means making basic decisions about how you will build trust in the community, understand the cultural context, and create relationships with participants. Your design should include a plan for introducing the study to the community or site, enlisting local field assistance, creating a comfortable and secure environment for interviews or focus groups, and managing the data. How you will train and monitor field staff is also part of the design. We discuss these in Chapter 5.

Designing the study also raises critical decisions about what kinds of data you will collect and how to collect data in a way that best matches the purpose and flow of the research. Whether your data will come principally from observation or from interviewing or group discussion (see Chapter 4), plan the study in such a way that you will be able to alter or modify the process as new information and questions emerge.

An important decision at this point concerns the degree of structure in the questions you will ask participants. Although open-ended questioning is a basic tool in qualitative research, questions can be asked in many different ways. You will need to decide at the design stage how much structure is appropriate for your purpose (Patton, 1990).

The first alternative, shown in Table 3.3, is an informal conversation with little or no preparation and sequencing of questions. This option is appropriate if your purpose is to explore a topic on which you have very little information. You do not know exactly what questions you will ask until you are prompted by clues from the participants and the study environment. A less structured approach is well suited to some participant observation studies because questions emerge naturally from what you are seeing and hearing (Patton, 1990). Thus, one question or observation leads to another as you build your understanding of the situation. However, the flexibility of this kind of questioning also tends to make it time-consuming. Moreover, it assumes a great deal of experience on the part of the interviewer and may increase the difficulty of the analysis. For less-experienced observers and for most in-depth interviews and focus group discussions, we recommend the more structured but still open-ended alternatives that follow.

The second option, a topic guide or outline, helps you focus the interview or group discussion without being tied to the specific wording or sequence of the questions. The expectation is that how questions are framed and the sequence in which topics are probed would change in dynamic response to the content and depth of information shared by the participant(s). The chief advantage of this technique is that data collection is systematic but gives you greater flexibility to adapt questions to participants and circumstances. It is a commonly used tool for gathering comprehensive information on specific research questions in a relaxed, conversational style. The resulting data are less comparable than in a standardized open-ended interview, but they may be more responsive to the way that participants naturally construct a situation. (See the discussion of construction of topic guides in Chapter 4.) However, the quality of the data arising from this approach is highly dependent on the interviewers' knowledge of the research area and their ability to listen carefully and think on their feet, framing questions in open-ended and nonjudgmental ways. Careful training with plenty of opportunity for experiential practice is usually required.

A third strategy, asking a predetermined set of open-ended questions, is the most standardized approach to qualitative data collection. If you choose this type of questioning, you lose flexibility but gain comparability and more straightforward analysis. This approach is especially useful for comparative studies when it is important to maximize common features while remaining sensitive to cultural differences among the study groups (Knodel, 1994). This format also lends itself to studies that are highly focused, for example, a program evaluation in which you want to interview several service providers with little time to spend on the interview (Patton, 1990). Structured questions may be a good strategy if you have multiple interviewers or focus group moderators with varying experience and different interviewing styles.

Analyzing the Data

Chapter 6 presents in detail the steps for analyzing qualitative data. However, certain aspects of data analysis will need careful consideration as you design your study or describe your analysis plan when writing a proposal for funding. Specifically, you should determine the following in the design phase:

- Who will conduct the analysis?
- What level of detail will be needed to respond to your research questions?
- Will the analysis be computer-assisted or manual?

If a computer will be used, decide in advance on a qualitative software package for text analysis. If you are combining qualitative and quantitative methods, you will want to have a clear plan of analysis for each and a strategy for interpreting the results in an integrated discussion.

Qualitative analysis can be a deeply personal and subjective exercise. For this reason, some qualitative researchers decide from a study's outset to use a team approach for analysis, involving data collectors as well as researchers more removed from daily field activities. The process of examining, negotiating, and incorporating multiple perspectives on data can strengthen their final interpretation. If using a team approach, anticipating the analysis process at the beginning is especially useful:

- Will all team members read and work on all the data, or will specific team members be responsible for different aspects of the investigation?
- Will team members work separately and then meet to share and reconcile their findings, or will the team conduct the analysis in group meetings?
- How will the team resolve differences of opinion?

For an expanded discussion of group analysis, see Chapter 5.

If only one person will conduct analysis, it is important to review the data as they are collected. If not actually collecting data, the principal investigator or analyst must at least have access to interim data in order to identify areas for clarification or further probing.

Another decision to make at the design stage is the form your data will take. The purpose of your qualitative study will imply a certain level of detail. For example, you may be able to explore broadly the different personal, relational, and institutional barriers to use of dual protection from pregnancy and STIs by summarizing preliminary information from other observations or from interviews or group discussions. On the other hand, if you want to use qualitative data to design interventions that increase individuals' skills in negotiating dual protection, a formative problem, you will want to know exactly how people do and do not express themselves in such intimate circumstances. Fully transcribed tapes of interviews, in addition to notes about nonverbal cues or body language, would be more appropriate. If you are embarking on a mixed-method study, you will also need to decide in advance how you are going to handle the data from different methods and coordinate the findings in an integrated discussion.

Finally, the level of detail you anticipate and, to a lesser degree, the number of people involved in analysis will influence decisions about the use of computers. Manual analysis is sufficient when your goal is to map out broad categories of information or when the volume of data is small. As the analysis becomes more complex (i.e., examining the nuances of language or comparing responses among a number of subgroups) and as the volume of data increases, a computer can greatly assist the analysis process. Again, if the analysts themselves will not be keying in data or operating analysis software programs, give some thought to how the data will be moved from field notes to data files to analysis procedures. Some software packages have special features to assist a team approach. (See discussion of specific advantages and disadvantages of different types of software packages in Chapter 6.)

Disseminating Results

In order for study results to be accessible to and used by others, you will need to build into your design a plan for dissemination, with a corresponding budget. Your study purpose has direct implications for how and to whom you should disseminate study findings and what approach should be taken in writing up qualitative data for wider dissemination in peer-reviewed journals. (See Chapters 7 and 8 for a fuller discussion.) Likewise, as you focus your research questions, consider the eventual audiences for your findings and plan the length and detail of your report, presentation, or manuscript accordingly. When you sit down to write, "you begin a systematic inquiry of what you already know, what you need to know, and what you are looking for" (Wolcott, 1990, p. 22). In short, outlining your study purpose and design can be done at the same time that you develop a tentative table of contents for your final report. This approach will sharpen your focus and help you sequence your material.

Research Ethics: Decisions for the Protection of Study Participants

Prior to initiating your research, your proposal will likely require review and approval by one or more ethics committees or institutional review boards (IRBs). (When conducting research in one or more international settings, you may need to obtain approval in your home country as well as each international site.) The purpose of IRB review is to ensure that your research is, first of all, worth doing—that it will contribute to the general advancement of scientific knowledge. Equally important, reviewers will determine whether you are adequately protecting the physical and social well-being of your participants. Your ability to conduct a study while respecting research ethics should be reflected in the research design.

Increasingly, qualitative researchers are required to describe in detail numbers and types of participants they will recruit, and specify recruitment strategies as well as data collection and analysis approaches in order for committees to determine whether there is adequate protection of human subjects. When developing your research proposal or your study protocol, provide specific plans but allow flexibility for adaptation in case recruitment or data collection strategies require modification. Possible approaches might include targeting a range (rather than a finite number) of interviews of FGDs, providing a list of topics to be covered during data collection, or noting that if a specified data collection approach—for example, use of FGDs—proves to be unacceptable to the study population, researchers will implement an individual interview approach instead. Building flexibility into your protocol will ensure that you benefit from the exploratory and iterative nature of the qualitative research approach. It will also save you from having to stop data collection and obtain additional ethical review approvals for amendments if your original plan does not prove viable.

Obtaining Informed Consent

All human research must be conducted with the informed consent of participants, but how it is implemented depends on the nature of the research and the type and degree of risk that participation entails. At its most basic, informed consent means that study participants understand the following:

- The purpose of the research
- How they were chosen to participate
- Data collection procedures, specifically what is involved for the participant
- Possible risks and benefits
- Assurances of confidentiality
- Voluntary participation
- Compensation for study participation, if relevant
- Whom to contact with questions and concerns

Risk to Participants

What kind of harm might come to a participant in a sensitive or controversial health study? Potential harm to study participants is not just physical but can also be psychological, social, economic, or professional. In fact, physical wounds may heal more quickly than wounds to a person's reputation or sense of security (Williamson, 1995). Because qualitative research designs may obtain detailed and at times deeply personal information from and about small numbers of individuals, they can raise ethical challenges. In strongly patriarchal societies, subordinate women may be especially at risk in studies of contraception, abortion, female circumcision, domestic violence, or any reproductive decision that might conflict with norms of behavior. Clandestine contraceptive users in Mali feared rejection or divorce if their husbands discovered their pills. Women in Haiti feared physical abuse if they demanded that HIV-infected partners use condoms. Brazilian adolescents suffering the consequences of unsafe abortion might have been arrested if discovered. Providers who reveal actions by their superiors that compromise service quality may endanger their jobs. Injection drug users willing to participate in research on social networking and addiction bear a double burden of risk, not only for their own safety but also for that of any users and dealers they identify in confidential interviews.

Consequently, in culturally sensitive studies, your ethical responsibility goes beyond the simple statement of informed consent. Moreover, many of the topics that commonly arise in public health research are likely to elicit delicate material—private and personal experiences, wishes, fears, even confessions—that the participant wants only the interviewer to hear. Avoiding deception, asking permission to record what they say, being willing to turn off the tape recorder, and being honest about the intended use of the research are all part of your responsibility to your participants, along with ensuring that they come to no emotional, physical, professional, or financial harm because they agreed to speak with you (Rubin & Rubin, 1995). The common practice of assigning identification (ID) codes to participants to protect personal identity can be explained as further assurance of confidentiality. Researchers should also make sure they are not under any legal constraints, for example, requirements to report certain kinds of illegal behavior. If they are, they must inform participants of these legal obligations.

Your first responsibility to your study participants is to assess the possibility that simply talking with you may pose a risk for some and to protect them from harm, even if it means changing the interview site or omitting material that might jeopardize the participant's safety. In contrast to IDIs, the use of FGDs poses unique ethical challenges for research, since there is no guarantee that individual participants will not share information they have heard during the FGD with others who were not present. When collecting data within a group setting, it is important to remind participants about the need to maintain others' confidentiality, as well as their right not to share private information during the discussion. We further discuss ethical considerations related to specific methods in Chapter 4.

The Signed Consent Form—Do You Need It?

How will participants indicate their consent? Most written study designs are expected to answer this question in detail. The signed consent form is a hallowed tradition of IRBs everywhere, but in some cases oral informed consent may be a more appropriate format. Examples are studies in which a breach in confidentiality could have profound repercussions for the participant, such as clandestine users of contraception, men who have sex with men in countries where same-sex behavior is criminalized, women who have undergone unsafe abortion, or unmarried adolescent clients of a family planning clinic. For a study of adolescent women admitted to a hospital with complications of abortion, for example, one IRB ruled that the parental consent requirement for participation in the study was inappropriate, because it could put the participant at greater risk than the study itself. Box 3.4 describes requirements for obtaining signed informed consent for U.S. federally funded research conducted both domestically and abroad.

BOX 3.4 SOME FEDERAL REQUIREMENTS FOR INFORMED CONSENT

Human subjects research supported by U.S. federal funds is required to be conducted in compliance with U.S. federal regulations (45 CFR 46). These regulations include several waivers related to informed consent:

- Waiver of documentation of informed consent (that is, no signature needed)
- Waiver of particular items from the list of required elements for informed consent
- Waiver of informed consent (usually only used for things like chart review studies or lab studies using stored specimens)
- Waiver of parental consent for minors

U.S. IRBs are constrained in the extent to which they can grant each of these types of waivers.

Most IRBs can be expected to waive the signature requirement if all three of the following conditions apply:

1. The only record linking the subject and the research is the consent document.
2. The principal risk would be potential harm resulting from breach of confidentiality.
3. The research presents no more than minimal risk of harm to subjects and involves no procedures for which written consent is normally required (Williamson, 1995).

Institutional review boards (IRBs), or protection of human subjects committees, are mandated by governments and research institutions to protect participants in research by reviewing proposals for compliance with internationally recognized guidelines.

When you encourage people to talk to you openly, you incur serious ethical obligations to them.

(Rubin & Rubin, 1995, p. 93)

As a substitute for signed consent, the interviewer may be asked to sign a statement for each participant confirming that the participant has read (or heard) and understood the statement and has given oral consent. However, regardless of the mechanism for obtaining consent, the study design should include a description of possible risk that could result from participation in the study, as well as the statement of informed consent exactly as it will be presented to the participant. Protecting human subjects should also include a referral plan or other response to possible harm should it actually occur in the course of the study. (See Appendix 2 for examples of consent forms used in qualitative studies of reproductive health.)

Other Considerations: Budget and Time

Ultimately, your research design will be determined in large part by the resources you can bring to it, including the kind of funding available and how urgently the information emerging from your research is needed. If you are a doctoral student with limited funding, you may choose to append a small qualitative study to a secondary analysis of an existing quantitative dataset. If your research is meant to provide feedback to an ongoing child immunization intervention or to inform the development of a new one, you may need to modify your data collection plans so they are implementable within the amount of time available. As you develop your research plans, it is essential to think carefully about the time as well as the human resources, materials, and other costs required to implement your research strategy, and to adjust your sampling strategy, choice of data collection methods, and analysis approaches to these realities. Budgets and timelines will be further discussed in Chapter 5.

Summary

A well-organized research proposal makes a strong argument to potential funders or your research advisors for the relevance and integrity of the research. Once funded or approved, the researcher will need to implement his or her study in a manner that ensures that the study's purpose and objectives are met. Whether the researcher meets or falls short of these objectives will be determined in large part by how well the study design matches its objectives.

In this chapter, we have provided guidance on the main design decisions, often detailed in a **research protocol**, which should be considered prior to initiating a study. They include decisions about who will participate in the study and which other data sources will help answer the research questions; what data collection methods to use and whether to use solely qualitative or mixed methods; and processes for analyzing and disseminating study results while protecting study participants.

Designing a qualitative or mixed-method study can be a highly creative process. No two researchers are likely to come up with exactly the same study design, even when given the same research topic as a starting point. Furthermore, one of the real strengths of a qualitative design is its ability to be adapted to pursue and deepen your understanding of emergent information. For that reason, it is important to remember that qualitative design is always a work in progress. Although a sound written design at your project's outset gives you and your reviewers a frame of reference, it is a plan, not a contract. It systematically details the problem driving the research and the strategy for solving it, but the design remains flexible to change, as repeated questioning and analysis in the field lead you to new questions and new ways to delve deeper. Such flexibility, ill-advised in most quantitative research, is a necessary feature of qualitative methodology. The researcher's ability—indeed, obligation—to examine data as they arrive, throw out invalid assumptions, restate questions, and shape the design as the study progresses will ultimately contribute to the vitality and credibility of the results.

Key Terms

1. **Research proposal:** A document, usually intended for submission to a potential funding source or other reviewer, that provides an overview of

a proposed study. The degree of detail depends on requirements of the funder as specified in a request for proposals, but at a minimum, the proposal should address the study's background and rationale, goals and objectives, and procedures for data collection and analysis.

2. **Mixed-methods research:** Pragmatic and intentional research strategy that employs both qualitative and quantitative approaches to data collection and analysis in order to obtain a more complete understanding of both the "magnitude" and "meaning" of a research topic (Creswell et al., 2011).
3. **Formative research:** Takes place before a program or another scientific investigation is undertaken for the purpose of defining the selected population, creating appropriate programs or research procedures, and ensuring that the program or study will be culturally relevant and acceptable.
4. **Descriptive research:** Provides information about a population, health system, or other phenomenon without evaluation, prediction, or intervention. A descriptive study may also be formative if it is a preliminary phase for the design of another study.
5. **Explanatory research:** Explains as well as describes phenomena of interest. Such research generally tests explicitly stated hypotheses and often employs experimental design and statistical analysis, but it may also include qualitative or other mixed-method approaches.
6. **Community-based participatory research:** A research process that emphasizes partnership, joint decision making, and co-learning on the part of researchers and practitioners or community members participating in the research. Inherent to participatory research methods is the goal of empowering communities to identify and address their own health concerns (Israel et al., 2008, p. 49).
7. **Research protocol:** This document differs from a research proposal in terms of intended audience and purpose. Specifically, the research protocol provides a more detailed description of the study design and methods, including procedures to be used in sampling, recruitment, data collection and management, data analysis, and protection of human subjects. This document is typically prepared for a scientific review body such as an institutional review board or ethics committee. The conduct of the research follows closely the approved procedures in the protocol. Any significant changes in data collection topics or methods may require further review by the original ethical review committee and often an amendment to the protocol.

Recommended Readings

Creswell, J. W., Klassen, A. C., Plano Clark, V. L., & Smith, K. C. (2011). *Best practices for mixed methods research in the health sciences*. Bethesda, MD: National Institutes of Health.

Maxwell, J. A. (2013). *Qualitative research design: An interactive approach* (3rd ed.). Thousand Oaks, CA: Sage.

Patton, M. Q. (2014). *Qualitative research & evaluation methods: Integrating theory and practice* (4th ed.). Thousand Oaks, CA: Sage.

Teddlie, C., & Yu, F. (2007). Mixed methods sampling: A typology with examples. *Journal of Mixed Methods Research, 1*(1), 77–100. doi:10.1177/2345678906292430

Review Questions

1. How is a study's purpose generally described in a research proposal or protocol? What information might be presented to support the rationale for the study?
2. How do broad research questions differ from those that might be included in an interview?
3. Why can it be helpful to include multiple data sources in a qualitative study? What are some of the challenges of doing so?
4. How would you compare and contrast some benefits of theoretical versus *a priori* sampling? Provide an example of when you might use each strategy.
5. What are some general strengths and weaknesses of individual versus group discussions?
6. Think of a research question that might be answered through a mixed-method study. Who (or what data sources) would you include in the study? What data collection methods would you use? How would you sequence your data collection activities? Why?

References

Albert, L. M., Akol, A., L'Engle, K., Tolley, E. E., Ramirez, C. B., Opio, A., . . . , & Baine, S. O. (2011). Acceptability of male circumcision for prevention of HIV infection among men and women in Uganda. *AIDS Care, 23*(12), 1578–1585. doi:10.1080/09540121.2011.579939

Castle, S., Konaté, M. K., Ulin, P. R., & Martin, S. (1999). A qualitative study of clandestine use in urban Mali. *Studies in Family Planning, 30*(3), 231–248.

Chambers, R. (1981). Rapid rural appraisal: Rationale and repertoire. *Public Administration and Development, 1*, 95–106.

Chambers, R. (1994). Participatory Rural Appraisal (PRA): Analysis of experience. *World Development, 22*(9), 1253–1268.

Creswell, J. W., Klassen, A. C., Plano Clark, V. L., & Smith, K. C. (2011). *Best practices for mixed methods research in the health sciences*. Bethesda, MD: National Institutes of Health.

Eng, E., & Blanchard, L. (1991). Action-oriented community diagnosis: A health education tool. *International Quarterly of Community Health Education, 11*(2), 93–110.

FHI 360. (2011). *The Darfur Community Strengthening Program: Engaging communities to create change in a conflict-affected environment*. Durham, NC: FHI 360's Center for Civil Society and Governance.

Flick, U. (1998). *An introduction to qualitative research*. Thousand Oaks, CA: Sage.

Glaser, B., & Strauss, A. (1967). *The discovery of grounded theory*. Chicago, IL: Aldine.

Guest, G., Bunce, A., & Johnson, L. (2006). How many interviews are enough? An experiment with data saturation and variability. *Field Methods, 18*(1), 59–82. doi:10.1177/1525822X05279903

Helitzer-Allen, D., Makhambera, M., & Wangel, A. M. (1994). Obtaining sensitive information: The need for more than focus groups. *Reproductive Health Matters, 3*, 75–82.

Horowitz, C. R., Robinson, M., & Seifer, S. 2009. Community-based participatory research from the margin to the mainstream: Are researchers prepared? *Circulation, 119*(19), 2633–2642. doi:10.1161/CIRCULATIONAHA.107.729863

Israel, B. A., Schulz, A. J., Parker, E. A., Becker, A. B., Allen, A. J., & Guzman, J. R. (2008). Critical issues in developing and following CBPR principles. In M. Minkler & N. Wallerstein (Eds.), *Community-based participatory research for health: From process to outcomes* (2nd ed., pp. 47–66). San Francisco, CA: Jossey Bass.

Kemmis, S., & McTaggart, R. (2008). Participatory action research: Communicative action and the public sphere. In N. K. Denzin & Y. S. Lincoln, *Strategies of qualitative inquiry* (3rd ed., pp. 271–330). Thousand Oaks, CA: Sage.

Knodel, J. (1994). Conducting comparative focus group research: Cautionary comments from a coordinator. *Health Transition Review, 4*(1), 99–104.

Mack, N., Kirkendale, S., Omullo, P., Odhiambo, J., Ratlhagana, M., Masaki, M., . . . & Corneli, A. (2013). Implementing good participatory practice guidelines in the FEM-PrEP preexposure prophylaxis trial for HIV prevention among African women: A focus on local stakeholder involvement. *Open Access Journal of Clinical Trials, 5*, 127.

MacQueen, K., Chen, M., Jolly, D. H., Mueller, M. P., Okumu, E., Hawley, M. H., . . . & Eley, N. T. (2012). *Willingness of Black young adults to participate in biomedical HIV prevention trials in Durham, North Carolina.* Poster presentation, XIX International AIDS Conference (AIDS 2012), Washington, DC.

Maxwell, J. A. (2008). Designing a qualitative study. In L. Bickman & D. Rog (Eds.), *The handbook of applied social research methods* (pp. 214–253). Thousand Oaks, CA: Sage.

Maxwell, J. A. (2013). *Qualitative research design: An interactive approach* (3rd ed.). Thousand Oaks, CA: Sage.

Morgan, D. L. (1998). Practical strategies for combining qualitative and quantitative methods. *Qualitative Health Research, 8*(3), 362–376.

Obermeyer, C. M. (1997). Qualitative methods: A key to better understanding of demographic behavior? *Population and Development Review, 23*(4), 813–818.

Patton, M. (1990). *Designing qualitative studies: Qualitative evaluation and research methods* (pp. 169–186). Beverly Hills, CA: Sage.

Patton, M. Q. (2015). *Qualitative research & evaluation methods: Integrating theory and practice* (4th ed.). Thousand Oaks, CA: Sage.

Rubin, H. J., & Rubin, I. S. (1995). *Qualitative interviewing: The art of hearing data.* Thousand Oaks, CA: Sage.

Shattuck, D., Kerner, B., Gilles, K., Hartmann, M., Ng'ombe, T., & Guest, G. (2011). Encouraging contraceptive uptake by motivating men to communicate about family planning: The Malawi Male Motivator project. *American Journal of Public Health, 101*(6), 1089–1095. doi:10.2105/AJPH.2010.300091 DOI:10.2105%2FAJPH.2010.300091#pmc_ext

Strauss, A., & Corbin, J. (1990). *Basics of qualitative research: Grounded theory procedures and techniques.* Newbury Park, CA: Sage.

Tashakkori, A., & Teddlie, C. (1998). *Mixed methodology: Combining qualitative and quantitative approaches.* Thousand Oaks, CA: Sage.

Tolley, E. E., Eng, E., Kohli, R., Bentley, M. E., Mehendale, S., Bunce, A., & Severy, L. J. (2006). Examining the context of microbicide acceptability among married women and men in India. *Culture, Health & Sexuality, 8*(4), 351–369.

Tolley, E. E, & Severy, L. J. (2006). Integrating behavioral and social science research into microbicide clinical trials: Challenges and opportunities. *American Journal of Public Health, 96*(1), 79. doi:10.2105/AJPH.2004.043471 DOI:10.2105%2FAJPH.2004.043471#pmc_ext

Tolley, E. E., Tsui, S., Mehendale, S., Weaver, M. A., & Kohli, R. (2012). Predicting product adherence in a topical microbicide safety trial in Pune, India. *AIDS and Behavior, 16*(7), 1808–1815.

Trow, M. (1957). Comment on participant observation and interviewing: A comparison. *Human Organization, 16*, 33–35.

Wallerstein, N. B., & Duran, B. (2006). Using community-based participatory research to address health disparities. *Health Promotion Practice, 7*(3), 312–323.

Weitzman, P. F., & Levkoff, S. E. (2000). Combining qualitative and quantitative methods in health research with minority elders: Lessons from a study of dementia caregiving. *Field Methods, 12*(3), 195–208.

Williamson, N. (1995). *Protecting study participants in social science research versus biomedical research* [unpublished manuscript]. Research Triangle Park, NC: Family Health International.

Wolcott, H. F. (1990). *Writing up qualitative research: Qualitative research methods* (No. 20). Newbury Park, CA: Sage.

Wong, C. M., & Noriega, S. (2013). *Exploring gender-based violence among men who have sex with men, male sex worker and transgender communities in Bangladesh and Papua New Guinea: Results and recommendations.* Durham, NC: FHI 360.

CHAPTER 4

COLLECTING QUALITATIVE DATA

THE SCIENCE AND THE ART

OBJECTIVES:

- To describe the three primary qualitative data collection methods (observation, interviews, and focus group discussions), including:
  - The type of information each method elicits
  - The mechanics of conducting each method
  - Logistical issues
- To describe additional structured data collection techniques (freelisting and pile sorts, photo narrative, vignettes, body mapping, social network analysis) and participatory methods

> ***Every interview is an interpersonal drama with a developing plot.***
>
> ***(Pool, 1957, cited in Holstein & Gubrium, 1999, p. 112)***

THREE PRIMARY METHODS FORM the bedrock of qualitative data collection: observation, in-depth interview, and focus group discussion. We distinguish *method,* a systematic approach to data collection, from *technique,* the art of asking, listening, and interpreting throughout the data collection process. Each of the three bedrock methods applies special tools and techniques for gathering data—the "basic units or building blocks of information" (Rossman & Rallis, 1998, p. 5). Qualitative research methods differ with respect to the relationship between the data collector and the participants. Observation varies from unobtrusive (nonreactive) techniques, where the observer's intent is to be unnoticed, to more interactive (participatory) techniques for observing social process. Many techniques used in in-depth interviewing and focus group discussion are designed to help study participants collaborate more actively with the researcher, generating rich, detailed data through expression of the participants' own views and experiences.

This chapter describes the qualitative researcher as observer, interviewer, and group moderator. For each approach to research we offer a variety of techniques, but our selection is not exhaustive. As you become more experienced in qualitative research, you will discover many more techniques of creative listening and learning. Working from an interpretivist or transformative perspective, you will focus on different issues, uncover new sources of data, and find more ways to enable people to tell their stories. But wherever you go, the basic principles of observing and interacting with individuals and groups will be the foundation on which you build your practice.

Observation

Observation is the oldest and most basic source of human knowledge, from casual understanding of the everyday world to its use as a systematic tool of social science. It is hard to imagine any field research, qualitative or quantitative, without an element of observation. Data collection does not begin and end with an interview. Interviewers and focus group moderators are also observers, noting body language, facial expression, and other nonverbal clues to subtle meanings. Qualitative researchers, particularly, must be acutely aware of context, observing the ebb and flow of activity around the study site. A chance conversation, an unexpected event, a spontaneous gathering—all may contain clues to understanding participants' expressions and meanings in the more formal interviews and discussions.

Depending on the purpose of your research and your own cultural, linguistic, and demographic background, you will have to choose (or recognize) whether you will be observing from an outsider's or an insider's perspective—or somewhere in between. Each approach has its place among the tools of scientific observation. Outside observers maintain greater distance in order to view events from their own perspectives. Inside observers reduce distance by joining activities and interacting with people in order to view events through the eyes and ears of a participant, although the researcher will always have an outsider's perspective to some degree. As a researcher you are unlikely ever to be a true insider unless you are a member of the study population. However, your own perspective as a trained observer enables you to listen, question, and interpret what you see. Indeed, one way to decrease the distance between the researcher and the subjects of the research is to work as a team with data collectors who are part of the local culture.

In this chapter, we present these two ways to observe as separate approaches. But in practice, most field observation involves skillful interplay of both. With experience you will learn to gauge the proper distance between yourself and your participants, knowing when to step back and when to join in.

Experienced observers use both qualitative and quantitative techniques, with qualitative observations differing from quantitative primarily in their focus on process and human interaction rather than numbers. For example, counting the numbers of clients in different health center clinics could reveal variation in clinic use. However, it would not capture the qualitative interaction between clients and providers in the same clinics, a finding that might help explain different patterns of clinic attendance. Regardless of how and what you observe, observations become data only when they are conducted according to the rules and conventions of scientific inquiry.

Unobtrusive Techniques

Following the early work of Eugene Webb (Webb, Campbell, Schwartz, & Sechrist, 1966), we use the term *unobtrusive*—also called nonreactive—to describe techniques in which the researcher collects data without interacting or reacting visibly to participants' activity. Next we describe **direct observation**, an unobtrusive technique.

Direct Observation

One strategy for observation is to remain on the fringe, watching people and events as unobtrusively as possible, observing without participating or actively eliciting data from research participants. Choose this technique if you want to see how something happens rather than how other people perceive that it happens, gathering your own impressions by direct observation instead of through the eyes and ears of study participants. Program evaluation and operations research often combine unobtrusive, direct observation with other measures—for example, in quality of care studies—to observe the client experience firsthand, including the dynamics of interaction between client and provider. In such a setting, you might want to know how clients are received and how long they wait, who directs the flow of conversation, how information is offered, how questions are asked and answered, and whether providers initiate counseling on particular topics of interest to your research problem. See Box 4.1 for guidance on how to conduct direct observations.

Unobtrusive observation is sometimes used to validate interview data or other information that study participants report. For example, family planning counselors may have told interviewers that they always provide clients with information on a range of contraceptive choices—an insider perspective. Direct observation by the researcher—the outsider perspective—could

BOX 4.1 GUIDANCE FOR CONDUCTING DIRECT OBSERVATIONS

Following are three steps for conducting observations:

1. Create a list of things to watch for during the observation.
   In many observation sites—a busy pharmacy, an active community center, a clinic full of people waiting for attention—the din of activity can be distracting. A list, as simple or detailed as you wish, will help you focus your attention. In the form of a checklist, it can also be used to document your observations. For example, during observations of health educators' talks about sexual health to female sex workers in Central America, a checklist was used to document which topics were covered in the talks.
2. Conduct the observation, being sure to take notes as discreetly as possible.
   Frantic scribbling of verbatim conversations and flipping notebook pages will only remind people that you are observing them and may raise anxiety about your intentions. To minimize note-taking, some observers use checklists with space for short, abbreviated comments. Others jot occasional notes on small cards, taking mental notes as much as possible. Taking notes on electronic tablets also may be a discreet option in some settings. You could also voice record your observations afterward, using a smartphone or other digital recording device.
3. Expand your notes as soon as possible after each observation.
   Incorporate mental notes and impressions, and reflect on what they have revealed about the research problem. Add interpretations, or tentative conclusions, to your notes. What you see and hear will almost always lead to new insights and new questions about relationships and events in the setting. In addition, incorporate the observation list into your notes and formulate new points to observe in the next session.

confirm their reports by noting the presence of a variety of contraceptives in half-empty boxes and colorful family planning posters on the walls, as well as witnessing actual counseling on the methods. Several days of observation might reveal that in practice, providers usually mention only one method to clients and have only that one in the supply closet. In the case of contrary evidence, the challenge to the qualitative researcher is to discover the reason for the apparent contradiction, for example, through **in-depth interviews** with clients, providers, and those managing family planning supplies.

The quality of the data will depend on your ability to watch and listen without interrupting the natural flow of activity. An observer almost always has some effect on the study situation because unless he or she is hidden behind a one-way vision mirror, as in some laboratory-controlled studies and market research, the observer's presence is noticeable. To minimize distortion of the observed behavior, an observer might be introduced simply as someone who is learning about health care in that area; the observer could then take a position behind the client–provider pair and observe silently from the sidelines. Longer periods of observation are usually more effective than shorter ones, because they allow people to become accustomed to the observer's presence and return more easily to their natural interaction. Familiarity and acceptance of the observer are key to reducing social desirability bias that might be attributed to your presence.

In addition to concerns about the effect of the observer on the interactions being observed, we would note that completely unobtrusive observation, where people are observed unaware, has ethical implications that should be carefully considered; this approach could be a breach of privacy, undertaken without the informed consent of the observed. Therefore, it may be more appropriate to start by introducing the observer to the observed.

Direct observation may also be used to learn about the field environment. For example, you could arrange for an informal tour of the setting to observe such things as the proximity of places where clients live to health facilities, roads, and water pumps; the presence of electrical wiring; or the type of roof or dwelling.

Interactive (Participatory) Techniques

Participant Observation

What is participant observation? Participant observation brings the researcher into direct interaction with people and their activities. As defined by anthropologist H. Russell Bernard (1995, pp. 136–137), participant observation "involves getting close to people and making them feel comfortable enough with your presence that you can observe and record information about their lives." As the foundation of cultural anthropology, this method has many uses in different domains of social science. "The thing to remember about participation," Bernard reminds us, "is that it belongs to everyone, positivists and interpretivists alike. . . . Whether your data consist of numbers or words, participant observation lets you in the door so you can do research."

Unlike nonreactive direct observation, in which you must be as unobtrusive as possible, in participant observation you will ask yourself: How can I get close to people? Will they share their lives, their thoughts, their activities with an outsider? In this more interactive approach, your responsibility is to stimulate conversation and behavior that will let you enter the culture as its members' guest. In initiating the observation, your challenge will be to adapt your interactive style to the participants' cultural style. For example, you would approach young schoolgirls differently from the way you might introduce yourself to commercial sex workers on the street. Experienced observers learn to present themselves in whatever way will put study participants at ease while simultaneously stimulating their interest in interacting with the observer and maintaining ethical standards by communicating their identity as a researcher. In some areas of research, including studies of sexual and reproductive health, the participant observer is more likely to remain an outsider on the inside, maintaining identity as a researcher but spending enough time in the cultural setting to know and understand people in the natural course of their lives.

The techniques for entering a culture are as many and varied as cultural variations themselves. The goal is to enable people to accept you and interact naturally with you for sustained periods of time. As they get used to your presence, they may act almost as if you were not there (Bernard, 1995, p. 136). Once accepted, you must continue to balance insider and outsider perspectives as you watch and listen to what unfolds. With practice you will respond naturally and flexibly to fluctuations in the research environment, always alert to unexpected events that could reveal important information on the cultural dynamics of the group.

To illustrate this process, imagine that you are going to study how women make health decisions for themselves and their families. Following preliminary introductions in the community, as described in Chapter 5, you obtain permission to join a local mothers' club. The group meets weekly to socialize and discuss their concerns as young mothers. At the first meeting you attend, you explain who you are and why you want to join them as an observer, sharing your own concern for issues the women believe are important. Until the women know and trust you, you probably do more listening than active participating. Remember that you are there as a researcher-observer, not masquerading as a mother in the group, although you may indeed be a mother. As the women become comfortable with your presence, you might begin to ask a few questions or steer discussion toward topics related to their health decisions. Participating will give way to more listening, with occasional questions to explore interesting leads. Be open also to questions the women might have about you and be willing to reciprocate by sharing some of your own life or research experiences. However, avoid becoming an authority in their eyes. Emphasis on common experiences, values, questions, and concerns will help to minimize the effect of your presence on the views the group expresses.

Between the club's weekly meetings, you might arrange individual visits with some of the members at their homes or informal visits to other places the women gather, such as a church group or local health center waiting area. Becoming known and accepted as a visiting member of the community will add to your sensitivity and effectiveness as a participant observer. As you piece together data from many conversations, you will notice how they converge around certain recognizable themes or perhaps reveal conflicting messages that suggest new directions to explore. In contrast to an interview, the participant observer's commitment to the study group is likely to be more intimate and sustained over a longer period. For understanding sequences and connections of events that contribute to health decisions, participant observation can be a powerful tool (Bogdewic, 1992).

In the scenario just described the researcher is a woman, but there are equally rich opportunities for men to conduct participant observation. Examples might be studies of AIDS awareness among male assembly-line workers, HIV risk among truckers driving long-distance routes through countries with a high prevalence of infection, and knowledge and attitudes of health risk among men who are migrant farmworkers. Although participant observers of the same sex may be able to put participants more quickly at ease when research topics are sensitive, same-sex research is not always a necessity. In numerous studies, observers have gained the confidence of both men and women in the study site and have skillfully integrated different gender perspectives in the analysis.

The ability to communicate in the local language or dialect is a valuable asset, but this is often not an option in cross-cultural observation. Although an experienced local assistant can help offset a language gap and offer cultural as well as linguistic interpretation, people from other cultures or who do not speak the language must realize that they are observing the scene from a greater distance, in addition to seeing it from their own cultural perspective. An alternative to "outsiders" collecting the data is to work in teams with trained data collectors who are members of the local community, even if they are not necessarily members of the sub-group under study. (We discuss the use of field teams in more detail in Chapter 5.)

The guidelines in Box 4.2 outline information field researchers needed in order to identify recruitment sites at bars and other establishments for an HIV-prevention study with women.

Documenting Participant Observation Through Field Notes

The importance of **field notes** that are clear, detailed, and descriptive cannot be overemphasized. The journalist's query—who, what, when, where, why, and how—is a useful guide to recording field observations. Suggestions for what to include in field notes also appear in Box 4.3. Make a practice of documenting conversations and events as soon as possible after they happen, and set aside time after every observation to complete your notes.

BOX 4.2 USING PARTICIPANT OBSERVATION TO IDENTIFY RECRUITMENT SITES AT BARS AND OTHER ESTABLISHMENTS FOR AN HIV-PREVENTION STUDY WITH WOMEN

Following is guidance provided to the field team for an exercise to identify places appropriate for recruiting women at high risk of HIV exposure.

1. List and briefly describe the location of each site for participant observation as you go along.
2. Number each site and indicate its location on a map. Identify streets, sectors, establishments, neighborhoods, or other identifying features near the site.
3. Talk to the patrons and staff of the establishment to learn more about the women who frequent the site, whether they are staff (e.g., bar girls/waitstaff) or patrons. During your conversations, try to learn the following information:
   a. Who are the women who come to the site? Include descriptions of age, where they are from, where they live, whether they have a stable residence in the area, where and how they solicit clients and other sex partners, and the types of clients and sex partners they have.
   b. How many women who engage in official or unofficial sex work are present at this site? Which days during the week and month are busy at the establishment? What times of day are busiest? Who is present during those times? When could the women be best accessed without interrupting their work?
   c. To what extent is stigma an issue, whether related to HIV, sex work, or other concerns?
4. Pay attention to how you, the researcher(s), were received at the site. Were you welcomed openly? Treated with reserve? Was there an atmosphere of distrust? What were any other reactions to you, positive or negative? How would you recommend approaching people (e.g., owners/managers, staff, patrons) in this site?
5. During the participant observation, also consider any potential barriers that may exist for recruiting and retaining women for a study in this community. Did you or your field team run into any problems, and if so, were you able to overcome those problems? What facilitators may exist for recruiting and retaining women for a study in this community?

Source: Based on guidelines provided by Kathleen M. MacQueen, FHI 360.

BOX 4.3 SUGGESTIONS FOR HOW TO WRITE FIELD NOTES FROM PARTICIPANT OBSERVATIONS

- Start each note with the date, time, location, and a brief description of the purpose or circumstance of the observation.
- State clearly the ages, sex, and number of people you have observed or conversed with.
- Describe the interaction, event, or process you observed or in which you participated, recalling the content of conversations.
- Record your thoughts and impressions (labeled as such) about what you observed or experienced.
- Develop working hypotheses based on the observation, perhaps compounded with previous observations.
- Plan next steps.

New field observers sometimes make the mistake of writing notes that are vague and imply judgment: "The unpleasant young man who came into the clinic was loud and impatient." Using descriptive terms can eliminate vagueness and reduce obvious bias.

> "The man who appeared to be in his early twenties approached the clinic supervisor and claimed in a loud voice that he had been waiting for 3 hours to see the doctor. The receptionist asked him to take a seat and told him the doctor would be with him shortly. The man shook his head forcefully and replied in a loud voice that he had been told the same thing twice already."

The second note presents a more vivid picture of the scene without the overlay of observer judgment. In this case, it would be equally important to include observation of objective facts, such as the actual amount of time the man had been waiting, the number of staff on duty, and the number and behavior of others who were also waiting. Notes on comfort, noise level, lighting, decor, posters, health information, and other descriptions of the scene will help you later analyze the observed behavior in relation to the context. The extra effort to capture the moment in detail can provide you with rich observational data that will be meaningful when you review your large accumulation of field notes. Appendix 3 provides examples of field notes from participant observations based on the guidelines in Box 4.2 for identifying recruitment sites for an HIV-prevention study.

Field notes may also be taken about observation of research participants during in-depth interviews and focus groups, using the same approaches described for observation.

As you record observations, keep asking new questions, and interpret what you have seen and heard based on what you currently know. Gradually, interpretations take the shape of tentative conclusions that add structure to what you are observing. This running account will help you organize your search more efficiently, building from concrete instances to more general understanding—the process of inductive reasoning characteristic of qualitative research.

Note that researchers using ethnographic approaches, such as in anthropological fieldwork, tend to use field notes from observations or participant observations in this iterative way by revisiting and reinterpreting notes from previous observations, often with the goal of developing their research questions. This is in contrast to many public health studies whose objectives have already been identified and that use observations for other goals related to achieving the research objectives, for example, to identify appropriate health clinics for studying patients with particular health conditions.

As we pointed out earlier, participant observation can begin from any theoretical perspective. It is important, therefore, to be keenly aware of your own orientation as an outsider and interpreter of the scene, documenting the distinction between what you see and what it means to you. Similarly, the observer's awareness of self in relation to the field of observation is critical to record. Qualitative researchers must frequently ask themselves two common reflexive questions: "What effect am I having on this scene?" and "How is what I observe affecting me, the observer?" Experienced participant observers learn to recognize the subtle interplay between the observer and the observed, and they make it part of the record as they interpret what they see and hear.

As your field notes grow, keeping them organized may become increasingly difficult. In Chapter 6, we will discuss techniques for coding text in large datasets, a process that can help the participant observer, as well as the interviewer, begin to analyze and interpret raw data while still in the field.

The Role of Key Informants in Participant Observation

Ethnographers have always relied on **key informants** to help them make sense of their observations and interactions in unfamiliar cultures. Key informants are insiders with special knowledge, status, or communication skills who are willing to share what they know with the researcher (Gilchrist, 1992).

They speak on behalf of others, expressing points of view that may be different from their own. They are not independent observers but rather "the voice of the people of concern" (Eng & Parker, 1994, p. 207).

Although researchers ask all qualitative research participants to share their knowledge and perspectives, a key informant in the tradition of ethnography sometimes has a different relationship to the researcher, providing information, introductions, and interpretation, often on a day-to-day basis, as well as access to observations that an outsider would not normally have. In an ethnographic or longitudinal study, you are likely to have more personal involvement with a key informant who becomes your trusted adviser and guide to the culture. Although your relationship to interview and focus group participants is one of mutual trust and rapport, the key informant partnership often includes a degree of collegiality not typical of most data collection. Why should a qualitative researcher develop a special relationship with a few people instead of regarding all study participants as equal collaborators? Pragmatic limits constrain the researcher (Gilchrist, 1992). One cannot be in all places at all times, observing everything and interviewing everyone. But most important, a researcher from the outside is unlikely to have the cultural perspective and community experience necessary to explore all aspects of the problem. A personal relationship with a key informant, developed over time, helps to ensure more efficient access to rich information.

Key informants might explain cultural norms that govern the health topic of interest, including the meaning of behaviors that seem to deviate from the norm. They will comment on your interpretation of conversations with others in the community and help you synthesize pieces of information from different sources. They might introduce you to other potential key informants, such as a youth leader, a member of a women's advocacy organization, or a community health worker.

Identifying Key Informants

Identifying key informants can be done informally or more systematically. A formal approach to identifying key informants is the quantitative cultural consensus model developed by Weller and Dungy (1986) and described in Bernard (2002). However, we advocate for a more informal approach in which you make inquiries of people you meet, asking them to help you identify individuals who are subject matter experts, in the sense that they belong to the community, have experience with the topic under study (e.g., is diabetic himself, or has had tuberculosis), or can help you get linked into a network of people by accompanying you in places where you might not gain access on your own. For example, you might begin a study of the influence of gender norms on HIV risk with participant observation in a community known through your review of statistical records to have a high prevalence of sexually transmitted infections (STIs). As you get to know people in the community, perhaps two or three stand out because they are particularly interested in the problem and are knowledgeable and articulate on topics concerning sexual risk. When you introduce yourself around the community, people may refer to such individuals as the ones who "know what's going on." You visit with each of them and find them willing to share what they know and take you to people and places that will help you understand gender relationships in relation to sexual risk in this community. These will be your key informants.

Working With Key Informants

As in all qualitative data gathering, it is important to formulate a basic set of questions to start the process. Although these questions could be written, you should incorporate them casually into conversations with key informants. Accompanied by your key informant, you might start with a tour of the facility or workplace you plan to study or a community or neighborhood where potential participants gather. Initial questions might be as general as these: Who comes here? What do they do? To whom do they talk? As you begin to make connections, your questions will become more focused on specific issues related to the study's purpose and context: Why do certain things happen? How do people deal with a new event or a stressful situation? In this way, a key informant can orient you to the study population in its natural environment. Interaction with key informants can range from informal discussion to later consulting them as sounding boards for data interpretation.

Information and insights gleaned from conversations with key informants should be documented, whether you record your thoughts using a smartphone or tablet device and later transcribe them, or you simply write detailed field notes soon after the interaction. Doing so will help you identify additional questions and keep a record of information your key informant has shared.

Many public health studies feature key informants in another, more formal role—as experts whose thoughts and opinions are solicited through formal interviews. For example, Eng and Parker (1994) used key informants to evaluate a health promotion program serving a rural poor county of the Mississippi Delta. In order not to interfere with the community's broader goals for local empowerment, lay community health advisors were asked to select 28 key informants for the study and conduct the interviews themselves. Speaking to familiar local people, key informants provided data on incidents associated with drug dealing. They also were able to identify related community-centered activity that demonstrated improvement in community competence to act on a public health problem.

Although we advocate use of key informants in some capacity in most studies, quantitative as well as qualitative, we caution that there are limits to the information that informants usually can provide. Key informants are not infallible. A trusted informant may be reluctant to admit not knowing something or may try to please you by telling you what he or she thinks you want to hear. Key informants also may have their own biased interpretations, especially if they come from ethnic, religious, or socioeconomic groups that are different from the study population. Just as you look at a situation from different methodological perspectives, you would be wise to have more than one key informant so that you are not dependent on one person's interpretations. You can then raise and discuss contradictions or new ideas with other informants until you have consensus on an issue or perhaps decide to look elsewhere for different insight.

Be sensitive also to comments made by community members about your close interactions with key informants and take steps to correct misperceptions. Always ask yourself how any key informant will affect your acceptance in the wider group. Although an informant may have much to offer, giving a single person extra attention could have negative consequences, engendering jealousy or suspicion in the group under study. Thus, it is always important to weigh the risks and benefits of developing a particularly close relationship with any individual in the setting.

Including Key Informants in Research Proposals and Protocols

If you plan formal interviews with key informants as part of your study, you will of course include this activity in your research proposal and protocol. If participant observation is part of your study, also include the use of key informants in your proposal's or protocol's Methods section. In this way, you will be able to compensate them for their time if it is appropriate to do so. Other ways to compensate key informants include substituting a donation to the organization of his or her choice, which may be appropriate in cases where the person has high status or is highly compensated in her professional role.

Strategies for Managing Bias and Maximizing Rigor in Participant Observation

Participant observation by definition entails subjective interpretation and, therefore, the potential for bias. However, there are a number of things you can do to keep subjectivity in control and maximize the rigor of observation data. Although it is important to become part of the group, be aware of the boundaries that distinguish your role as researcher-observer. For example, young staff conducting work in an HIV surveillance study were chosen in part because their youthfulness would help them blend in and build rapport with the young research participants. However, because their work would include observation of drinking and sexual behavior in bars, they benefited from careful guidance by supervisors on the limits of their participation (C. Woodsong, personal communication, February 2001).

Another strategy for enhancing the rigor of a participant observer study is the careful documentation we have discussed. At the end of a long day in the field, it is an easy pitfall not to document what you have observed. But by neglecting to take this important step, you risk losing what you may have learned or keeping valuable information only in your own mind, unavailable to the rest of the team. Lost data can have serious consequences in potential misinterpretation of other data and can lead to erroneous or incomplete conclusions. It also leaves you vulnerable to claims that your research may not be reliable. By creating an audit trail (see Chapters 5 and 6), you will document your observations and conclusions in such a way that other researchers will be able to reconstruct the process that has led you to your results (Morse, 1994). Participating in the creation of an audit trail can be a valuable learning experience for all members of the research team.

Other techniques to maximize the rigor of observation data include making comparisons among multiple observers or coders and verifying results with additional observations or semi-structured interviews with other key informants. However, as we emphasize throughout this text, discrepant findings do not necessarily mean methodological weakness; they may be a reflection of multiple realities, contradictory but valid perspectives and experiences in the study population.

Interviews and Focus Groups

Developing Interview and Focus Group Topic/Question Guides

Experienced qualitative data collectors often gather meaningful data with little more than a set of topics as a guide; the research questions are clear in their minds, and the techniques of qualitative data collection are their normal ways of working. By the time they are ready to conduct interviews or focus groups, topics of conversation flow easily from the research questions. **Interviewers** may also have memorized the list of topics to cover and be able to direct conversation spontaneously from one topic to another, stopping to clarify points or probe comments or perhaps return to earlier questions as needed to ensure that participants have gone as far as they can with each topic.

However, there are also circumstances in which a more explicit set of interview or focus group guidelines is preferable, such as for semi-structured interviewing or focus group moderating. For example, institutional review boards (IRBs) sometimes want to see and approve the specific questions and their translations, if applicable, rather than only the topic domains. You may also want to compare the answers to particular open-ended questions across a large number of interviews or focus groups and across research sites. In addition, you may want to ensure some degree of uniformity in which questions are asked when multiple research staff members are collecting the data. Writing down suggested follow-up questions and probes may also be helpful when the research staff may not all have the same degree of in-depth knowledge about the research topic. Finally, researchers new to these techniques will benefit from a more structured set of guidelines. Box 4.4 outlines the process for constructing a semi-structured question guide.

BOX 4.4 PROCESS FOR CONSTRUCTING A SEMI-STRUCTURED QUESTION GUIDE

COMPOSE RESEARCH QUESTIONS

Reread the research protocol at least once, concentrating especially on the research objectives and associated problem statements. Decide which objectives can be addressed in each type of data collection category. Then turn the problem statements into a short list of broad questions that reflect what you want to learn in the study and in the particular interview or focus group category. Interviewers should commit this list to memory. For example, "I want to know how people in this community (e.g., policymakers, women with young children, men) would react to a campaign to encourage handwashing. What factors would encourage or discourage handwashing?"

IDENTIFY TOPIC DOMAINS AND SUBTOPICS

Subtopics are variations on the more general topic domains. There may be more than one topic domain in a single research objective, and each topic domain may have several subtopics. For example, a topic domain might be "acceptability of dual method use (DMU)" while subtopics could include "understanding of DMU, experience with DMU, and perception of partner's opinion."

DECIDE ON A SEQUENCE

Arrange topic domains and subtopics in a logical sequence that suggests a natural flow for discussion. The pattern and sequence of themes do not have to follow the order of research objectives as they are described in the research protocol.

(Continued)

BOX 4.4 PROCESS FOR CONSTRUCTING A SEMI-STRUCTURED QUESTION GUIDE (Continued)

DEVELOP SPECIFIC QUESTIONS

Each topic domain or subtopic may have three kinds of questions: a main question, follow-up questions, and probes. The main question introduces the topic domain. Follow-up questions get more specific and take the discussion to a deeper level. Probes go even deeper, seeking clarification and asking for more detail.

PREPARE OPENING AND CLOSING STATEMENTS

Compose text that lets participants know that the interview or focus group discussion is beginning or has ended. The opening statement includes an explanation of the project and the ground rules of the interview or focus group. Prior to the closing statement, it is appropriate to ask participants if they have any questions for you. Then the closing statement thanks participants for sharing their insights and experiences and reminds them again of the confidentiality of the data.

Many researchers prefer a semi-structured **topic guide** with questions that reflect the initial themes and subthemes contained in the basic research problem. This kind of tool may be a set of standardized open-ended questions, with examples of how questions can be worded, as well as serving as a reminder of the material to cover (see Box 4.4). The topic guide can also suggest follow-up questions for various possible responses and examples of probes to elicit information at greater depth. If you will be presenting vignettes or other scenarios to stimulate ideas, you should include them in the guide.

Interviewers are encouraged to use their own words in the interview but to keep firmly in mind the purpose of each question and its relation to the research problem, referring to the guide as needed. Interviews and **focus group discussions** can take many paths, moving toward and sometimes away from the key problem. Organizing the topic guide around a few central questions can help keep you oriented in the right direction, following possible new leads but always returning to the study's purpose.

Although we urge all interviewers and focus group moderators to state questions in a natural way and not to read semi-structured guides as they would the questions on a structured survey or questionnaire instrument, many will feel more confident with some specific questions to help them manage the interview or discussion. Several examples of topic guides are shown in Appendix 4.

Asking Qualitative Research Questions

A carefully defined research problem is an invitation to examine the issue with more specific questions. There are many kinds of qualitative questions, as outlined in Box 4.5. The research problem will determine whether your design should focus on people's experiences, actions, and behaviors; on their

BOX 4.5 TYPES OF QUALITATIVE RESEARCH QUESTIONS

Type of Question	Purpose	Examples
Experience/behavior questions	Intended to elicit descriptions of experiences, behaviors, actions, activities; what a person has done, seen, heard, or thought.	How did you introduce your partner to the idea of using a condom as well as the IUD? If I were present when you talked to your adolescent son about HIV, what would I hear?
Opinion/value questions	Aimed at how people interpret specific events or issues; answers reflect a decision-making process and may reveal goals, opinions, norms, intentions, desires, and values.	What do you think about a girl your age getting pregnant? In the reorganization of this health service, what programs do you think should have highest priority? In your opinion, who should have the final say in decisions about how many children to have?
Feeling questions	Probe emotional responses to experiences; typically spontaneous, often not the result of a decision, often non-rational; may emerge in responses to other kinds of questions.	How did you feel when you learned you were HIV positive? How do women react to situations where they fear physical violence?
Knowledge questions	Intended to discover what people consider factual information—what people think is true. Interviewer records but does not correct misinformation, except at the end of the interview.	What are some ways that a person can get HIV? Tell me about some different kinds of family planning you know. If a man and woman have just had unprotected sex, is there anything they can do to avoid a pregnancy?

Source: Adapted from Timyan (1991).

opinions and values; on their feelings or emotional responses; or on what they know or believe to be true in certain situations. Most qualitative studies combine two or more of these elements. Note that some of the questions in Box 4.5 could be asked from either a qualitative or a quantitative perspective.

A quantitative interviewer might suggest several topics and ask respondents to rate their importance. Qualitative questions give participants more freedom to structure their answers as they wish. For example, a health department might want to know what its family planning program can do to reduce rates of unwanted pregnancy in the local adolescent population, suggesting a need for formative research. Stated this broadly, though, one could do little except speculate on a possible solution.

First, you would need to break the big question into specific, researchable questions:

- What are actual rates and trends in adolescent pregnancy?
- What services do local family planning clinics offer young people?
- At what age do adolescents become sexually active?
- What are contraceptive use rates among teenagers?

Much of this information can be obtained from records, surveys, and other quantitative sources. It is valuable information for describing the extent of the problem, constructing the context, and understanding the problem of unwanted pregnancy in this population.

As you continue to explore the problem, however, you probably will want to know where adolescents themselves stand on this question. An interpretivist perspective can guide you in articulating additional, specific questions:

- How have adolescents experienced reproductive health services?
- How have young people understood the information they have received about sex and sexual health?
- How do young couples negotiate sexual protection?
- What do early sexual relationships mean to adolescents in terms of costs and benefits?
- What has happened when adolescents have tried to reduce their risk of pregnancy or STIs?

Adopting a transformative perspective, on the other hand, you might decide to examine the meaning of negotiation in relation to the balance of power in the partner relationship and the ability of adolescents to participate in decisions affecting their health.

Questions like these call for a qualitative approach, because in different ways they ask why adolescent pregnancy in this community is so high. They expand and elaborate on the original research question—how to reduce adolescent pregnancy—by addressing some of the underlying dynamics of adolescent sexual experience. They also have the potential to elicit a range of information, including knowledge, experience, opinions, and feelings, as well as their social context—types of questions that are summarized in Box 4.5.

However specific such questions seem in the beginning, later data collection may uncover material that leads to new and more insightful questions, which in turn may suggest even more ways to understand and articulate the nature of adolescent pregnancy. What do clinic personnel believe is their responsibility to young people who want contraceptive advice? To what extent do young women discuss pregnancy and disease prevention with their partners? Such is the iterative nature of qualitative research at the level of problem definition. Even after the data collection begins, you may find that you continue to refine and build on your research questions in the light of new insights.

Conducting in-depth interviews with different participant groups can be important for illuminating multiple perspectives and will give you a more complete picture of your research topic. For example, Case Study 4 in Appendix 1 describes the different perspectives obtained from women and their partners regarding contraception and fertility desires.

A source of formative questions not to be overlooked is stakeholders in the project—individuals and groups who understand the context of the problem and whose own goals will be served by the results of the research. For example, researchers in Mali had not been aware that service providers were worried that so many women were coming to the family planning clinic in secret. Asking practitioners "What information would help you provide better service?" can generate new questions that will lead to more relevant and useful conclusions.

Leaders of women's advocacy groups can also be a valuable source of collaboration if your research problem is consistent with their agenda for women. In our experience, advocacy organizations often lack the resources to conduct research and are eager to share their own knowledge as insiders to develop mutually rewarding research questions.

When you take your research questions to the field, remember that in the iterative process of qualitative inquiry, your design work may not be finished. Qualitative research problems are often deeply stratified, composed of layers of meaning that have not been accessible to or addressed by other methods in the past. Thus, it may take several iterations before the experienced researcher is satisfied with a set of research questions that will tap the problem's underlying dimensions. The natural evolution of a qualitative research question is a growth process in which a basic question (for example, "Why are people not coming to this clinic?") can continue to generate new and more refined questions. On the other hand, the tendency of good research questions to grow and multiply must not imply design without form. Vigilance is needed to ensure that emerging research questions retain an internal consistency and a clear relationship with the basic problem or purpose of the research.

Framing Qualitative Questions

Whether in individual interviews or group discussions, qualitative questions are informal, nonjudgmental, and open. Speak clearly but casually, avoiding any suggestion that one answer might be more desirable than another. Inexperienced interviewers often use words that inadvertently suggest answers. The question "Do you believe all those things people are saying about immunization causing harm to young children?" suggests that they really are not true. Asking participants to simply comment on what they have heard about immunizing children is a more open invitation to express a candid opinion. Sometimes interviewers ask a yes-or-no question with an immediate follow-up question for more detail, but in general, it is advisable to avoid dichotomous wording and emphasize open-ended questions that encourage participants to interpret questions themselves.

Although we refer to qualitative interviews as conversations, most interviews and focus group discussions follow a pattern that comprises three kinds of questions: **main questions, follow-up questions**, and **probes** (Patton, 1990; Rubin & Rubin, 1995). The pattern is flexible but helps the interviewer or **moderator** cover the topics in sufficient depth to make the most of the opportunity to gather the rich information that participants can offer.

As Box 4.6 illustrates, the pattern begins with a clear idea of the topic or the direction you want the question to take. Because you will already have explained in a general way the purpose of the interview, you do not have to repeat the topic to the participant with each question. Main questions come from the themes and subthemes of the research problem. They introduce topics to be discussed in the form of questions. If one theme of a program evaluation is client perception of services, you might begin by asking, "What has been your experience with this health center?" Or for a study of women's vulnerability to HIV/AIDS, "How do you manage to protect yourself from infection?" Main questions are open enough to encourage spontaneous response but specific enough to keep the dialogue focused. If the discussion moves too far from the topic, you may want to repeat the main question, perhaps in a different way, to get back on track. However, be aware that getting off track may be a clue to

BOX 4.6 LEVELS OF INTERVIEW QUESTIONS IN A QUALITATIVE STUDY OF EMERGENCY CONTRACEPTION (EC)

Qualitative interviews typically begin with a few broad questions and then move to more specific questions, following participants' clues and encouraging depth and detail. The direction and pattern of movement can vary, depending on how the participant responds to the issues.

Topics	Main Questions	Follow-Up Questions	Probes
Knowledge	Can you tell me what you know about EC?	What have you heard from others? In your opinion, are these things true?	Anything else about EC?
Source of information	Where did you hear about EC? What did this person say about it? Who else is talking about EC these days?	How did you happen to be discussing it?	Tell me more about that. Can you give me some examples?
Experience	Do you know anyone who has used EC? Have you used EC yourself?	Why did you decide to use it? What was using it like for you? Were you glad or sorry you had tried it? What made you glad or sorry?	Who influenced your decision? Why did you decide that way?
Opinion	What do you think are the advantages and disadvantages of EC?	How could EC help or harm someone like yourself? How do you think others would react to your use of EC?	What are some ways EC could help or harm a person? What about your husband/partner/mother-in-law?
		Do you think women you know would want EC to be available? Why or why not? Would you want EC to be available for yourself? Why or why not?	What would women say if it were offered to them? What about men? What are some reasons that people you know might not want to use EC?

a different way of looking at the problem or an idea you might want to pursue or return to later in the interview.

Main Question Your main questions should reflect the logical flow you anticipate in the conversation, moving from easy and least threatening questions to more complex and interesting issues as you build rapport. However, as experienced interviewers know, this sequence may be logical only to the researcher. Participants often answer a main question before you have asked it. You must then decide quickly whether to continue with that topic or suggest coming back to it later. Or the participant may reconstruct the meaning of the question in a different way, requiring flexibility to keep the discussion focused while encouraging the participant to express his or her perspectives and experiences. Interviewers and moderators often ask the most important—and perhaps more difficult—questions more than once, from different angles and at different points in the interview. Through experience you will learn how to move around among the main questions, pursuing each to its logical conclusion while not neglecting questions or new ideas.

Follow-Up Questions A follow-up question moves the interview or discussion to a deeper level by asking for more detail. Follow-up questions are a natural part of any conversation. They suggest to the speaker that the listener is interested enough in what the speaker has just said to want more information. To some extent you can anticipate follow-up questions in advance, but even in a standardized open-ended format, you cannot know exactly what they will be until participants respond to the main questions. In the example in Box 4.6, a participant might have answered the first question by saying, "Well, I hear emergency contraception can prevent pregnancy." You would then ask for detail on what the person has heard and whether she or he knows it as fact (a knowledge question).

Probes A probe is a kind of follow-up question that takes the discussion into still deeper territory, with or without specific reference to the topic. For example, the interviewer might say, "Please tell me more about that" or "Then what happened?" or "I don't think I know what you mean—can you explain?" As you gain experience, you use these conversational devices naturally. They tell the participant that you are listening closely and that what she or he has said is important. They also indicate to the participant the level of detail you want and enable you to clarify points or pursue new ideas in a conversational manner. Note, however, the importance of maintaining a comfortable balance between too much detail and not enough. Insufficient probing could suggest boredom, but aggressive probing might be intrusive (Rubin & Rubin, 1995). Through experience and careful listening, you will know how to probe sensitively and when to stop.

In-Depth Interviews

In-depth interviews are typically an exchange between one interviewer and one respondent and may be unstructured or semi-structured. Scholars have called this kind of intensive, one-on-one interviewing a "conversational partnership" (Rubin & Rubin, 1995, p. 10), "conversation with a purpose" (Burgess, 1984, p. 102), and a "social encounter" (Holstein & Gubrium, 1999, p. 106). These terms reflect the uniquely interactive nature of qualitative interviewing, differentiating it from the standardized survey interview. In most survey research, the interviewee is expected mainly to respond to structured questions.

In unstructured interviewing, the interview is more informal, guided by a few broad topics rather than a detailed guide with specific questions. However, there are many ways you can create structure without compromising the open exchange that is the hallmark of most qualitative techniques. In unstructured interviewing, qualitative researchers encourage study participants to take a more active role in determining the discussion's flow. Interviewer and participant are collaborators, "working together to achieve the shared goal of understanding" (Rubin & Rubin, 1995, p. 11). In a relaxed and comfortable setting, the conversation generates empirical data by enabling participants to talk freely about their lives (Holstein & Gubrium, 1999). A qualitative unstructured interview should not be a mechanical reading of standardized questions; collecting information-rich data requires mental agility, sensitivity, and practice.

Semi-structured interviews use interview guides with open-ended questions written out, to be asked in a more or less ordered sequence. This style of interviewing may be a better fit for team-based data collection on large projects, where several different interviewers will be collecting the data, perhaps in different research sites and in different languages. It is also appropriate if you want to be sure that interviewers ask the same questions in all interviews to produce comparable data (Bernard, 2002). On the other hand, overly strict fidelity to an interview guide can compromise the flexibility needed for the interviewer to follow the respondent's lead into uncharted territory, thus risking loss of important information. The experienced interviewer seeks a balance, able to cover the questions in the guide while staying alert and responsive to new clues and unanticipated directions. As discussed later, being able to respond on the spot with effective follow-up questions is a vitally important skill in both unstructured and semi-structured interviewing.

There is also a hybrid style of interviewing in which you or the trained interviewers in your team may ensure that all broad topics or specific questions under each topic are covered over the course of the interview, but not necessarily in a particular order.

Stages of the Interview (and Focus Group Discussion)

A particularly versatile format for in-depth interviews and focus groups in applied behavioral health research is the semi-structured approach we introduced earlier. Interviewers typically use a written set of flexibly worded topics or questions that keep the conversation guided and on track but without imposing boundaries on the participant's style and expression.

Rubin and Rubin (1995) describe this type of in-depth interview as a series of stages:

- Creating natural involvement
- Encouraging conversational competence
- Showing understanding
- Getting facts and basic description
- Asking difficult questions
- Toning down the emotional level
- Closing while maintaining contact

Although these stages are presented here for in-depth interviews, they are easily adapted to focus group discussions as well.

Creating Natural Involvement (Rapport Building)

Beginning with an informal chat is a good way to build rapport, setting the stage for the relaxed atmosphere you want to create for the interview. It helps to be able to comment on events or situations that are familiar and important to the respondent. If possible, link the purpose of the interview to some common experience, for example, "A young man in my office passed away from AIDS the other day. It has been hard for all of us who knew him." Or in a study of children's antisocial behavior and the mass media, the interviewer might begin, "I find it difficult to know how to respond to the violence my children see on television and on the streets." Sharing experience is a way of expressing the bond that you hope will develop into the conversational partnership that will generate the information you seek. Women interviewing women, or men interviewing men, may find common ground in gender, for example, in family relationships, childbearing, job seeking, or other experiences in the context of being a woman or a man. Expression of concern about the widespread prevalence of a common problem like adolescent pregnancy or a debilitating chronic disease may also be a springboard to the conversational partnership. Such common ground can be drawn upon throughout the interview process to continue building rapport.

During the informed consent process, you will have explained clearly what the study is about and why the respondent has been asked to participate. You will also have clarified the participant's rights and responsibilities and the voluntary nature of participation, as well as provided contact information for someone who can answer questions about the study, such as the investigator or ethics committee representative. Finally, you will have obtained the individual's informed consent to continue.

As you begin to develop rapport, you will move into a more formal introduction, explaining who you are and what you want to know. You might remind the participant that he or she may choose not to answer any question for whatever reason. The respondent meanwhile will be assessing you, trying to decide what you really want and whether you can be trusted. It is important to show that you are genuinely interested, that you do not come with a judgmental attitude, and that you will honor his or her confidentiality and trust.

Encouraging Conversational Competence

In the first few minutes of the interview encounter, you set the tone for the conversation that follows. People often agree to participate in an interview but are insecure or skeptical that they would have anything to offer. The interviewer's job is to give participants the sense that their opinions and experiences are important to the study. Starting with easy, nonthreatening questions allows them to feel sure about what they know and pleased to have an appreciative ear. Participants familiar with survey interviews may instantly adopt a compliant role, offering impersonal, monosyllabic answers to questions. It is therefore critical to dispel as quickly as possible the notion of passivity or subordination to the interviewer.

As you develop your own qualitative style, the language you use should help to establish you as a partner rather than an interrogator. "I'm hoping you will help me understand how women make choices about pregnancy." "I'd like to explore with you what it means to be the mother of a large family." "When it comes to housing and feeding the family, we men have a lot of responsibility. Let's talk a little about where the paycheck goes." "I know that as a grandmother you care very much about how the children are raised," and perhaps later, "I'm wondering how you feel about circumcising the girls." Whether or not you agree with the participant's views, your manner should reflect great interest and compassion. As they come to trust you and the confidentiality of the interview, participants will welcome a sympathetic listener; they will become more personally invested in the topic and will move with you to deeper levels of their experience. The interviewer-partner does not coax answers from the respondent but enters actively into the discussion in a way that explores incompletely articulated thoughts and encourages new directions (Holstein & Gubrium, 1999).

Showing Understanding

As the interview progresses, you can encourage openness and depth by showing that you understand and empathize with what the respondent is telling you. When a mother of six in a very poor village was telling the interviewer how hard it was to have so many children, the interviewer responded, "Yes, I can imagine life is very hard for you right now. How do you keep your children looking so healthy?" The question builds rapport by showing that the interviewer understands and by reinforcing the respondent's competence in her role as a mother. Emotional support comes through in a sympathetic tone of voice, responsive facial expression, murmurs, and gestures—all of which suggest acceptance of the person. It is not necessary to relate one's own personal experiences or to approve of everything the individual has done. Your role is to put the conversational partner at ease to share life experiences without fear.

Getting Facts and Basic Descriptions

Once the partnership is established and conversation flows easily, you are getting into the heart of the interview. Now you can encourage longer answers by asking the partner to tell you about an incident or describe a typical encounter related to the topic of the research, following it up with simple, direct questions. At this stage of the interview, you focus on descriptive material, holding any delicate or emotionally charged questions for later.

A topic to introduce at this stage might be how household decisions are made about adopting cleaner-burning cook stoves to replace cook stoves that pollute the air inside of living spaces and result in respiratory health problems. A woman may talk about how couples make decisions, perhaps including men's ultimate decision-making authority. From here, the interviewer can channel the conversation toward the challenge some women have in making their voices heard and influencing men's decisions. The exchange may prompt the interviewer to explore gender relations and dynamics. As a skilled listener, the interviewer will be alert to clues that the participant is ready to move to more sensitive levels of discussion.

Asking the Really Difficult Questions

Save your most difficult questions until you sense that your conversational partnership is relaxed and trusting. Be aware not only of your partner's stage in the process but also of your own comfort with the relationship and your readiness to raise issues that may take considerable skill to manage. Researchers in health behavior must frequently discuss topics that lie outside normal discourse with strangers. In varying degrees, open discussion of sex is taboo in virtually all cultures; women, especially, may be socialized to strict norms of sexual privacy. As you enter this stage of the interview, it is important to respect the fact that you may be violating certain expectations of behavior and to be especially sensitive to the conversation's effect on your participant. Remember that you can ask and repeat important questions at different points in the interview. Repeating a difficult question later in a different way gives the participant a chance to think about it and offers you an opportunity to ask it from a different angle.

When the research problem requires you to ask difficult questions, there are ways to soften their impact. You may need to remind your respondent that the interview is confidential, that no names are recorded, and that identification will not be revealed. It also helps to acknowledge the sensitivity of the topic with a simple comment like "I know this is a hard thing to discuss—I really appreciate your sharing."

Another way to show responsiveness and empathy is to use familiar words and expressions in the conversation—an advantage of the informal style of qualitative interviewing. Telling a story or showing a picture that illustrates the topic is a way of depersonalizing a difficult area without sacrificing spontaneity. When you ask respondents to talk about an issue through fictitious characters, you are allowing them to control the extent to which they disclose information about themselves. If necessary for the research, the interviewer might ask if the picture or story is like anything in their own lives, but qualitative interviewers who have used this technique usually find that the respondent shifts spontaneously from the impersonal third-person to the first-person expression of self.

Hesitation may not mean embarrassment but may be simply a pause that reflects difficulty understanding the question. It can also mean that the respondent, especially if a woman, has never been asked her opinion on any topic. We have found that women in some societies are so unaccustomed to being consulted on matters of fertility that it may take several interviews before they are able to participate fully in the interview conversation.

Toning Down the Emotional Level

When participants have been open with you on sensitive or embarrassing topics, they may begin to feel uncomfortably exposed. As the interviewer you may need to help restore the sense of privacy that enabled them to share their lives with you in the first place. Again, you can simply remind them of the confidentiality of the information. When toning down the emotional level of the conversation, the researcher can turn the interview around and ask if the participant has questions to ask or has answers to other questions.

But sometimes it is difficult to move away from interview conversations that have stirred up strong emotions. If the conversation is upsetting to the participant, you can decide to change the topic or discontinue the interview. An alternative is to allow participants to ventilate their feelings until they become calmer or until you can shift naturally to a more neutral topic. A risk that qualitative interviewers often face is that they may learn more than participants want them to hear (Alty & Rodham, 1998). The more comfortable the respondent is with you, the more easily she or he will disclose information not meant to be shared. You may hear such off-the-record comments after the interview or focus group has ended. The interviewer's ethical response to material that seems to go beyond the participant's original informed consent is either to interrupt the conversation at that point or to ask the participant whether those remarks can be included in the transcript. It might be important to have these comments in your personal notes to help you understand the meaning of broader issues. However, if the participant does not want them shared, your ethical obligation is to indicate clearly in your notes that they should never be quoted in full or described in publications.

To some extent we can predict topics that are potentially embarrassing or disturbing: drug or alcohol addiction, sexual preference if not in the open, acts of violence, sexual intimacy, abortion, infidelity, and contraception that may be in conflict with religious beliefs or cultural norms. Other topics may evoke painful emotion, for example, loss of children or experience with rape or spousal abuse. Or a topic may have political sensitivity that you as an outsider have not guessed. In short, you need to be always on the alert for change in the tone of the interview conversation that could suggest that you are entering a vulnerable area. Rather than risk further discomfort for your respondent, avoid the question if it is not essential to the purpose of the research. If what you need to know is whether infidelity is a common experience for women in the community, it is not necessary to probe the marital relations of your conversational partner. If you ask her about women in general, she is free to illustrate her response with her own experience only if she wishes to do so.

On the other hand, qualitative researchers must be prepared to answer another important but often overlooked ethical question: What is the responsibility of the interviewer when a study participant asks for help? Even if violence is not the topic of the research, questioning women on gender decisions may suddenly evoke personal accounts of an abusive relationship. You will want to research appropriate referral services prior to beginning data collection.

The interviewer must be prepared for such unanticipated disclosures, balancing the requirements of the interview with ethical responsibility for the participant's well-being. In one country where we experienced this scenario, we were able to refer vulnerable women to a local intervention program for abused or neglected women by handing all participants a card at the end of the interview with the name, address, and phone number of a women's counseling center. Other examples include a participant's fear of having an STI or disclosure of recent untreated complications of an unsafe abortion. In such situations, the interviewer's ethical responsibility is to refer the person to a sympathetic social service or health practitioner. Not all problems will have such convenient solutions, but interviewers must be prepared to identify distress and respond with empathy and appropriate referral.

Closing While Maintaining Contact

Once the participant has accepted the role of conversational partner, it can be difficult to terminate the conversation. You will need to express thanks for the time taken to share valuable information, perhaps reiterating the confidentiality of the record. In case you need to return later to ask the participant to confirm or elaborate on a statement, it is wise to ask permission to call on the person again and verify contact information. Although the interview has ended, informal conversation usually continues. Be alert to casual banter, because it may contain unexpected clues or new leads to answering the research question. Unless participants indicate that parting comments are off the record, make notes on your observations at the moment or as soon as possible.

Focus Groups

A focus group is "the use of group interaction to produce data and insights that would be less accessible without the interaction found in a group" (Morgan, 1988, p. 12). The methodology of focused group interviews was first developed for social science during World War II by sociologists studying military morale and the impact of propaganda materials on public opinion (Merton, Fiske, & Kendall, 1990). Sociologist Harold Blumer (1969, p. 41) later used focus groups in a series of drug studies, remarking that "a small number of... individuals who are acute observers and who are well-informed... brought together as a discussion and resource group, is more valuable many times over than a representative sample." Focus group discussion has also proved a useful tool for marketers studying consumer opinion on commercial products.

Unlike simple group interviews in which several people may be interviewed at once for convenience, focus groups depend as much on the exchange of ideas among participants as they do on answers to specific questions from the person leading the focus group. This person is called the **moderator**, underscoring the role of guide and facilitator in the group process. There is also a **notetaker** who may play a role in the informed consent process with participants, in addition to taking detailed notes during the discussion and typically operating the recording equipment.

Moderating a focus group has much in common with in-depth interviewing. Introducing topics with main questions, asking more specific follow-up questions to elicit more detailed information, and probing the meaning of responses are as important in focus group discussions as they are in individual interviews.

When to Use Focus Groups

In recent years, focus group methodology has been applied increasingly to research in population and health. Its use by researchers and consultants in these areas has shed new light on, for example, people's understanding of risk factors for heart disease, diabetes, and HIV; socioeconomic influences on health decision making; perspectives on health in the school curriculum; and attitudes toward community health interventions. Focus groups are equally useful for formative research and for evaluation of outcomes. On the other hand, indiscriminate use of focus groups by researchers with little experience in qualitative methods or focus groups, in particular, sometimes creates confusion about how and when to use them. In practice, focus group discussions are only one of a growing number of qualitative methods, and they are valuable in situations where the most rewarding data will come from interaction in a group (Morgan, 1988).

As we discussed in Chapter 3, there are relatively clear indicators for choosing a focus group over an individual in-depth interview. Groups can be highly effective sources of data for studies that focus on social norms, expectations, values, and beliefs. Especially rich topics for focus groups are those that stimulate people to share their own ideas and debate others' views. Focus group discussions thrive on controversial topics. However, it is critical to the quality of the data that participants be well versed in the topic, either through personal experience or a vested interest arising from a particular role or position. In Case Study 11 in Appendix 1, personal experience with the topic was ensured by researchers showing focus group participants videotaped public service announcements and a documentary before asking them then to react to the videos.

Composition of Focus Groups

Most focus groups are relatively homogeneous, composed of people who are similar with respect to characteristics related to the topic. A study of breastfeeding practices might start with people of childbearing age, but it could soon become apparent that women feel uncomfortable speaking with men about these issues. Or in some cultures, younger women are often reluctant to express their views in the presence of older women. Mothers may be unwilling to listen to women who have not borne children. Both sex and age often become defining variables when assigning people to discussion groups. Similar constraints may divide members of different ethnic groups, rural residents from urban, educated people from nonliterate, professional and technical workers from manual workers. Or it may be important to the research design to segment participants for the sake of stratification in analysis, the ability to compare and contrast the views of different subsets of the population (see Chapter 6). As the study progresses, you may find it advisable to expand the sample if emerging data suggest tapping new or different sources of information, or if additional stratification of participants is warranted. Box 4.7 offers guidance for deciding how many focus groups to conduct, based on stratification of participant groups and other factors.

BOX 4.7 DECIDING HOW MANY FOCUS GROUPS TO CONDUCT

There are three factors to consider in deciding how many focus groups to conduct, all of which are related to study design.

1. By how many demographic variables do you wish to stratify the focus groups and why?

   A good rule of thumb is to conduct is at least two focus groups for each defining demographic variable. For instance, if the groups are divided only by sex, four groups may be sufficient. However, in practice, focus groups are seldom divided on only one variable, and the necessary number of groups quickly multiplies. If two age categories (e.g., younger and older) are added, the number of groups jumps to eight. Adding an education variable with three categories will bring you to 24 groups. And if you decide to conduct the study in three locales—rural, urban, and peri-urban—you will need 72 discussion groups, an unwieldy sample size for most field studies. To limit the number of focus groups to a more manageable size, consider which variables may possibly influence people's perspectives on your research questions. Then limit your stratification to only those variables. Also consider the feasibility of recruiting individuals who meet the criteria.

(Continued)

BOX 4.7 DECIDING HOW MANY FOCUS GROUPS TO CONDUCT (Continued)

2. What financial and human resources do you have available?

   The lesson many qualitative researchers have learned is the need to balance the number of variable subsets (e.g., sex, age, residence) against the resources (e.g., time, money, personnel) available for recruiting participants, conducting the focus groups, and transcribing, translating, coding, and analyzing the data. This equation takes you back to the study design. If you have more groups than you can handle, the chances are that your study design is too complex for the resources at your disposal. You may need to revisit the study objectives and focus them more tightly. Remember that establishing a comfortable balance between the number of focus group discussions and available resources should take place at the design stage, not once you are in the field.

3. What time resources are available?

   How much time you have available to conduct your study affects how much data you will be able to collect, transcribe, translate (if applicable), and analyze. A typical schedule for conducting focus groups is not more than one group per day. Transcription of focus groups may take as many as one to three additional days, depending on whether the transcript is being typed or handwritten and whether simultaneous translation is included. A two-hour discussion is likely to generate 25 to 50 pages of transcript. A set of 72 discussions could yield as many as 3,600 pages to code and perhaps translate by the end of the study. Simple arithmetic demonstrates the importance of selecting criteria carefully to include variables essential to sound design while keeping the size of the dataset within limits established by the research.

For most purposes, groups of 8 to 10 participants are sufficient to stimulate good but manageable discussion for the moderator, who must keep the discussion focused while encouraging everyone to take part. The smaller the group, the less likely that discussion will express wider norms, values, or opinions. On the other hand, a large group is not only difficult to manage, but may also provide incomplete data if reticent members defer to their more voluble peers.

Although you hope that everyone in the group will contribute freely and openly, it is important to select individuals who are not likely to dominate the discussion or inhibit others' participation. This is less about discerning people's personalities than about considering their roles and status in that community. For example, if the study design calls for the opinions of people in positions of authority—the company manager, a hospital director, or a community official—consider including them in individual key informant interviews rather than as focus group participants alongside health service clients. Alternatively, you might decide to invite these authorities, or a subset of them, to take part in separate focus groups; however, busy schedules often do not allow for such individuals to take part in focus groups.

Should focus group participants be strangers or friends? Writers on focus group methodology often emphasize the importance of anonymity among participants, on the premise that one can speak more freely with strangers than with people one knows and will meet again. However, in many settings, especially in developing countries, it is neither feasible nor advisable to expect a group of strangers to participate in a discussion. It may be difficult to find participants who are not already acquainted. In some cultures, women, and sometimes men, are uncomfortable sharing their perspectives with people they do not know. The researcher therefore must base this decision on local norms of interaction. Under no circumstances should you ever allow observers or interested bystanders to listen to the discussion; doing so would violate confidentiality and possibly inhibit open discussion.

Protecting Confidentiality in Focus Groups

In order to protect confidentiality, participants' real names should never be used during focus groups. To assure focus group participants that their identities will be kept confidential once focus groups are transcribed and analyzed, the codes or numbers assigned to participants (see Box 4.8) can be used in place of their names. An alternative is to ask participants to choose pseudonyms, but this approach sometimes leads to participants who know each other to use real names by mistake. Whichever you choose to use, numbers or pseudonyms are a reminder that a system is in place to protect the anonymity of anything participants say. Sometimes participants refer to each other by the numbers they are wearing, even when they know each other by name: "I agree with eight that . . . "

The Moderator's Role: Facilitating the Discussion

As we have seen earlier in this chapter, qualitative interviewing requires a high level of interpersonal skill to develop a conversational partnership. Similarly, the focus group moderator's special task is to create a group of conversational partners and to listen with nonjudgmental interest while keeping the discussion focused and moving. Whether in the individual interview or group discussion, the responsive interviewer or moderator shows interest, curiosity, empathy, and encouragement but also must be flexible, creative, and able to tailor questions and comments to each person's unique responses

BOX 4.8 COLLECTING BACKGROUND INFORMATION FROM INTERVIEW AND FOCUS GROUP PARTICIPANTS

A brief sociodemographic or background profile on each interview or focus group participant can provide valuable information for later analysis and presentation of the findings. Knowing something about the individuals whose comments are recorded on the transcript will help you describe your sample, interpret what participants have said, and analyze emerging themes in the light of contextual differences and similarities. Background information can also enliven publications and reports by bringing alive the people behind the findings: "A 30-year-old factory worker and mother of six commented that..."

The information collected should be brief and clearly related to the research problem, for example, sociodemographic characteristics such as age, education, occupation, marital status, or family size. In clinical research, qualitative investigators sometimes use information from the sexual and reproductive history to help them understand their data: age at first pregnancy, use of contraception, number of pregnancies and live births, desired number of children, and so forth.

The rules in collecting background data are simple:

- Keep it relevant.
- Keep it short.
- Keep it confidential.

If sociodemographic or other data will enhance your analysis, collect it after participants provide their informed consent and before the interview or focus group discussion begins. Remember to keep the background form simple; two pages or less of easy, short-answer or multiple-choice questions are usually sufficient to record a few relevant facts. Participants may provide the data by completing the forms themselves or responding orally to a researcher. Even in a focus group study, this is not a group exercise; it is done individually to preserve confidentiality and anonymity. The forms are identified only by participant codes that correspond to the unique code number that each individual participant is assigned to use during the discussion. By attaching the code to the participant's words in the transcript, it is possible to link sociodemographic data with individual focus group speakers. Store the completed forms securely, in a location accessible only to the researchers and their assistants.

BOX 4.9 CHARACTERISTICS OF A GOOD INTERVIEWER OR MODERATOR

- Ability to feel at ease and to put others at ease
- Ability to build rapport and project unconditional respect and acceptance of others
- Ability to convey warmth and empathy
- Good verbal and interpersonal skills
- Good listening skills
- Ability to project enthusiasm and genuine interest in others
- Awareness of own nonverbal reactions, using body language to project positive responses
- Ability to interpret and explore what people say in light of the research problem, as opposed to providing rote responses
- Ability to interpret and explore local cultural references and nuances

Source: Adapted from Debus (1986).

(see Box 4.9). A topic guide or semi-structured **question guide**, introduced earlier in this chapter, is an important tool for keeping the discussion focused while encouraging participants to speak naturally and spontaneously.

Facilitating a focus group discussion on a sensitive topic is never easy, but moderators who are new to qualitative data collection can find that hearing all points of view and keeping the discussion on track can be especially challenging. It is not unusual for an interviewer to begin a qualitative project with a strong background in survey work. Many find it difficult at first to replace the structure of a quantitative interview with the flexibility that qualitative research demands—asking open-ended questions, probing answers, and following the participants' lead while keeping the discussion focused on the research problem. Common errors in moderating a focus group discussion appear in Box 4.10.

As in the in-depth interview, depending on the cultural context and the sensitivity of the topics to be discussed, it may be more acceptable to focus group participants if the moderator and notetaker are the same sex as the participants. If women are not accustomed to expressing their views to men,

BOX 4.10 COMMON ERRORS IN FOCUS GROUP MODERATING

Common errors that appear in focus group transcripts are the following:

- Allowing one or two participants to dominate the discussion or not enabling reticent participants to speak
- Remaining too long on a topic, continuing to repeat questions even after participants have nothing additional to say
- Using the same words to repeat a question instead of rephrasing it
- Repeating the original question rather than probing about what has just been said or noticing new ideas and asking participants to elaborate
- Interrupting people who begin to express a different point of view by repeating the original question as if the speaker were not addressing it
- Accepting comments on what people should do without probing what they actually do and why there is a difference
- Not probing the logical conclusions of ideas ("If that, then what?" or simply, "Why?")
- Not probing assumptions to see where they come from ("Why do people say that?")
- Letting a good question drop if it is not answered immediately
- Failing to explore vague or nonspecific terms or to clarify vernacular expressions that may not be familiar to the researchers
- In studies about sexual and reproductive health, allowing the group to talk only about married (or more stable) relationships and ignoring casual (less stable) unions
- Asking leading questions that might bias the answers. Following are examples of leading probes *not* to use:
  - Do you mean . . . ?
  - Is that the only thing you can think of?
  - You do not mean that . . . ?
  - Don't you think that . . . ?
  - Would you agree that . . . ?

(Continued)

- Nonleading probes are usually open-ended inquiries such as the following:
  - How do you mean?
  - In what way?
  - What else?
  - There is no hurry. Take a moment to think about it and tell me all that comes to your mind.

even the most skilled male moderator may inhibit discussion. Other characteristics will depend on the topic of discussion and cultural norms that prescribe who can discuss what with whom. Similarly, respondents in developing countries who have had little opportunity to know Westerners may be uncomfortable with a U.S. or European interviewer. Productive interaction may therefore depend on cultural similarity and the ability of researchers and participants to understand each other's language and perspectives.

The Focus Group Notetaker's Role: Documentation

The notetaker has the role of recorder-observer of the focus group. To ensure accurate data and to facilitate analysis, qualitative researchers usually audio record their focus group discussions. Although videotaping would capture more nonverbal expression, participants may find the camera more intrusive than a simple audio recorder. For most data collection, we therefore recommend digital voice recorders. Even so, overreliance on the recorder is a common pitfall with negative consequences when technology fails. Therefore, a team of two trained moderators is needed, one to guide the discussion and the other to act as notetaker who will monitor the recorder while recording on paper as much of the discussion as possible (Hogle, Stalker, Hassig, Henry, & Young, 1994).

Although verbatim text from transcripts will be of great value in the analysis, notes on the discussion are also important. The skilled field researcher learns to take good notes unobtrusively and to expand them quickly after the focus group, regardless of whether the discussion has been recorded. In case of an inaudible recording, a power failure, or lost data, the researcher will have recorded on paper enough of the discussion to preserve the raw data. In addition to copious notes on the verbal process, the notetaker also enters observations that will enrich the transcript with nonverbal messages that have a bearing on the discussion. For example, expanded notes might state that

"Participant 6 appeared angry and left the group" or that "the group seemed much amused by this remark."

It is the notetaker's responsibility to associate the speaker code (i.e., number or letter) with what the person says. The notetaker follows the discussion carefully, indicating the code number or letter and the first few words of each comment; these are usually enough to identify the speaker when the notetaker's observations are transferred later to the transcript. It is not essential to identify every comment, and in fast-paced discussions, such precision is often impossible. However, to the extent you are able to identify who said what, you will have a richer analysis and a livelier presentation of the data, because you can amplify comments from the transcript with information about the speaker. (We discuss integrating participants' comments and characteristics into publications and reports in Chapter 8.)

Conducting the Focus Group

Steps to conducting focus groups are outlined in Box 4.11 and are elaborated here for points on which further detail may be useful.

As participants enter, the moderator and notetaker collect the sociodemographic data from each participant individually and privately. Participants are then directed to refreshments and to chairs arranged in a circle. The moderator sits with the participants in the circle, with the notetaker just outside the circle to avoid distracting the group. The audio recorder is placed where it can easily record the discussion but will present as little distraction to participants as possible. We generally do not recommend passing a microphone around to each speaker, although this approach may be used when the meeting place has a lot of background noise or the centrally located recording device is weak.

The moderator welcomes the group and introduces her- or himself and the notetaker, explaining the role of each. The moderator also explains the purpose of the recorder: to enable the researchers to capture ideas that emerge from the discussion without identifying the speakers by name, as well as to ensure that all contributions are documented. Participants are assured that written reports will not include names and that recordings will not be shared outside of the research team. Participants should also understand that there are no right and wrong answers and that all opinions are welcome.

Then begin the process of administering informed consent. Read and review the informed consent document with the group, and make certain that everyone has the opportunity to ask questions. If you find that someone does not understand a point fully, review that part of the consent form again until you are sure that confusion or misconceptions have been cleared up. Obtain consent from the participants as a group. We recommend recording the consent to have an additional record of participants' consent. At the end of the

BOX 4.11 STEPS TO CONDUCTING A FOCUS GROUP

BEFORE LEAVING FOR THE FOCUS GROUP SITE

- Review notes, including notes from focus groups you conducted earlier for the study, including any team debriefings.
- Review study protocol and topic/question guide.
- Gather materials: Prepare digital recorder, extra digital recorder, extra batteries, notepads, pens, labels, name tags, topic/question guides; gifts, snacks, or travel reimbursements for participants; and any other materials you may need, such as pictures to stimulate conversation, chart paper, and so on.
- Test digital recorder.

AT THE SITE BEFORE DISCUSSION BEGINS

- Set up the room. Arrange chairs or mats in a circle. A table may or may not be present, depending on cultural norms of conversation.
- Set up the refreshments. These should be available before the focus group discussion begins.
- Test the recorder.
- Greet the participants.
- Collect sociodemographic data from each participant.
- Ensure that participants help themselves or are served the refreshments.
- Make labels with numbers corresponding to data sheets if you are using them to identify individual speakers during recording and note-taking.

STARTING THE DISCUSSION

- Introduce yourself and the notetaker.
- Describe the use of the digital recorder, and remind participants that notes will be taken.
- Summarize the purpose of the study.

(Continued)

BOX 4.11 STEPS TO CONDUCTING A FOCUS GROUP (Continued)

- Review the statement of informed consent. Make sure that everyone understands. Obtain consent from the group (often oral consent, rather than written).
- Encourage confidentiality. Ask participants to guard the confidentiality of others in the group.
- Describe the focus group discussion process. Emphasize that there are no right or wrong answers; all present should participate; all should respect the opinions of others; and that all should help to keep the discussion on track.
- Review the ground rules of the focus group, including not speaking out of turn and silencing mobile phones. Invite participants to suggest additional ground rules.
- Advise the group of the anticipated length of the discussion, recommended as a maximum of 1.5 hours. Invite questions.

CONDUCTING THE DISCUSSION

- Begin with warm-up or ice-breaker questions.
- Be aware of who is talking and who is not. Do not allow one or two individuals to dominate; bring silent participants into the discussion.
- Begin with the first substantive topic and questions.
- Use broad, open-ended questions. Avoid yes-or-no or short-answer questions in a questionnaire format. Frame the discussion with more general questions and encourage participants to raise issues that are important to them.
- Always probe. On some occasions, moderators may want to probe for additional information when a participant's initial answer appears incomplete. Probing does not mean suggesting a more interesting answer. Probes that suggest answers are leading probes and must be avoided.
- Do not hesitate to use silence (waiting expectantly while a speaker thinks through her idea) and nonverbal prompts (raising your eyebrows, nodding your head, saying "hmmm," and so on). They tell the respondent that you are listening and interested in whatever she has to say.
- Note any questions that the group does not seem to understand, as well as questions that stimulate good discussion. If necessary, revise the topic guide after the session for future discussion.

(Continued)

- Record body language and other nonverbal communications. The participant's tone of voice or physical movements may communicate more than she is actually voicing. An idea stated forcefully or even angrily might emphasize the strength of a participant's convictions. A hesitant manner might suggest the participant is not sure about the idea she is stating or that she anticipates disagreement from others in the group. Rivalries or one-upmanship between group members may also be communicated nonverbally. Such dynamics should be noted. Body language and nonverbal communications should also be noted.
- Use the guidelines flexibly; return to topics that were not fully discussed or that needed more thought.

END OF THE DISCUSSION

- Thank the participants.
- Explain how the discussion information will be used.
- Remunerate discreetly. Distribute travel reimbursement, small gifts, or honoraria if used.
- Collect the digital recorder and written notes.

AFTER THE DISCUSSION

- Expand your notes in outline form. The notetaker and moderator should do this together, immediately following the session if possible, or at least on the same day as the focus group discussion. Record in writing any nonverbal data.
- Transcribe the recording. This may take 8 to 12 hours for each hour of focus group recording, depending on whether you are simultaneously translating the data and how much overlap there was when speakers were talking. The task may be shared or rotated from notetaker to moderator. Develop a system to transcribe as quickly as possible. Make sure to label each electronic document for each data collection event with a unique identification code in the header or footer of the document. This code can also be used in the file name so that files can be easily identified.
- Review the transcribed notes. Add the researcher's comments in parentheses. These could include observations about the group, remarks to probe in later discussions, or methodological problems.

process, remind participants of the group's responsibility to guard the confidentiality of the discussion.

It is important for participants to understand the general goals of the discussion, but "clarifying goals does not necessarily mean revealing . . . the questions under study. Clarifying goals does mean communicating to participants what you want to know from them" (Basch, 1987, p. 416). Indeed, in an overly informed group, members may obligingly supply the answers they think you want to hear, regardless of their truth. Once the participants generally understand the topic and procedure, the moderator may then ask them to introduce themselves, although if anonymity in the group is important, introductions can be replaced with informal conversation and nonthreatening questions to put the group members at ease and encourage them to talk among themselves.

The moderator then asks participants to accept ground rules, such as speaking one at a time, not interrupting each other, silencing mobile phones, and speaking clearly and slowly so that the recorder can pick up even the most subtle remarks. Participants should be asked to suggest additional ground rules, which will reinforce the idea that their contributions are a valuable part of the research process. The moderator encourages participants to speak freely, addressing questions any way they want, while at the same time reminding them that discussions sometimes wander off track and may need to be refocused. This can be a difficult course to steer but may be greatly facilitated by a well-designed yet flexible topic guide, as discussed earlier in this chapter.

Following this warm-up period, introduce the first topic. The moderator should observe the group closely, watching for signs that some participants might merely be agreeing with others rather than voicing opinions of their own. Other signs of potential problems in the group process are participants who are unenthusiastic, aloof, confused, overly positive, or excessively negative; are highly critical of others; or attempt to control the discussion with their own points of view. Early identification makes it easier to respond effectively to these problems. For example, a domineering participant might be seated next to the moderator to discourage eye contact, or the moderator might remind the group that ground rules include respectful listening.

Ending the Focus Group

At the end of the discussion, the moderator may ask the participants to summarize what they have said, adding any comments they want to include. Or the moderator might supply the summary, beginning with "Since we are almost out of time, I will try to summarize what you have told me." The summary is a chance to clarify issues and give the group a sense of work accomplished. Participants are able to restate points and correct any misunderstandings the moderator may have. The notetaker then turns off the recorder. Most groups conclude with light refreshments, which local assistants can organize.

Some researchers include a debriefing with participants at the close of the discussion, inviting feedback on the discussion experience. Did they feel included? Were they comfortable with the topics? Do they think the group fully explored the topics? Were there topics or questions that the group should have discussed but did not? Can they think of how the discussion should have been conducted differently? Debriefings can be useful not only for evaluating and revising the discussion protocol, but also for providing additional context in data analysis. They also are an important learning resource for the field team.

The question of reimbursement to participants frequently arises in focus group research. Should participants be reimbursed for the time they contribute to discussing the research questions? A rule of thumb on this issue is to take local customs and expectations into consideration. If people have come to expect payment for their participation in research, then it is appropriate to pay them according to the local scale.

Structured Data Collection Techniques

It is often the case that individuals or groups will be able to organize and articulate their thoughts more easily if they have a concrete reference point. There are a number of ways to add this kind of structure to interviews and focus groups without compromising flexibility and spontaneity. Centering a question on an image or task adds a tangible dimension to an otherwise abstract issue. Framing potentially uncomfortable issues in a less personal context also is helpful. For example, the interview or focus group guide might start a topic with a statement of presumed fact: "We have heard that women are not going to the clinic for prenatal care. Can you comment on that?" or "A woman in another village told us that she had been beaten several times by her husband. Are you familiar with such a problem in your own community?" This indirect structure is likely to elicit a more open response than "Why did you not attend the antenatal clinic?" or "Have you ever experienced domestic abuse?"

The following techniques for adding structure to data collection can be used with almost any qualitative method, particularly when you are interested in helping a group to center on specific research issues, as in focus group discussions and participatory action research.

Freelisting and Pile Sorts

An old technique with application to qualitative research in public health is **freelisting with pile sorts**. For these combined techniques, the researcher asks participants to make a list of all instances of some phenomenon. Items on the categories list are then transferred to cards that participants sort into piles according to their own criteria and labels. This approach is based on the principle that people make sense of their worlds by grouping their observations and experiences in classes known as domains. A **cultural domain** is "a set of items or things that are all of the same type or category" (Schensul, LeCompte, Nastasi, & Borgatti, 1999, p. 115). How people assign items to domains indicates to the researcher how they interpret the meanings of these items in their own lives.

For example, if you are interested in popular perceptions of STIs, you might ask participants in a study to list all the diseases and symptoms they can think of and organize them in groups according to common characteristics. The common denominators they use can tell you a great deal about the meanings people attach to STI symptoms. You may discover that people classify symptoms according to traditional notions of cause and effect, attributing some to transcendent causes, whereas others sort the cards into piles that represent biomedical, environmental, or political explanations.

To take this example a step farther, you might want to explore possible links between cultural definitions and choice of provider by using pile sort. To use this technique, you could ask participants to group the items in help-seeking categories, including different types of healers as well as peer consultation, self-help, or no action at all. Whether you are collecting data from individuals or groups, this technique lends itself well to qualitative exploration, because in probing the logic behind participants' assignments of items to categories, the researcher may uncover reasons for popular perceptions and behaviors that might not otherwise be apparent. This is also an example of a situation in which interviewers or moderators must be prepared to devise questions in the moment, based on the participants' freelisting and pile sort responses. (See Case Study 12 for another example of how a pile sort can be used.)

The lists that participants create are themselves an important linguistic tool if they provide insight into cultural expression on topics related to the research problem. For example, public health researchers conducting a formative study of neonatal mortality in Guatemala wanted to understand how local people expressed the topics and feelings surrounding the loss of a child in their idiom. Inviting women to tell their stories, the researchers identified a list of words. They asked women then to sort the words into like piles, explaining similarities and differences among them. The result was a taxonomy of indigenous expressions that the researchers could use to develop culturally sensitive tools for collecting data. Through a better understanding of linguistic expression, they learned, for example, that many of their participants associated neonatal deaths with the lunar eclipse, referring to the lost child as "el niño eclipsado" (Patricia Bailey, personal communication, 2004). Most participants enjoy sorting items into categories and then talking about their decisions. The process itself can be interesting and the outcome motivating, as people begin to reinterpret familiar experiences in new ways.

Photo Elicitation

As its name implies, the **photo elicitation** technique uses photographs as part of qualitative interviews and focus group discussions. When using this technique, the interviewer or moderator presents a visual aid such as a photograph or poster and asks participants to talk about what it means to them. (See Appendix 2 for a topic guide that incorporates pictures and a pile sort exercise.) In a study of Latina women's perceptions of the quality of prenatal care, participants were shown photographic prompts—pictures taken in a clinic setting with actors posing as staff and clients (Bender, Harbour, Thorp, & Morris, 2001). An interviewer asked participants to describe each photograph, including how the woman in the photo was feeling. She then asked the participant if the photograph reminded her of any experience she had had and, if so, to tell the story of that experience. As these researchers point out, photographic prompts allow the participant to talk about herself in the third person, projecting experiences and opinions that may not be socially desirable onto the subject in the photograph.

Other photo elicitation studies involve participants themselves providing photos that they then talk about during an interview. For example, in a qualitative study with formerly homeless men and women with serious mental illness, participants brought 18 photos representing positive and negative aspects of their lives and narrated what the photos meant during an individual interview (Padgett, Smith, Derejko, Henwood, & Tiderington, 2013). (See Appendix 4 for an example of topic guides that incorporated photo elicitation.)

Photovoice

Photovoice—providing research participants with cameras to capture strengths and problems in a community and then asking the participants to explain what the pictures represent—is another way of using photos in qualitative studies, often as part of participatory research and community empowerment projects (Bender & Castro, 2000; Carlson, Engebretson, & Chamberlain, 2006; Hergenrather, Rhodes, Cowan, Bardhoshi, & Pula, 2009; Wang, 1999; Wang & Burris, 1997). In their review of 31 studies that used photovoice, Hergenrather et al. (2009) identified 10 best-practice steps in implementing the technique: (1) identification of a community issue; (2) participant recruitment; (3) photovoice training; (4) camera distribution and instruction; (5) identification of photo assignments; (6) photo assignment discussion; (7) data analysis; (8) identification of influential advocates; (9) presentation of photovoice findings; and (10) creation of plans of action for change. They note that effective questions are critical for eliciting narratives and reactions about the photos. In addition, write-ups of findings should include explicit descriptions of data analysis, as well as project evaluation and the impact of studies that incorporate photovoice (Catalani & Minkler, 2010). While it is possible to use visual data analysis methods to analyze photos, frequently the textual data from discussions about the photos are the focus of the analysis.

This technique is especially well suited to inquiries from a transformative perspective, because it has the potential to give voice to people who may not be heard otherwise. For example, in 2010, photovoice was used to understand the perspectives and challenges of children in Lira, Uganda, who were living on the streets, outside of family care. Children were provided with cameras to capture what they felt was important for others to know about their lives, including why they were living on the streets, as well as their hopes and dreams for their lives. In-depth interviews were then conducted so that researchers could learn more about what was in the photos the children had taken, and the photos were placed in a sequence that told a story (i.e., storyboarding). Finally, a poster was designed for each child that triangulated the results of photovoice, the interviews, and storyboarding. The posters were later hung in locations around the community. The photographic record empowered these vulnerable children to communicate with stakeholders in the community about issues that affected their everyday lives (Lisa Albert, personal communication).

In another example, photovoice was used to engage young people from a public housing community in Durban, South Africa, in addressing needs related to health and quality of life in their community. An international health research project provided cameras to a group of local high school students to capture their perspectives on things, people, and places they encountered daily in their community, which suffers from poverty and unemployment. Importantly, the research team had strong existing ties with the community (including school leaders) and a commitment to community engagement. Local university student researchers were given intensive training in photovoice methods, and the high school students were trained in practical photography skills. The young photographers completed an analysis worksheet for every image, including information on why they took the photo and what it meant to them as community members. During the same time period, the research team conducted in-depth interviews of community residents. The culmination of this three-pronged inquiry was a community gathering attended by parents, community elders, and municipal and school officials. The young photographers presented their photos, which revealed in graphic detail that the community soccer field was central to their daily lives and social interactions. The photos were hung in the local high school, and

a video of the project was posted online. Local housing officials soon took notice, and the city's plans to turn the soccer field into a parking lot were called off. Creating and presenting a photographic record had empowered these vulnerable children to engage with stakeholders in the community on matters that affected their everyday lives. It then led directly to an urban planning decision that tangibly improved the health of the community and set a precedent for other communities to follow (Dehmer, 2014; Mosavel, Marks, Dehmer, & Borcheller, 2014).

Vignettes

Another way to elicit perceptions in interviews or focus groups is by telling a story or presenting a **vignette** that is fictitious but is designed to include issues at the heart of the research problem. Vignettes are often used in quantitative research but are also a useful qualitative technique, particularly for sensitive topics. Researchers present the vignette—which can be in the form of a written story, a video, or a picture—and then ask participants to react to the story, its characters, and/or the situation, such as by asking them what the character would or should do in that situation and why. This could be followed by asking what the participants themselves would do and why.

When developing the vignette, care should be taken to ensure that the gap between the life experiences of research participants and the characters in the story is not too great; otherwise, participants may not be able to relate to the scenario (Hughes & Huby, 2002).

A focus group study of sexual decision making and HIV/AIDS risk in Haiti presented the topic through the story of an imaginary young woman, Joujou, who believed she was at great risk of acquiring HIV from her partner, René (Ulin, Cayemittes, & Metellus, 1995). Issues to be explored were embedded in a culturally familiar context of women's economic dependence and sexual subordination. When she discovers that René has other sexual partners, Joujou must decide how to protect herself. The interviewer then opens the discussion to the group, inviting their ideas and suggestions, and prompting them to think beyond their initial reactions with such questions as "How do you think René would react to that?" or "How can Joujou support herself and her children if she leaves him?" Participants in both men's and women's groups quickly recognized Joujou's dilemma and entered into vigorous discussion of alternatives and their consequences for women's lives. As in Bender and Harbour's photo narrative study (Bender et al., 2001), storytelling relieved the pressure of self-disclosure by asking people to comment on the problems and decisions of another person, albeit a person like themselves.

Note that when used in focus groups, these techniques elicit participants' perceptions of cultural norms, views, and behaviors of people like themselves but are not a dependable record of case-based behavior. As discussion builds, speakers frequently identify with the photo or story actors, switching easily from third-person to first-person narrative. Nevertheless, in most instances, only the individual interview and similar techniques, with or without additional structure, can fully capture individual perceptions and behavior.

Body Mapping

Body mapping is a technique in which participants draw maps of the human body. It has frequently been used as a therapy tool to help people living with HIV and people suffering from post-traumatic stress disorder to reflect on their experiences (Crawford, 2010; Solomon, 2002). As a research tool, it has been used to study, among other things, the health impacts of employment insecurity (Wilson et al., 2011) and the effects of occupational hazards (Gastaldo, Magalhães, Carrasco, & Davy, 2012). For example, in a study in Canada with foundry and insulation workers, researchers used body mapping to explore the health impacts of past exposure to asbestos. After workers had drawn maps of their workplaces and exposures to asbestos, they then documented their health problems on life-size body maps using dot stickers that were color-coded according to type of health problem. Once completed, the body maps showed clusters of dots representing respiratory disease, cancers, and cardiovascular disease. The findings were ultimately used as evidence in what proved to be successful worker compensation claims (Keith & Brophy, 2004).

The technique is also particularly useful in studies of people's perceptions of reproductive anatomy and physiology, fertility awareness, and other reproductive health issues, as it may be a more comfortable means of expression for participants who are reticent to speak openly about sexual matters. As a visual representation of the participant's understanding of reproductive function, the participant's drawing, or body map, can then become the focus for in-depth conversation with the interviewer.

For example, a participatory action project in Zambia used body mapping to understand how Zambian youth conceptualize the reproductive system (Shah, Zambezi, & Simasiku, 1999). The researcher asked small groups of adolescents divided by age and sex to make simple sketches of the human body to show how the reproductive organs function. The researcher then asked each group to label the body parts and explain their functions, prompting them with questions such as "How does a woman get pregnant?" or "How can pregnancy be prevented?" Researchers were able to identify gaps and distortions that could be addressed through intervention. As the author of this report points out, body mapping can be combined with other qualitative methods or expanded into picture stories, or cartoons, as the basis for discussing sexual relationships. Although semi- and nonliterate people will not be able to write labels on their maps, research has shown that they can participate in a body-mapping project, interpreting their drawings orally to the researcher (Shah et al., 1999).

In similar uses of body mapping, researchers sometimes chose this technique to study women's perceptions of maternal morbidity. Women will express themselves more easily about reproductive risk if they can talk as they draw in organs on a female figure. As the women describe each organ, how it works, and how it can fail, researchers are able to identify, for example, cultural perceptions of cause and effect, as well as local patterns of help-seeking for symptoms that participants identify.

Social Network Analysis

Social network analysis is based on the premise that individuals seldom make decisions in isolation. Through network research we are able to explore attitudes, beliefs, and actions of individuals in the context of group affiliations. Tracing a person's social network helps the researcher understand what people do and think in relation to group norms and expectations. It also reveals how people, as well as ideas and information, circulate in and among different groups. Discovering the social network can be a first step in developing effective interventions to reduce behavior that puts people's health at risk.

Social network research has been used extensively to study risk behavior associated with sharing drug injection equipment and engaging in unprotected sex with HIV-infected partners. For example, in 2009, a network study of injection drug users in Ho Chi Minh City, Vietnam, sought to determine the feasibility of identifying sexual networks that included acutely infected persons and recent seroconverters in a geographically defined catchment area (Thanh, Moland, & Fylkesnes, 2009). In-depth interviews were conducted with individuals who tested as negative for HIV, as having a recent HIV infection, and as having an established infection to explore how voluntary testing and counseling experience, as well as knowledge of personal HIV status, affected respondents' behavior and relationships. The study was ultimately able to identify and characterize the sexual networks of men and women at high risk of HIV through injection drug use and sex work.

Social network analysis begins by identifying the members of the network.

- What sets these people apart from nonmembers?
- What qualities do they share?
- What brings them together, and how strong is the bond?

The task is to determine the criteria for inclusion or exclusion and establish network boundaries. This process may be as easy as obtaining a class roster or list of employees, or it may be as difficult as patiently tracking down individuals through participant observation and key informant interviews. Researchers can discover clues to network boundaries by asking people what makes a member. Having defined the network and identified its members, the investigator proceeds to explore the meaning of the relationships among network members through in-depth interviews and participant observation.

In northern Thailand, where unwanted pregnancy and STI rates among young people are high, researchers turned to social network analysis to help develop new programs to reduce sexual risk (Bond, Valente, & Kendall, 1999). The research team used a technique called snowball sampling, a respondent-driven approach that enabled them to identify the social networks they would study. The team randomly selected two young women at public dormitories, workplaces, and entertainment venues and asked each to name five friends they frequently went out with at night. These friends were contacted and asked to name five more friends. When no new names were mentioned, the process stopped, yielding three networks of affiliated youth at each site. In-depth interviews with individual network members explored cultural norms and behavior related to friends and romantic partners. Discovering sexual linkages led to identification of youth subcultures, communication channels, and patterns of risk behavior that varied among the networks. With this information as a base, program planners could then work with natural peer leaders to establish an outreach program that focused on healthier sexual decisions among different categories of youth at risk. Although the number of members in any one network may be small, the Thai example illustrates that knowing the network's characteristics can help researchers and program planners understand the health risks of its members.

Social network studies often combine qualitative and quantitative techniques in the same research design. From a quantitative perspective, investigators use surveys and statistical analyses to measure relationships within, and linkages between, networks. Computer software for quantitative network analysis enables the researcher to characterize, quantify, and create visual images of these relationships (Borgatti, Everett, & Freeman, 2001). Qualitative analysis takes a more holistic approach in order to explore the meaning and context of the network relationships in their natural setting. Combining quantitative and qualitative methods is a powerful strategy, not only for studying network characteristics but also for understanding the diffusion of ideas and behaviors within and among networks.

Summary

Collecting qualitative data is a process of bringing what you want to learn together with what you observe and what participants know and have experienced (Rubin & Rubin, 1995). This chapter has emphasized the concept of partnership in participant observation, qualitative interviewing, and focus group discussion. Although we advocate a semi-structured topic guide to help the interviewer or moderator keep the research problem in focus, flexibility is critical. Successful data collectors are prepared to adapt the tool and their personal styles to the discussion's natural flow, wherever it takes them, as long as they are learning and addressing the objectives of the interview or focus group. Qualitative interviewing and moderating therefore demands versatility and sometimes quick change when the mood of the discussion shifts or unexpected but important content interrupts the planned sequence. Similarly, participant observers return to the field each day open to new and possibly surprising discoveries.

Whether in observation, interview, or group discussion, researchers often feel bombarded with stimuli. Participants eager to share their experiences and ideas can quickly overwhelm an inexperienced data collector with valuable information. Careful planning and meticulous record keeping can help the investigator manage information overload. The conceptual framework, imprinted in the mind of the interviewer or observer, is a valuable compass, helping to keep a firm grasp on the research's purpose and main questions and to locate what participants say or do in the emerging picture. Because even the most experienced qualitative researcher does not expect to remember all the details of what happens in the field, clear transcriptions and detailed field notes are key to skillful management of large amounts of information that otherwise will be lost to science.

Each interview, each focus group discussion, each trip to the field can be an adventure. You will not know in advance exactly what will emerge, but with a clear sense of direction, flexibility, and enthusiasm for the unknown, your discoveries can become valuable contributions to qualitative understanding of many public health issues.

Key Terms

1. **Direct observation:** A method that involves watching people and events as unobtrusively as possible, without participating or actively eliciting data from research participants.
2. **In-depth interview:** An exchange between one interviewer and one respondent that may range from unstructured to semi-structured.
3. **Participant observation:** A qualitative method that involves interacting with people so that you can learn about and document their lives (Bernard, 1995).

4. **Field notes:** Clear, detailed descriptions of direct or participant observations that do not imply judgment about what has been observed. Field notes are also used to describe nonverbal information about participants in in-depth interviews and focus groups.
5. **Ethnographer:** A social scientist, usually an anthropologist, who studies culture by direct observation and interview.
6. **Key informants:** Insiders with special knowledge, status, or communication skills who are willing to share what they know with the researcher (Gilchrist, 1992).
7. **Interviewer:** Researcher who leads the interview exchange with the respondent.
8. **Topic guide** or **question guide:** Explicit set of guidelines for interviews and focus groups that may range from a list of topics to specific questions and probes to cover during data collection.
9. **Focus group discussion:** A moderator-led exchange of ideas between several research participants and between participants and the moderator that produces a range of responses.
10. **Main questions:** Open questions that come from the themes and subthemes of the research problem and introduce the topics to be discussed.
11. **Follow-up questions:** Open questions that follow the main question and ask for more detail.
12. **Probes:** A type of follow-up question that asks for even further detail.
13. **Moderator:** Researcher who leads the focus group discussion with the group of respondents.
14. **Notetaker:** Researcher who documents focus group discussions and operates recording equipment.
15. **Freelisting with pile sorts:** When the researcher asks participants to make a list of all instances of a phenomenon and then to sort the instances into piles based on their own categories and labels.
16. **Cultural domains:** A set of items that are all of the same type or category.
17. **Photo elicitation:** A technique in which the interviewer or moderator presents a visual aid, such as a photograph, and asks the participant(s) to talk about what it means to them; participants may also supply the visual aids.
18. **Photovoice:** A technique that is typically part of participatory research and community empowerment in which researchers provide participants with

cameras to document phenomena in their community and then ask them to explain what the pictures represent.

19. **Vignette:** A short, fictitious story, which in qualitative research is often about a sensitive topic, that is told to participants to elicit their reactions.
20. **Body mapping:** A technique in which research participants draw maps of the human body to help them reflect on their experiences with and knowledge about health issues.
21. **Social network analysis:** A technique in which social networks are traced to help the researcher understand how people react to group norms and expectations, as well as how people, ideas, and information circulate in and among different groups.

Review Questions

1. What are the three main methods of data collection in qualitative research?
2. What are some structured data collection techniques that might be used for orienting participants around a given topic?
3. What is the difference between direct observation and participant observation? When might you use each one?
4. What are the seven stages of the interview and focus group? For the topic of your choosing, develop an in-depth interview or focus group guide that takes these stages into account.

Recommended Readings

Appleton, J. V., & Cowley, S. (1997). Analysing clinical practice guidelines: A method of documentary analysis. *Journal of Advanced Nursing*, *25*(5), 1008–1017. doi:10.1046/j.1365-2648.1997.19970251008.x

Barter, C., & Renold, E. (1999). *The use of vignettes in qualitative research*. Social Research Update: 25. Department of Sociology, University of Surrey: Guildford, England.

Bernard, H. R. (1998). *Handbook of methods in cultural anthropology*. Lanham, MD: AltaMira Press.

Bernard, H. R. (2002). *Research methods in anthropology: Qualitative and quantitative approaches* (3rd ed.). Lanham, MD: AltaMira Press.

Collier, J., & Collier, M. (1986). *Visual anthropology: Photography as a research method.* Albuquerque: University of New Mexico Press.

De Munck, V. C., & Sobo, E. J. (1998). *Using methods in the field: A practical introduction and casebook.* Lanham, MD: AltaMira Press.

Denzin, N. K., & Lincoln, Y. S. (2000). *Handbook of qualitative research* (2nd ed.). Thousand Oaks, CA: Sage.

DeWalt, K. M., & DeWalt, B. R. (2010). *Participant observation: A guide for fieldworkers.* Walnut Creek, CA: AltaMira Press.

Guest, G., Namey, E. E., & Mitchell, M. L. (2013). *Collecting qualitative data.* Thousand Oaks, CA: Sage.

Hughes, R. (1998). Considering the vignette technique and its application to a study of drug injecting and HIV risk and safer behaviour. *Sociology of Health & Illness, 20*(3): 381–400. doi:10.1111/1467-9566.00107

Hughes, R., & Huby, M. (2002). The application of vignettes in social and nursing research. *Journal of Advanced Nursing, 37*(4), 382–386. doi:10.1046/j.1365-2648.2002.02100.x

Jorgensen, D. L. (1989). *Participant observation: A methodology for human studies.* Newbury Park, CA: Sage.

Lee, R. M. (2000). *Unobtrusive methods in social research.* Philadelphia, PA: Open University Press.

Mack, N., Woodsong, C., MacQueen, K. M., Guest, G., & Namey, E. (2005). *Qualitative research methods: A data collector's field guide.* Research Triangle Park, NC: Family Health International. Available at: http://www.fhi360.org/sites/default/files/media/documents/Qualitative%20Research%20Methods%20-%20A%20Data%20Collector%27s%20Field%20Guide.pdf

Rubin, H. J., & Rubin, I. S. (1995). *Qualitative interviewing: The art of hearing data.* Thousand Oaks, CA: Sage.

Spradley, J. P. (1980). *Participant observation.* New York, NY: Holt, Rinehart, & Winston.

References

Alty, A., & Rodham, K. (1998). The ouch! factor: Problems in conducting sensitive research. *Qualitative Health Research, 8*(2), 275–282. doi:10.1177/104973239800800210

Basch, C. E. (1987). Focus group interview: An underutilized research technique for improving theory and practice in health education [review]. *Health Education Quarterly, 14*(4, Winter), 411–448. doi:10.1177/109019818701400404

Bender, D. E., & Castro, D. (2000). Explaining the birth weight paradox: Latina immigrants' perceptions of resilience and risk. *Journal of Immigrant Health, 2*(3), 155–173. doi:10.1023/A:1009513020506

Bender, D. E., Harbour, C., Thorp, J., & Morris, P. (2001). Tell me what you mean by "si": Perceptions of quality of prenatal care among immigrant Latina women. *Qualitative Health Research, 11*(6), 780–794. doi:10.1177/104973230101100607

Bernard, H. R. (1995). *Research methods in anthropology: Qualitative and quantitative approaches* (2nd ed.). Walnut Creek, CA: AltaMira Press.

Bernard, H. R. (2002). *Research methods in anthropology: Qualitative and quantitative approaches* (3rd ed.). Lanham, MD: AltaMira Press.

Blumer, H. (1969). *Symbolic interactionism: Perspective and method.* Englewood Cliffs, NJ: Prentice Hall.

Bogdewic, S. P. (1992). Participant observation. In B. F. Crabtree & W. L. Miller (Eds.), *Doing qualitative research: Vol. 3. Research methods for primary care* (pp. 47–70). Newbury Park, CA: Sage.

Bond, K. C., Valente, T. W., & Kendall, C. (1999). Social network influences on reproductive health behaviors in urban northern Thailand. *Social Science & Medicine, 49*(12), 1599–1614. doi:10.1016/S0277-9536(99)00205-1

Borgatti, S. P., Everett, M. G., & Freeman, L. C. (2001). *UCINET V Network analysis software manual.* Harvard, MA: Analytic Technologies.

Burgess, R. G. (1984). *In the field: An introduction to field research.* London, UK: Allen & Unwin.

Carlson, E. D., Engebretson, J., & Chamberlain, R. M. (2006). Photovoice as a social process of critical consciousness. *Qualitative Health Research, 16*(6), 836–852. doi:10.1177/1049732306287525

Catalani, C., & Minkler, M. (2010). Photovoice: A review of the literature in health and public health. *Health Education & Behavior, 37*(3), 424–451. doi:10.1177/1090198109342084

Crawford, A. (2010). If "the body keeps the score": Mapping the dissociated body in trauma narrative, intervention, and theory. *University of Toronto Quarterly, 79*(2), 702–719. doi:10.1353/utq.2010.0231

Debus, M. (1986). *Handbook for excellence in focus group research.* Washington, DC: Academy for Educational Development.

Dehmer, Z. (2014). *Building global bridges* [video]. Available at http://www.vimeo.com/91845721

Eng, E., & Parker, E. (1994). Measuring community competence in the Mississippi Delta: The interface between evaluation and empowerment. *Health Education & Behavior, 21*(2), 199–220. doi:10.1177/109019819402100206

Gastaldo, D., Magalhães, L., Carrasco, C., & Davy, C. (2012). Body-map storytelling as research: Methodological considerations for telling the stories of undocumented workers through body mapping. Available at http://www.migrationhealth.ca/sites/default/files/Body-map_storytelling_as_reseach_LQ.pdf

Gilchrist, V. J. (1992). Key informant interviews. In B. F. Crabtree & W. L. Miller (Eds.), *Doing qualitative research: Vol. 3. Research methods for primary care* (pp. 70–89). Newbury Park, CA: Sage.

Hergenrather, K. C., Rhodes, S. D., Cowan, C. A., Bardhoshi, G., & Pula, S. (2009). Photovoice as community-based participatory research: A qualitative review. *American Journal of Health Behavior, 33*(6), 686–698. doi:10.5993/AJHB.33.6.6

Hogle, J., Stalker, M., Hassig, S., Henry, K., & Young, L. (1994). *Conducting effective focus group discussions.* Arlington, VA: Family Health International.

Holstein, J. A., & Gubrium, J. F. (1999). Active interviewing. In A. Bryman & R. G. Burgess (Eds.), *Qualitative research: Vol. 2. Methods of qualitative research* (pp. 105–121). London, UK: Sage.

Hughes, R., & Huby, M. (2002). The application of vignettes in social and nursing research. *Journal of Advanced Nursing, 37*(4), 382–386. doi:10.1046/j.1365-2648.2002.02100.x

Keith, M. M., & Brophy, J. T. (2004). Participatory mapping of occupational hazards and disease among asbestos-exposed workers from a foundry and insulation complex in Canada. *International Journal of Occupational and Environmental Health, 10*(2), 144–153.

Merton, R. K., Fiske, M., & Kendall, P. L. (1990). *The focused interview: A manual of problems and procedures* (2nd ed.). New York, NY: Free Press.

Morgan, D. L. (1988). *Focus groups as qualitative research.* Newbury Park, CA: Sage.

Morse, J. M. (1994). Designing funded qualitative research. In N. K. Denzin & Y. S. Lincoln (Eds.), *Handbook of qualitative research* (pp. 220–235). Thousand Oaks, CA: Sage.

Mosavel, M., Marks, M., Dehmer, Z., & Borcheller, L. (2014). *The space between.* Richmond, VA: Virginia Commonwealth University Department of Social and Behavioral Health.

Padgett, D. K., Smith, B. T., Derejko, K. S., Henwood, B. F., & Tiderington, E. (2013). A picture is worth . . . ? Photo elicitation interviewing with formerly homeless adults. *Qualitative Health Research, 23*(11), 1435–1444. doi:10.1177/1049732313507752

Patton, M. Q. (1990). *Qualitative evaluation and research methods* (2nd ed.). Newbury Park, CA: Sage.

Pool, I. S. (1957). A critique of the twentieth anniversary issue. *Public Opinion Quarterly, 21,* 190–198. doi:10.1086/266700

Rossman, G. B., & Rallis, S. F. (1998). *Learning in the field: An introduction to qualitative research.* Thousand Oaks, CA: Sage.

Rubin, H. J., & Rubin, I. S. (1995). *Qualitative interviewing: The art of hearing data.* Thousand Oaks, CA: Sage.

Schensul, J. J., LeCompte, M. D., Nastasi, B. K., & Borgatti, S. P. (1999). *Enhanced ethnographic methods*. Vol. 3 in J. J. Schensul & M. D. LeCompte (Series Eds.), *Ethnographic toolkit*. Walnut Creek, CA: AltaMira Press.

Shah, M. K., Zambezi, R., & Simasiku, M. (1999). *Listening to young voices: Facilitating participatory appraisals of reproductive health with adolescents*. Washington, DC: FOCUS on Young Adults.

Solomon, J. (2002). *"Living with X": A body mapping journey in time of HIV and AIDS. Facilitator's Guide*. Psychosocial Well-being Series. Johannesburg: REPSSI.

Thanh, D. C., Moland, K. M., & Fylkesnes, K. (2009). The context of HIV risk behaviours among HIV-positive injection drug users in Viet Nam: Moving toward effective harm reduction. *BMC Public Health, 9*(98). doi:10.1186/1471-2458-9-98

Timyan, J. (1991). *Guidelines for gathering qualitative data for HAPA PVO grants project evaluation*. Baltimore, MD: Johns Hopkins University, Institute for International Programs, School of Hygiene and Public Health.

Ulin, P. R., Cayemittes, M., & Metellus, E. (1995). *Haitian women's role in sexual decision-making: The gap between AIDS knowledge and behavior change*. Research Triangle Park, NC: Family Health International.

Wang, C. C. (1999). Photovoice: A participatory action strategy applied to women's health. *Journal of Women's Health, 8*(2), 185–192. doi:10.1089/jwh.1999.8.185

Wang, C. C., & Burris, M. A. (1997). Photovoice: Concept, methodology, and use for participatory needs assessment. *Health Education & Behavior, 24*(3), 369–387. doi:10.1177/109019819702400309

Webb, E. J., Campbell, D. T., Schwartz, R. D., &Sechrest L. (1966). *Unobtrusive measures: Nonreactive research in the social sciences*. Chicago, IL: Rand McNally.

Weller, S. C., & Dungy, C. I. (1986). Personal preferences and ethnic variations among Anglo and Hispanic breast and bottle feeders. *Social Science and Medicine, 23*(6), 539–548. doi:10.1016/0277-9536(86)90146-2

Wilson, R. M., Landolt, P., Shakya, Y. B., Galabuzi, G., Zahoorunissa, Z., Pham, D., . . . , & Joly, M. P. (2011). *Working rough, living poor: Employment and income insecurities faced by racialized groups in the Black Creek area and their impacts on health*. Toronto, Canada: Access Alliance Multicultural Health and Community Services. Available at http://www.wellesleyinstitute.com/wp-content/uploads/2011/12/Access-Alliance_Working-Rough-Living-Poor-Final-Report-June-2011-E-version.pdf

CHAPTER 5

LOGISTICS IN THE FIELD

OBJECTIVES:

- To describe the significance of establishing community links with stakeholders, partners, and advisory committees in the community where the research will be conducted
- To describe methods for building rapport, forging relationships, and fostering partnerships in the community where the research will be conducted
- To provide guidance for building and training an effective research team
- To provide tools and techniques for conducting research activities in the field
- To discuss ethical concerns that may arise while conducting research in the field

DRAWING ON THE experiences of many qualitative researchers, this chapter takes the reader through the transition from study design to implementation in the field. In the following pages, we help you create a research-friendly environment by addressing some of the pivotal decisions and tasks that may affect the study. No single text can anticipate all the logistical issues in any study, whether establishing initial contacts, identifying and involving key stakeholders, assembling and training a field team, or recording and managing data while protecting the confidentiality of participants. In this chapter, we offer the reader a logistical toolbox from which to address many of these questions. However, the experienced researcher knows to "expect the unexpected" and is ready to improvise when the toolbox does not have the answer.

Most qualitative research is interactive—composed of many face-to-face, often intimate, conversations with study participants. Ideally, we would spend long periods of time in the community or other setting, getting to know the people informally in their everyday lives. Researchers who are able to live in

Reason and logic are needed to chart your way through the woods ... painstaking planning, analysis, and execution, testing the ground every step of the way. [But] human compassion and understanding are also necessary throughout the journey.

(Fetterman, 1991, p. 87)

the research site during the study have found that participating in local events, observing both the routine and the exceptional, adds a great deal to their understanding of the social context. Yet practical limits on time and resources may be constraints. In large studies you may also be supervising the work of trained assistants who collect the data. In such circumstances, it is crucial to find ways to stay as close as possible to the field by, for example, paying frequent visits to the site, talking with local people, reviewing transcripts, and questioning data collectors about their observations and progress. If you are working across national, cultural, or language barriers, you may have

BOX 5.1 DEVELOPING A RISK MANAGEMENT PLAN

Depending on the size and complexity of your study and study team, you may find it useful to develop a **risk management plan** prior to implementation in the field. This does not necessarily refer to "risk" in the legal sense, but to logistical barriers or resource limitations that may arise and threaten successful implementation. A risk management plan typically includes:

- Procedures for identifying, evaluating, and responding to potential risks
- A thorough, prioritized list of possible risks, identified by the team prior to study implementation
- Plans for monitoring the study for new risks that might emerge

When predicting risk with your team, think about things that may affect your field implementation activities, schedule, and/or budget, such as: local holidays, events, or elections; unanticipated training needs; need for additional or replacement equipment for data collection; severe weather; staff illness or departure; scheduling difficulties with study participants and/or stakeholders; delays in obtaining ethical and/or community-level approvals; or study participant recruitment difficulties. The list of risks should be as comprehensive as possible, with the understanding that some may inevitably be overlooked.

a counterpart who will be your interpreter and guide. In any case, you or that colleague has to be there—listening, questioning, hearing, observing.

Although in this chapter we cover day-to-day issues in implementation, every field experience has its unique challenges, some predictable and some not. However, potential risks usually can be averted or managed if a plan is in place to identify, prioritize, and address them as needed (see Box 5.1). Ultimately, a well-thought-out risk management plan will help the team manage complications in the field more efficiently and respond effectively to schedule delays, budgetary pressures, and any other impediments to successful field implementation. The Centers for Disease Control and Prevention (CDC) offers templates for developing a risk management plan and risk log that can be accessed in their templates library online (CDC, 2010).

Introduction to the Community: Building Rapport

Research textbooks that go from study design to data collection often fail to provide directions through the maze of introductions and permissions, formal and informal, which are necessary for bridging the divide between researcher and study participants. **Rapport building** with the community and key **stakeholders** is essential to the success of your whole project. Winning the trust of the community means listening to many voices, understanding people's perhaps different perspectives, and engaging with them on their own terms. Imagine that you were planning to conduct qualitative research on human trafficking among young women. It might be important to demonstrate rapport with NGOs involved in social protection and human rights leaders or local social welfare officials to gain their approval. They, in turn, can help you win the trust of the local community.

A critical component of interpretive understanding is knowing the study participants' world or the social context in which they live. Pay attention to district medical officers, community officials, heads of organizations, and traditional and other local leaders, because they may have their own vested interests in your presence as well as your findings. Some may be protective of their constituents; others may fear possible negative consequences from your research. Still others may expect unrealistic support from you on some local issue. As part of rapport building, take the time to explain the purpose and implementation of the study, turning potential adversaries into partners and ensuring that expectations for your study and time in the community are clear. Having a clear, concise study brief may be helpful for this purpose. Such a brief could be printed (one page or front and back) for easy distribution to community members, or it could be electronic and housed on a study website.

It should include a brief description of the research goal and objectives, funders, partners, and study activities. The LinCS 2 Durham Project (see Case Study 3 in Appendix 1), which worked to build partnerships between scientists, community organizations, and citizens in Durham, North Carolina, developed a website with a page dedicated to project information that served as an excellent example of an electronic study brief (FHI 360, n.d.). Keep in mind that community leaders not only control access to the study site, but once they trust you, they can provide valuable access to and understanding of local culture, customs, and personalities.

Stakeholders

Most investigators start with introductions to district administrators; medical and nursing directors; gender, minority, and youth advocates; as well as religious leaders, teachers, traditional leaders, or others invested in the program or community. Stakeholders may also be external to the community, such as the funder, the sponsor, or the investigator's university or employer. Some questions you may consider as you develop a list of stakeholders and community leaders to whom you will introduce yourself and the study include the following:

- Who may be impacted by this research and the outcomes, positively or negatively?
- Who may have the influence to affect community participation in the research?
- Who may have a specific interest in the research topic either directly or indirectly?
- Who are potential funders/investors with interest in the research?
- Are there other researchers working in the community currently or recently?

Do not overlook informal leaders, including influential women in the community and people who may not occupy positions of formal authority but tend to be consulted by others who know and respect them.

Visit these individuals, making appointments if possible, to introduce yourself and your study. In some communities you may be expected to present yourself to a governing council who, along with the mayor or administrative head, will decide whether to approve the activity you propose. Similarly, a clinic director might ask you to explain your ideas to a board or to the clinic staff.

Community leaders and local officials frequently take their cues from their constituents in deciding what stance to take on a proposal coming to them from the outside.

Remember that getting appointments and permissions can be time-consuming. The data collection schedule you developed for your study probably has little relevance in the time frames of most community leaders and administrators. Take possible delays into account when you plan the study (see Box 5.1 for more information on risk management), and regard this introductory phase as a vital part of the research process. Approached this way, an otherwise frustrating delay can become an opportunity to become better acquainted with the research site.

As you navigate your introductions and begin to build relationships, you may consider maintaining a **stakeholder register** to help you and your team track these relationships. A stakeholder register may take the form of a table that includes the following information for each stakeholder:

- Name
- Organization
- Contact details
- Stakeholder type
- Preferred method of communication
- Frequency of communication
- Role in the community
- Role in the research (if any)
- Interests
- Expectations
- Influence

If the network of stakeholders is particularly complex, you may want to create a diagram incorporating arrows to show relationships between stakeholders, organizations, community members, and the research team. These documents should be updated throughout the duration of the research because new stakeholders may emerge and relationships may evolve (MacQueen et al., 2012).

Family Influences

Family members are also stakeholders and should be given special consideration because individuals' decisions to participate in your study may depend on their influence. Many research problems in sexual and reproductive health involve culturally sensitive material; women whose independence is limited by their subordination to more powerful family members may be fearful of consenting to participate in such a study. If they do consent, they may feel limited in how much of their lives they reveal without danger of recrimination. The same caveat applies to women in casual unions with sexual partners. In authoritarian relationships like these, the researcher may have to present the purpose of the study to a head of household, whether husband, father, mother-in-law, or unmarried partner. If so, the presentation should be honest but relatively general, with firm insistence on the privacy of the interview. Another approach to winning cooperation of powerful family leaders is to invite them to share their own views on the topic in separate, and equally confidential, interviews—whether or not such an exchange is part of your study design. Showing respect for the opinion of an otherwise resistant person not only involves him or her in a positive way but may also offer interesting insights that you might have missed.

On the other hand, in studies of particularly sensitive issues, full disclosure on the topic of the research may put the participant at risk in his or her family or community. In such a circumstance, your ethical priority is to protect the participant. In a study that included clandestine users of contraception in Mali, researchers and providers alike were careful to help participants maintain secrecy from husbands who, the women felt, might punish them for attending a family planning clinic or even participating in the study (Castle, Konaté, Ulin, & Martin, 1999).

Involving Policymakers and Change Agents

Research can often influence policy or the way services are delivered. If your intent is to link your study results to local policies and programs, it is important to include policymakers, service providers, and NGOs early in the design and implementation. For example, ask staff of the Ministry of Health to orient you to particular resources and needs of the study population; meet with a member of Parliament who has a special interest in the problem you plan to study; introduce the study to the district commissioner or other local or traditional authority; or discuss the study with medical and nursing officers in charge of health services in the area. Invite suggestions for implementation, and be open to possible new ways of articulating the research question for a better fit between the purpose of your study and policymakers' goals for improving the population's well-being.

Establishing reciprocity by including stakeholder questions not only facilitates access to the study population but also may result in a stronger research design with findings more relevant to the problems and the institution's policy needs. As cited earlier, when one of the authors introduced a proposed study of contraceptive decision making among women to the administrators of a family planning clinic in Bamako, Mali, they said they would like to know more about how women involve their husbands in the decision. The research team therefore introduced partner negotiation as a major topic in the interviews and later shared the results with the entire staff. Similarly, NGOs often can use research findings to develop advocacy messages. Invite leaders of local gender or youth advocacy organizations to contribute to the research design by suggesting questions that would help them serve their constituents' needs. You are not obligated to use stakeholders' questions, but if they are relevant to the basic research problem, you will win cooperation and respect by finding ways to obtain the information they need.

Project Advisory Committees

An effective vehicle for mobilizing the interest of policymakers and community leaders is the project advisory committee. Depending on the nature of your study, you may want to establish an advisory group of influential people who will meet periodically to review progress on the study and give advice on implementation issues. Such a group might include representatives from local and central government, schools, churches, women's advocacy organizations, youth groups, and other organizations. Because advisory committee membership may imply special privilege, it is best to include as broad a representation as possible so that selection of members does not seem to favor only one segment of the community.

Advisory committee members customarily do not participate directly in the design and conduct of the research. Their role is to advise. It should be clear from the outset that their purpose is to provide valuable consultation and review, not to make research decisions. Different members of the committee may take on different roles related to their interests and expertise, but typical activities might include reviewing protocols, suggesting culturally appropriate ways to ask questions, identifying key messages in the findings, linking results to recommendations, and participating in dissemination plans. You can help to ensure that these influential people will promote and use study findings if you begin by formulating clear research questions that address policy or programmatic issues, explaining or demystifying the research methods, and providing a role for stakeholders in the process.

Developing the Field Team

Never underestimate the value of local assistance. Including people from the study site in your field strategy not only helps in day-to-day management but also enhances community rapport and increases the professional team's understanding of the site. Professional data collectors and local assistants will work well together if they appreciate the complementary roles that each can play.

Field Assistants

When introducing the study to the community, identify a few local people who are especially interested in the project, who know the community, and who are willing to work with you. They will be your local field team. In Chapter 4 we discussed the role of key informants—people with special knowledge and insight into the phenomenon you are studying. The local assistants who help you implement the study should also be honest informants on the local scene and channels of information to their peers. But whereas a key informant is primarily a confidante and guide to the culture, local assistants are there mainly to help you with practical arrangements. They might be lay church leaders, community workers, or simply individuals who are well known and respected by their peers. As a general rule, it is advisable not to seek assistance from people who are controversial or in positions of authority in the group. Examples of people not to include on the field team might be the mayor or a member of his or her family, a prominent traditional healer or shaman, or the medical officer in charge of the health center. These individuals might provide valuable information, but other participants may perceive them as intimidating or coercive. Confidentiality issues may also arise.

The role of the local field team might include interpreting the study to people in the community, helping identify respondents who meet the sample selection criteria, welcoming participants (focus group members or interviewees), organizing refreshments, distracting curious visitors during interviews or focus group discussions, or reminding individuals in the sample to come on time to the interview site. Local team members must not be present during interviews or focus group discussions and must not have access to data in any form. They should be strongly encouraged to respect the privacy of people in the study sample who have agreed to participate.

Local team members will know they play a vital role, especially if they are welcome to attend meetings of the whole team and if they receive a stipend consistent with the local pay scale. They may also appreciate a simple certificate or letter that documents their experience on your project. The certificate might be used to secure similar positions in the future.

The Professional Field Team

Field Supervisor

As researchers we usually are outsiders, educated in research methodology but naive to the sociocultural matrix in which we conduct our studies. The gap may exist not only across countries but even within a country, where socioeconomic, professional, or other differences can create communication barriers. When these situations occur, a field supervisor can be an invaluable counterpart, a skilled assistant who understands the cultural context, is fluent in the local language, and has experience in qualitative techniques. Working closely with the researcher, this individual can help coordinate and supervise much of the data collection. Needless to say, the field supervisor must be a person whom interviewers and other members of the team, as well as participants and community leaders, like and respect. A field supervisor who helps you gain access to information and serves as a cultural interpreter can also be a valuable key informant.

Interviewers, Moderators, Notetakers

Ideally, interviewers, focus group moderators, notetakers, and other staff are trained in a social science and experienced in qualitative data collection. Unfortunately, such individuals often are in short supply, because few universities around the world provide training in qualitative research. However, we have found that less-experienced people with strong interpersonal skills and readiness to apply new interactive techniques can learn to collect excellent qualitative data. Because the task of a qualitative interviewer is to become a conversational partner with the participant (Rubin & Rubin, 1995), personal attributes are important. A warm, empathic manner; sensitivity to different perspectives; and an ability to listen carefully and ask insightful questions are characteristics of a good interviewer, whether educated in the social sciences or not (see Box 4.9).

It is also important to know where potential interviewers would fit in the community structure. If interviewers or supervisors differ significantly from study participants with respect to distinctive characteristics such as education, economic status, or religious affiliation, they must be able to minimize the difference in status through an interpersonal style that is friendly and nonjudgmental. Would-be interviewers who, for whatever reason, are unable to put participants at ease, accept individual differences, or respond appropriately to the changing dynamics of the interview or group discussion will not be effective.

Data Manager

Depending on the size and complexity of your study, it may help to specifically identify a data manager. If data collection is limited, the data manager could also be an interviewer, but with the added role of monitoring data and data processing throughout the study. If the study is using mixed methods and includes a quantitative component, it is highly recommended to have a data manager. The data manager should be mainly responsible for establishing the systems that facilitate data collection, processing, and security. More specifically, the data manager will be responsible for organizing the data collection and processing schedule and assignments, receiving data once they have been collected, logging and securing data, and tracking data as they are shared among team members throughout the processing steps (transcription, translation, quality control review, and eventually analysis). The data manager may also be responsible for communicating necessary changes to the overall data collection schedule or to procedures and data collection methods between the principal investigator and the data collectors.

Training

Unless you are collecting all the data yourself, you will need to conduct a training workshop for your interviewers, focus group moderators, observers, or other field staff. Most teams will benefit from at least 1 week of comprehensive training (see Appendix 5 for a sample training agenda) before they enter the field, but training and monitoring are a continuous process, even as data collection proceeds.

You may find that your study is the first time that otherwise experienced field staff have been exposed to qualitative principles and techniques. Survey interviewers are available in most countries, but we have often noticed that those with more experience with structured protocols have the most difficulty being effective as in-depth interviewers and focus group moderators. When interviewers have been trained to phrase questions exactly as written and assign answers to preconceived response categories, as in a multiple-choice format, they do not easily adapt and modify questions, probe answers with new questions, and control, but not dominate, a guided conversation or focused discussion. A tendency of experienced survey interviewers is to use a topic guide as if it were a questionnaire, asking questions verbatim, shifting topics too quickly, and forgetting to follow leads to deeper and richer sources of information. Similarly, field staff who have been reared and educated in relatively authoritarian families and societies may need considerable guidance in nondirective, nonjudgmental interviewing styles. This task is made all the more difficult by the same cultural constraints on participants who may have trouble being conversational in an interview. The interview may seem like a formal interaction or even a duty. An excellent resource for training field staff is *Qualitative Research Methods: A Data Collector's Field Guide* (Mack, Woodsong, MacQueen, Guest, & Namey, 2005, pp. 37–45). In Module 3, the authors present useful tips for effective interviewing, such as becoming familiar with the research documents, practicing interviewing, and practicing using the equipment. Specific interviewing skills highlighted include the following:

- Rapport building
- Emphasizing the participant's perspective
- Adapting to different personalities and emotional states
- Asking one question at a time; asking open-ended questions
- Avoiding leading questions
- Verifying unclear responses
- Asking follow-up questions and probing

In addition to orientation to the research objectives and materials, training must include instruction in the elements of conversational style and nondirective interviewing, with ample demonstration and practice. A goal for successful data collection will be sufficient familiarity with the research questions so that the interviewer can engage a participant in creative dialogue without having to read aloud from the guide and without losing sight of the central research problem. Experienced qualitative data collectors can also benefit from a refresher course on the use of qualitative techniques, including formulating questions, following leads, effective probing, noting silences, and identifying field problems. Trainees will catch on to the conversational style more quickly if they can keep the main research topics in their heads; you may even consider listing these topics at the top of each interview guide as a quick reference for interviewers.

The Training Plan

The following are research ethics training curricula that may be used for training study teams:

- *FHI 360 Research Ethics Curriculum, 2nd Edition*
- *CDC Scientific Ethics Training*
- *CITI Responsible Conduct of Research Training*

We have found that the best training approach is practical and experiential, with liberal use of role-playing and simulated data collection. A typical training program might take a week or longer if the field schedule allows, depending on the complexity of the research problem and the trainees' skill levels (see Appendix 5). It usually begins with a thorough orientation to the research problem and purpose (consider 1 to 2 days for this), followed by careful review of the protocol, study procedures, and interview guide(s) (consider 3 or more days for this). The training agenda should include ample time for practicing interviewing skills and for **pilot testing** the data collection tools (see discussion of pilot testing later in the chapter). When interviewers have a good understanding of the topics covered in the interview guides and plenty of practice with interviewing skills, they will be better prepared to ask appropriate follow-up questions or probes, ask for relevant clarifications, and understand and interpret nuanced responses. It is also important to plan time to review the basic concepts of research ethics. Typically, training participants would be asked to complete required training on the ethics of research with human subjects prior to attending the training, but a review of the basic concepts is essential.

Also include in the training sessions a brief overview of data analysis, and in some settings, special training for staff who will help with the analysis. Understanding how the data will be analyzed reinforces for interviewers the importance of rapport in the interview partnership, as well as the importance of careful probing and flexible use of the interview or focus group guide. A simple explanation of coding and searching (see Chapter 6) will help interviewers understand that information will not be lost if it emerges out of the expected sequence of the interview.

In general, training topics are likely to include, but should not be limited to, the following:

- Study topic background and context
- Research ethics and informed consent
- Sampling, recruitment, eligibility assessment, compensation procedures

- Roles of the interviewer, moderator, and note taker
- Different moderator or interviewer styles
- The art of probing data
- Ways to encourage discussion participation
- Instruction in observing nonverbal cues
- Managing problems that arise in the interview or group
- Methods for closing the interview or discussion
- Mechanics of recording, translating, and transcribing the sessions
- **Data management** and security
- Training on data analysis, as necessary

Skills Practice

Devote several days in the training program to practice of interviewing and observation skills, beginning with role-playing and group feedback. As trainees become more proficient, consider bringing in outsiders to play participant roles in mock interviews or discussions. Actor-participants could be prompted ahead of time to simulate problems that commonly arise in interviews or groups, such as the argumentative participant, the silent participant, or the focus group member who dominates the discussion. Feedback from the group will help trainees gain confidence in handling these and other, often unanticipated, situations. If the team includes interviewers with qualitative experience, these individuals can assist with training, helping the less experienced at the same time they are reviewing qualitative techniques themselves. You might pair new interviewers with more experienced ones in role-playing, switching roles as the less-experienced person becomes more comfortable with interview skills.

As you observe these practice sessions, take notes on the process to share with trainees. For example, note when an interviewer misses a cue to another question or fails to probe a provocative comment. Trainees can also listen for gaps in the interview and prompt each other. If possible, record and transcribe the practice interviews and distribute copies to the trainees to illustrate the interviews' strengths and weaknesses. Group critique of both novice and experienced interviewers' practice sessions is also helpful. Exercises like these can build confidence while underscoring the importance of attentive listening and flexibility in adapting the guide to the interview's conversational flow. The investigator may wish to observe skills practice directly and note the level of each trainee's proficiency. This assessment will help determine how best to use trainees in the field. Finally, consider inviting a few more candidates to the training than will be needed for actual data collection activities, with the understanding that a few participants may decide that they do not want to join the study team, or you may determine that a few participants do not have the skills necessary to conduct the research.

Sensitive Topics

When writing the protocol, the investigator must consider sensitivities related to the subject matter and participants of their proposed research and the environment in which they are conducting it. Institutional Review Board (IRB) reviewers will assess the risks and ethical issues of the research before any field implementation can occur, but, ultimately, the researcher is responsible for ensuring that participants are treated humanely and are kept safe while the research is in progress. Therefore, it is crucial that the investigator and the study team members understand any sensitive issues around vulnerable populations such as minors; lesbian, gay, bisexual, transgender, and intersex persons; participants at risk of physical or sexual abuse; or participants engaging in illegal activities such as drug use or sex work. The investigator and team members are strongly encouraged to seek guidance and resources from experts who work with sensitive issues prior to beginning any fieldwork that is potentially sensitive. For example, the World Health Organization (2007) offers extensive guidance on best practices for conducting ethical and safe research with women and children who have experienced violence and abuse. The investigator and study team must also be aware of the local environment and laws; for example, in some countries, homosexuality, prostitution, abortion, and drug use may be illegal, and exposure of participants' engagement with such activities may put them at significant risk. Furthermore, it may be mandated that abuse of minors or other abuse cases be reported to authorities. These types of laws should be taken very seriously, and participants should be informed beforehand if you are required to report certain things to the authorities. Consider whether it is necessary to include questions in your interview guides that may elicit responses from participants that might reveal illegal activities or instances of abuse, abortion, drug use, and so forth.

In a study that took place in Bangladesh and Papua New Guinea, researchers wanted to learn more about the extent and nature of gender-based violence experienced by men who have sex with men, male sex workers, and transgender communities. Due to the criminalization of homosexuality, as well as social and political discrimination against these sexual minorities, the research team had to be very discrete in their recruitment processes.

When topics are sensitive, in-depth interviews can offer greater privacy and may therefore be preferable to focus group discussions. In this case, the research team collaborated closely with local community-based organizations and NGOs in order to recruit groups of participants who were already familiar with each other. Ultimately, the team determined that these pre-established relationships between participants allowed them to hold focus group discussions more safely and securely (see Case Study 7).

In consideration of such sensitive issues, a critical component of interviewer training is recognizing and responding to clues that a participant may be at significant risk. In qualitative research, the interviewer as a conversational partner cannot be impersonal and uninvolved. Confronted with disclosure of domestic violence, child abuse, or any threat to participants' well-being, interviewers who collect sensitive data must learn how to give a caring and helpful response without jeopardizing the quality of the interview. They should also be prepared to offer referrals for participants in need of counseling or other assistance. (See Chapter 4 for the interviewer's responsibility when a participant asks for help.)

Selection of the research team should ensure that data collectors or other field personnel will not bring personal biases to the research activities. It is critical to train the team and assess team members' abilities to handle sensitive topics in a neutral manner such that the participants are not subjected to judgment from your own team.

Field Materials

Provide members of your field teams, both professional and local, with written instructions, flow charts, checklists, diagrams, or summaries of the steps in the data collection phase. Such written communication might include the following:

- An overview of the project, with the main research goals highlighted
- A summary of ethical standards for the study
- Detailed task descriptions for the local field team and for each professional role (e.g., focus group moderator, notetaker, in-depth interviewer, field supervisor, or translator)
- A checklist of items needed for each data collection event
- A flow chart of the steps involved in sampling, recruitment, eligibility assessment, data collection, and data processing

- A calendar with daily activities such as team meetings, training, pretests, and scheduled interviews or focus group discussions
- An activities schedule, including a time frame for collecting data and completing transcriptions or translations if done in the field
- A sample introduction to the project
- Names and phone numbers of researchers who can answer questions and provide additional information about the project

You might also give copies of some of these materials to interested local leaders, especially if they are supervisors of individuals on your field team and have granted them time off for participation in the study.

Incorporating all of these documents into a master study manual (hard copy and/or electronic), which is kept with the data or study manager for reference, is very useful. Data collectors can always refer to the manual for further information or make additional copies of documents that they may want to have with them in the field.

Pilot Testing

The pilot test is a dress rehearsal for all members of the field team in a mock venue with characteristics of the actual research setting. As in all social research, it is important to ensure that a research team has tested interview and focus group guides or topic lists, observation guides, photographs and stories, or other tools of data collection in a group of trial participants similar to the participants in the actual study. If the study design includes subsamples of the population, each should be represented in the pilot test. Held at the end of interviewer training, a comprehensive pilot test gives data collectors additional hands-on experience and even more familiarity with the project. Interviewers who participate in this phase often add valuable suggestions for strengthening data collection materials and processes.

Pilot testing informed consent materials is as important as finding out whether participants will understand the interview questions. The pilot should therefore include an introduction to the project and an explanation of informed consent, worded as data collectors will present it to study participants. Is the language clear? Do participants understand the purpose of the research and the part they are expected to play? Are both women and men sufficiently assured of confidentiality to participate without reservation? If not, revise the statement until the researcher is confident that no one is taking part in the study without adequate knowledge of its purpose, expectations, and possible risk.

Ideally, pilot interviews or focus group discussions should be recorded and transcribed exactly as they will be in the study. If possible, allow time to analyze the data using whatever computer software or other approach you have chosen. Analysis of test data will point to any need for further revisions of the topic guides, instruments, or data collection process. It also enables the researchers to assess interviewing skills and retrain interviewers.

As part of the pilot test, researchers should also conduct a trial run of administrative procedures for managing data and protecting the confidentiality of interview or focus group discussion recordings or other raw data in the field.

On the basis of these trial results, rethink your data collection techniques. Are you tapping the issues most relevant to the research problem? Are trial participants understanding and responding openly to these issues? Are interviewers tactfully probing responses and giving participants opportunities to think creatively about the questions? Review of pilot data can be an excellent team-building exercise, involving all members of the professional team in reviewing and revising the data collection process.

Field Logistics

Before starting to collect data, there are other logistical issues to consider. Many will have been resolved at the research design stage. Often, however, questions emerge that are specific to the field setting and that may require some rethinking of the logistical plan. When such questions arise, the lead researcher can benefit greatly from the insight and experience that local team members bring to the study. Issues for review might include the following:

- Feasibility of sampling, recruitment, eligibility assessment, compensation, and data collection procedures
  - As planned in the protocol, will these procedures be feasible in the real-world setting, and specifically in the local context? How will privacy and confidentiality be maintained through these procedures?
  - Are recruitment procedures appropriate for sensitive populations? Will recruitment procedures allow recruitment of desired target populations and research naïve populations?

- Technology-related issues
  - What type of technology will be used for data collection? Will the technology be acceptable to study participants (is it discrete or obtrusive)? Are there power, service, and access issues to consider for the technology (do you need back-up batteries or power sources)? How will data be

downloaded from the device and how often? Data not backed up or downloaded might be lost or shared outside the team. Have you tested the equipment prior to any data collection event? Do you have a back-up device? If the technology is of value, is there a risk of it being stolen? For more on technology in qualitative methods, see Box 5.2.

BOX 5.2 TECHNOLOGY AND QUALITATIVE RESEARCH

With telephones, mobile phones, tablets, and the Internet in this digital age, we are surrounded by technologies that can greatly enhance our field research and data collection activities. However, technology should not be incorporated into research without awareness of ethical and logistical issues that could critically impact your research.

The portability and convenience of mobile phones and tablets make them great tools for digital audio and video recording, photography, and typed or verbal field notes. Telephones and computers, whether stationary or mobile, can be used for in-depth interviews and focus group discussions. The Internet also allows for IDIs and FGDs to be held by video conference, thus retaining the richness of non-verbal cues that are an important component of face-to-face interviews. Technology provides us with both synchronous (real-time) and asynchronous (occurring at different times) options for communication with research participants. Real-time communications can be phone conversations, online chats, online video or audio conferencing. Email and discussion boards are examples of asynchronous communications.

While these technological options can make it cheaper, faster, and easier to incorporate hard-to-reach and hidden populations into your research, there are serious privacy and ethical concerns. Special consideration must be given to informed consent procedures when technology will be used for data collection, and lead investigators should request privacy and security statements from any Internet or social media platform they intend to use. Be prepared that the IRB may pay particular attention to ethical issues surrounding use of technology for recruitment purposes and may require a special "social media management plan" in the research protocol if you plan to use social media in any way. When selecting research participants, recognize that technology may not appeal to audiences who are not tech-savvy, and it may even increase resistance among those who are already distrustful of researchers. Finally, research teams should always have contingency plans to address potential issues with Internet accessibility, power and charging limitations, and the security of electronic equipment.

- Transportation and safety of data collectors
  - Will the location of data collection pose an expense or safety issue to data collectors? Will the data collection site be conducive to a good interview (consider noise, lighting, and privacy)?
- Scheduling
  - Is the proposed schedule feasible? Have holidays and other potential schedule delays been factored into the schedule?
  - Has sufficient time for data collection, transcription, translation, and other processing steps been allotted (see discussion of timelines later in the chapter)? These things often take much more time than we anticipate! Especially at the beginning of the study, consider budgeting extra time for processing and review of the initial transcripts, followed by feedback from the project leader on the quality of the data and any suggestions for improving the data and data collection procedures.

In general, these procedures and logistics will already have been discussed and planned as the protocol was developed, but once in the field, what was planned may not be realistic. If the pilot testing is carried out in a realistic setting equivalent to that of the actual data collection, it may become clear which parts of the plan are feasible and which may need modification. But the project leader and study team members should think carefully about these things in advance so as to avoid any major issues in the field that may, in the end, lead to added expense for the study, timeline delays, or misunderstandings that could jeopardize the project.

Supervision and Monitoring

Have a plan for monitoring data collection and providing continued support to the field team. The researcher or a field supervisor should review all recordings or transcripts as soon after the interview as possible to pick up potential weaknesses that could affect the quality of the data. If the principal investigator is not in the field with the data collection team or the data will ultimately be analyzed by team members who are not in the field, they should also be given the opportunity to review transcripts, especially early in the data collection process, in order to provide feedback to improve future interviews. If the researcher's or field supervisor's presence is not distracting to the participants, he or she should also sit in on some of the interviews, perhaps in the role of notetaker, in order to provide consultation later to the interviewer or moderator.

Even the most experienced qualitative data collectors benefit from field supervision. Because the qualitative interview is not bound by a structured questionnaire, the interviewer is responsible for guiding the conversation, responding creatively to clues to new information, and helping each respondent to express him- or herself openly. Unless you are doing your own interviewing, you will need to review recordings and, if feasible, observe interviews from time to time. If you are not fluent in the language of the interview, your field supervisor can be an invaluable aid in the monitoring process.

To ensure protection of study participants, review with the entire team, including local field assistants, the importance of respecting privacy and confidentiality. Pilot testing and discussion of the informed consent process are natural ways to remind data collectors of possible risks of participation. Moreover, interviewers and moderators who come from the same culture as participants may be able to heighten the researcher's awareness of sensitive areas in which participants might be especially vulnerable. Discuss with data collectors how they will resolve situations that arise in the field, for example, family members who insist on being present in the interview or individuals who seem not to respect the confidentiality of other participants in a focus group discussion. Although you cannot control what focus group participants tell others after they leave the site, most will welcome a basic rule for trusting and respecting each other's confidence, especially if they have helped to formulate the statement. Asking participants as well as staff to sign a confidentiality pledge will reinforce the message.

Researchers in the field must be always on the alert for ways to help data collectors improve or alter the process for more relevant information. Reviewing fieldwork as it happens helps you ensure quality and enables you to modify the process or address possible new questions or interesting ideas as they emerge. For most interviewers and moderators, probing beneath the surface is an especially difficult aspect of data collection. Valuable information can be lost if data collectors miss opportunities to probe significant comments. Chapter 4 summarizes some of the common errors that occur in moderating focus groups and how the moderator might have avoided them.

Generating Data Files

Take seriously the adage "Your research is only as good as your data." Because how you document your data will be a clue to their trustworthiness, we advise great care in creating and managing data files (see previous section on assigning a data manager to ensure data quality). You can record an interaction with handwritten notes while or soon after it happens, but audio recordings may provide a more complete account. Others will be able to review the recordings and decide whether they would draw the same conclusions from them.

Using a computer to store and manage text facilitates the process of revising and updating your coding system as you review the data. We also recommend that you and your team agree upon procedures for establishing an audit trail to document any revisions that are made to data, the codebook, or any other study documents that may be altered in any way. Even with a small number of transcripts, it will be impossible to remember if, how, and why a transcript or code was revised once you are deep into the analysis or paper writing (see Chapter 6 for more details about audit trails). You should also consider mechanisms for protecting the integrity of electronic data once it is cleaned and finalized for analysis.

Yet despite the value of recorded data, you must also collect it in as unobtrusive a way as possible. We try to use a small table microphone that we place slightly out of the line of vision between interviewer and respondent. As soon as you introduce yourself and the study, explain the purpose of the microphone and ask permission to use it. We have found that participants usually forget the microphone quickly and may even be pleased that the researchers value what they have to say enough to record it. However, if at any point during the session a participant requests not to be recorded, you should turn off the recording device and resume recording only when the participant agrees (see previous section on Field Logistics). Good note-taking would obviously be an important alternative at this point.

Although recording devices are very useful, they should not be the only data record. The field notes that you generate from your observations or spontaneous conversations are also valuable data, complementing the records of interviews or focus group discussions that you transcribe from recordings. Notes entered in brackets in the transcript are a good way to flag interesting observations or draw attention to contradictory responses. Analogous to the numbers generated in quantitative research, data from all these sources may be handwritten, typed, or entered in a computer file. But be cautious: Observations that remain in the researcher's mind will not be part of the research.

Transcription and Translation

Transcribe recordings as soon as possible after the interview or discussion. If recordings are left to be reviewed only after fieldwork is over, you surely will miss subtle, nonverbal points as well as the opportunity to clarify ambiguities, investigate new leads, and follow up on emerging hypotheses. Transcription services are available to take the drudgery out of this often lengthy and tedious process, but only the researcher can add nonverbal data, such as a tone of voice or facial expression, that could affect how you interpret the text.

Interviewer input is especially important in transcribing group discussions. In our experience, it works best for the moderator and the notetaker to transcribe each recording together, putting the spoken messages together with coded speaker identifications and nonverbal clues that the note taker has recorded as the discussion develops. The notetaker's skill as observer and recorder of group process is obviously critical to the transcription's quality.

When scheduling your fieldwork, allow 2 to 3 hours of transcription for each hour of focus group discussion, or plan to conduct your interviews or discussions in the mornings and work on transcription in the afternoons. Immediate recall is essential for capturing subtle nuances, verbal and nonverbal, in qualitative responses.

Good transcription is time-consuming, and inexperienced researchers are sometimes tempted to cut corners by summarizing, rather than transcribing, the data. But language gives us important clues to meaning. How people say things is often as important as what they say. For insightful and powerful analysis, we advise taking the time to create verbatim transcriptions. A question often arises whether the transcription should faithfully replicate slang, jargon, obscenity, or incomplete or ungrammatical sentences exactly as spoken on the recording. For the purposes of most qualitative research, the transcript should be a faithful reproduction of the popular idiom, because that is how people express themselves. Even a pause in the conversation may be worth noting, because it may mean that the participant is tentative or unsure about what he or she is saying. And what about those grunts, sighs, and barely audible murmurs that punctuate most conversations? Researchers vary on this issue and must decide whether such utterances are extraneous or might be further clues to the meaning of the data. Consider using a predetermined transcription format that specifies how each transcriptionist should handle these components of the interviews. An excellent resource is the transcription protocol in McLellan, MacQueen, and Neidig's *Beyond the Qualitative Interview: Data Preparation and Transcription* (2003).

Notes and bracketed comments on the data collection process can be very useful. For example, the researcher might note in brackets that a particular question was loaded—phrased in such a way as to elicit a specific response. Methodological notes are red flags that alert the researcher later to points at which bias may be influencing the data and questions might have to be modified. Some qualitative data analysis software programs include the option of annotating or flagging text with such notes or comments.

Translation of vernacular expression is always challenging. Ideally, transcription and translation will be done at the same time, with input from the interviewer who collected the data for the transcript. Even if this degree of coordination is not feasible, the translator should work closely with the transcriber, trying to stay as close as possible to the original meaning. However, some words simply have no translation. Many idioms and metaphors are culturally specific, and concepts that fit one culture's conceptual framework may have no parallel in another. Describing symptoms and diseases is a case in point, because even when similar terms are used for an illness, they may have different meanings in different cultures. The best solution is to use the word or phrase that comes closest and to include the original word in parentheses. If you have more than one translator, it helps to develop a vocabulary list so that there is agreement on terms to be left in the local idiom and to ensure that all staff fully understand the meaning of each term. Inclusion of particularly expressive terms from the original language enriches the transcript and may lead to discovery of new themes or ways of constructing familiar concepts. If meaning is not easy to understand in a long, discursive response, the translator might then paraphrase it and enter it in the transcript in brackets with a note. Chapter 8 provides more detail on transcribing and translating data. Remember that all proper names and references to people, places, and/or organizations that may identify the interviewee should be deleted from all transcripts before they are shared with anyone outside of the study team.

Data Management and Storage

The researcher or field supervisor's job will be facilitated by a well-articulated plan for handling data as they are collected. Someone must be in charge of assigning identification codes to all individual records, including recordings, transcripts, demographic information sheets, and quantitative data if collected as part of the study (see Data Manager section earlier in the chapter). Store the documents in a secure location that can be accessed only by the researcher or field supervisor.

Preparation for efficient data management includes setting up a filing system with a place for each component of the study, for example:

- The original proposal
- Protocols developed for data collection
- Field notes
- Maps of the study community
- Topic guides

- Informed consent forms
- Sociodemographic data sheets
- Codebooks
- Instructions for data collectors and local field assistants
- Interview or focus group transcripts
- Other study materials

A good filing system will help ensure that important documents are not lost and that all materials will be at hand when you need them for analysis and writing results. An additional useful resource for data management practices is Module 5 of *Qualitative Research Methods: A Data Collector's Field Guide* (Mack et al., 2005).

Timelines and Budgets

Achieving an accurate estimation of time needed for data collection is never easy, but in qualitative research it is especially challenging. First, a qualitative interview or discussion is by definition flexible and open-ended. A session of 1 to 1.5 hours is a comfortable time frame for most participants; but as experienced interviewers know, much depends on how the guided conversation develops (remember to account for time for the informed consent process, too—pilot testing will help you estimate the time needed for this step). On the one hand, even with skillful encouragement, participants occasionally have little to contribute. More often, however, as trust builds, so will the momentum and intensity of the interview or discussion. Participants will become more animated, and you will begin to hear the experience you are seeking and possibly the emergence of new themes in your inquiry. The interviewer must also be alert to participant fatigue, including distractions or loss of interest, and conclude the interview while it is still a positive experience. A thorough pilot test will help you gauge how long to stay on any one topic and how to move ahead without rushing participants. But however carefully you plan, expect to find many variations in the ways that different individuals and groups will respond to the study.

Other issues to consider when estimating your time in the field are the supervisory needs of data collectors, the time required to transcribe recordings, and the importance of preliminary data analysis. The less experienced the interviewer is in qualitative techniques, the more time that person will need with a supervisor. Additional assistance may be needed to ensure accurate and ethically derived information.

Inexperienced qualitative researchers sometimes pack each day in the field with more interviews or focus groups than they or their interviewers can comfortably manage. If the team will be doing transcription or translation in the field, you may need to allow several hours for this task on the same day as the interview, depending on the interviews' length and the team's experience. A common time frame for a focus group study calls for one group discussion each morning: approximately 1.5 hours of discussion with time left for gathering and concluding activities. The afternoon is then devoted to transcription and translation, a process that typically takes 3 to 4 hours for each recorded session. On the other hand, if participants are employed outside the home or otherwise occupied during the day, it may be more convenient for them to meet in the late afternoon or evening. In that case, use the daytime hours for transcription, translation, and review of data. Be flexible to adapt the schedule to the needs of the men and women in the study. Remember also to include in your estimate an interviewer fatigue factor. Qualitative interviewing is intense and tiring; too tight a schedule may exhaust interviewers or moderators, with a negative impact on team morale and the quality of the data.

Finally, as we will again emphasize in Chapter 6, the researcher should try to plan time in the schedule to listen to recordings or read transcripts while still in the field. Preliminary review and analysis are important elements that distinguish qualitative research from other, more structured, investigations.

As Box 5.3 illustrates, estimating costs is an essential part of the research plan. It may be helpful to start by consulting budgets from similar studies in comparable populations, if available. Identify the largest costs and then break them down to smaller components. For example, define the timeline, major activities, and team structure first, and then continue to smaller units. Box 5.3 offers guidance. (See Appendix 6 for an example of a budget shell for qualitative research.)

It is difficult to predict what everything will cost, and your budget may need alteration as the research proceeds. If feasible, include a contingency line to cover unexpected costs that might surface later. Ultimately, the keys to effective budget development and management are to ensure that the budget is reviewed on a regular basis and that shortfalls or underspending are assessed and adjustments are made. The study team should also be consulted regularly to identify emerging costs that may affect the budget. Remember that timeline, budget, and research activities are interrelated, so changes to any of them will have implications for the others.

BOX 5.3 ILLUSTRATIVE BUDGET CONSIDERATIONS

Timeline: How many months/years will the research take? Will there be extended stretches of time such as holidays, elections, other seasonal changes that will affect the timeline? Have you considered adding contingency time, if feasible?

Team Structure: Who will comprise your team? Will you need subcontractors, consultants, supervisors, data collectors, moderators, notetakers, transcriptionists, translators, analysts, data managers? How many? What will be each team member's level of effort, and will they receive benefits as part of their compensation? How will staff compensation change over time if the study has a multiyear timeline?

Activities: Will you have travel costs? Will you have costs associated with obtaining IRB approvals? What are the costs associated with training the team? Will there be community introduction meetings before research begins? Will you conduct participatory observation, focus group discussions, and/or in-depth interviews? Will you need to rent space for data collection activities, for a study office, or for secure data storage? Will you provide compensation and/or refreshments to research participants? What activities will be planned for dissemination (don't forget costs associated with publishing study results and attending conferences)? What equipment and supplies are needed for these activities (e.g., digital recorders and batteries, office supplies, laptops, data entry or analysis software, transcription machines)?

Summary

Many research methods texts offer readers copious instructions on what to do and relatively little advice on how to do it. Their argument might be that because no two field experiences are the same, each investigator must negotiate the terrain individually, tailoring implementation to available resources. This caveat is valid. However, with careful planning, review of lessons learned, and a strong foundational knowledge of the research topic and context, the prudent investigator can anticipate and avoid many potential roadblocks. Applied diligently and appropriately, the following tools and guidance introduced in this chapter will help ensure successful implementation:

- Anticipate possible road blocks by developing a risk management plan with your team.

- Introduce the team to the community and stakeholders early and appropriately, and use local resources to navigate the context. Practice diplomacy and respect for cultural differences.
- Assemble and train a team of effective managers, assistants, interviewers, facilitators, note takers, and community liaisons who are detail oriented, who are sensitive and active listeners, and who will uphold an uncompromising code of ethics for the protection of participants and their families.
- Be meticulous about organizing field materials and practicing field procedures and data collection techniques before proceeding with research activities.
- Plan supervision and monitoring in advance of data collection. Have a back-up plan for retraining staff or adjusting field activities if it becomes necessary to do so.
- Maintain thorough and detailed data management and tracking practices. A good record system is critical for ensuring that essential study documents are maintained securely and that participant confidentiality is honored.
- Timelines and budgets must be planned realistically, reviewed regularly, and revised appropriately throughout the life of the study. Lessons learned and documentation from previous studies will contribute to a successful outcome.

A strength of qualitative research is that the researcher is continuously reviewing and evaluating the work in progress, clarifying questions, sharpening tools, and adapting techniques to new discoveries. We therefore urge researchers to be diligent about keeping ahead of the data collection, listening and observing, and reviewing notes and transcripts as they are generated. In sum, be constantly on the alert to correct possible weaknesses, ask new questions, and strengthen the research process as it unfolds.

Key Terms

1. **Risk management plan:** A document describing how risk management will be implemented. The plan includes the risk register a list of possible risks to the activities, including their probability, impact, mitigation, and the responsible party for addressing each risk (Project Management Institute, 2013).
2. **Rapport building:** Creating dynamics between the interviewer and participant that are positive, relaxed, and mutually respectful (Mack et al., 2005).

3. **Stakeholders:** A person or group at the local, national, or international level who can affect or be affected by the research (MacQueen et al., 2012).
4. **Stakeholder register:** A document identifying all study stakeholders and essential details for each stakeholder, such as contact information, type of stakeholder, role in community, interests, expectations, and potential influence (Project Management Institute, 2013).
5. **Pilot testing:** The process of conducting practice interviews or focus groups for the purpose of refining qualitative data collection skills as well as ensuring that the interview questions are appropriate and feasible for the intended audience and setting.
6. **Data management:** Specific steps and procedures for tracking, storing, and processing data throughout the life of the study to preserve and secure the data.
7. **Audit trail:** A set of documents that enables the researcher and others to track the research process from design through data collection and conclusions. It may include the research protocol, data collection tracking logs, field notes, and other materials.

Review Questions

1. Describe the importance of building rapport and identify three different types of constituents who are critical to the rapport-building process in the local context.
2. List at least five important interviewing techniques or skills that are essential for effective interviewing.
3. Identify several potentially sensitive issues that may arise during your research activities. What are some critical considerations for handling such sensitive issues?
4. What are some key strategies for planning effective and efficient field logistics, timeline, and budget?

Recommended Readings

Ellsberg, M., & Heise, L. (2005). *Researching violence against women: A practical guide for researchers and activists.* Washington, DC: World Health Organization, PATH.

Guest, G., & MacQueen, K. M. (2007). *Handbook for team-based qualitative research.* Lanham, MD: AltaMira.

References

Castle, S., Konaté, M. P., Ulin, P. R., & Martin, S. (1999). A qualitative study of clandestine contraceptive use in urban Mali. *Studies in Family Planning, 30*(3), 231–248. doi:10.1111/j.1728-4465.1999.00231.x

Centers for Disease Control and Prevention. (2010). CDC UP templates. Available at http://www2a.cdc.gov/cdcup/library/templates/default.htm#.VZ11RaPD_cs

Centers for Disease Control and Prevention. (2015). *Scientific ethics training*. Atlanta, GA: Office of the Associate Director for Science. Available at http://www.cdc.gov/od/science/integrity/hrpo/training.htm

CITI Program. (n.d.). *Responsible conduct of research*. Available at https://www.citiprogram.org/index.cfm?pageID=265

Fetterman, D. M. (1991). A walk through the wilderness: Learning to find your way. In W. B. Shaffir & R. A. Stebbins (Eds.), *Experiencing fieldwork: An inside view of qualitative research* (pp. 87–96). Newbury Park, CA: Sage. doi:10.1111/j.1728-4465.1999.00231.x

FHI 360. (n.d.). *About LinCS 2 Durham*. LinCS 2 Durham HIV Prevention Project. Available at http://lincs2durham.fhi360.org/about_lincs2durham.html

Mack, N., Woodsong, C., MacQueen, K. M., Guest, G., & Namey, E. (2005). *Qualitative research methods: A data collector's field guide*. Research Triangle Park, NC: Family Health International. Available at http://www.fhi360.org/resource/qualitative-research-methods-data-collectors-field-guide

MacQueen, K. M., Harlan, S. V., Slevin, K. W., Hannah, S., Bass, E., & Moffett, J. (2012). *The stakeholder engagement toolkit for HIV prevention trials*. Durham, NC: FHI 360. Available at http://www.fhi360.org/resource/stakeholder-engagement-toolkit-hiv-prevention-trials

McLellan, E., MacQueen, K. M., & Neidig, J. L. (2003). Beyond the qualitative interview: Data preparation and transcription. *Field Methods, 15*(1), 63–84. doi:10.1177/1525822X02239573

Project Management Institute. (2013). *A guide to the project management body of knowledge (PMBOK guide)*. Newtown Square, PA.

Rivera, R., & Borasky, D. (2009). *Research ethics training curriculum* (2nd ed.). Research Triangle Park, NC: Family Health International.

Rubin, H. J., & Rubin, I. S. (1995). *Qualitative interviewing: The art of hearing data*. Thousand Oaks, CA: Sage.

World Health Organization. (2007). *Ethical and safety recommendations for researching, documenting and monitoring sexual violence in emergencies*. Geneva, Switzerland.

CHAPTER 6

QUALITATIVE DATA ANALYSIS

OBJECTIVES:

- To show how qualitative analysis is guided by the research purpose, conceptual framework, and topic guides
- To describe five interrelated steps in qualitative analysis—reading, coding, displaying, reducing, and interpreting—and provide examples of data analysis products related to each stage
- To identify approaches to qualitative analysis that ensure rigor and increase credibility
- To describe how qualitative analysis may complement quantitative analysis

IN ALL SOCIAL RESEARCH, whether qualitative or quantitative, the investigator systematically examines data to discover patterns and in some cases to identify cause-and-effect relationships. The process must be well documented so that others can follow it, understand the decisions that have been made along the way, and independently verify the results. This is the heart of data analysis.

In important ways, qualitative and quantitative data analyses diverge. Quantitative analysis is basically *deductive*, that is, researchers have carefully structured their questions, identifying key explanatory variables and expected outcomes in advance. They either identify and control for contextual variables or consider them outside the study's scope. Data collection and analysis remain distinctly separate phases of quantitative research. Data are most commonly expressed in numbers. Analysis emphasizes prediction and testing of relationships between variables, using statistical methods.

The core requisites for qualitative analysis [are] a little creativity, systematic doggedness, some good conceptual sensibilities, and cognitive flexibility.

(Huberman & Miles, 1994, p. 17)

In contrast, qualitative studies are *inductive,* designed to explore and account for broader psychological, social, political, or economic circumstances in which research questions are framed. As earlier chapters have emphasized, qualitative researchers typically begin with more general, open-ended questions, moving toward greater precision as detailed information emerges. Though previous research and theory may suggest certain constructs in a conceptual framework, for example, the need to consider how health policies influence health outcomes, their definitions and relationships may at first be only tentative. As data are collected, the meanings of these ideas or concepts begin to take shape, making preliminary analysis a necessary part of data collection.

Qualitative analysis identifies ideas and findings as they emerge from the textual data. New findings merge into themes, which may become new hypotheses or new research questions as the analysis continues. Thus, an emergent process begins in the field and often continues to completion of the study. This chapter shows the reader how to process and interpret raw data—perhaps several hundred pages of transcripts, field notes, or other media—to locate themes that address research questions and raise new questions or theoretical issues.

As described in Chapter 1, qualitative research is iterative rather than linear; the researcher queries or reflects on the data as it is being collected. Preliminary analyses may give rise to additional questions, identification of new participants, or changes in data collection approaches. In other words, the qualitative researcher is engaged in analysis from the moment he or she begins collecting data through to the point that study findings are written up or disseminated to intended audiences.

Throughout this iterative process, it is important to keep the research purpose in mind. Mining qualitative data for its intrinsic meanings is enhanced by first revisiting the study objectives and theoretical or conceptual frameworks before proceeding to **coding**, **data display**, **data reduction**, and other steps that comprise qualitative analysis.

Consider, for example, formative research that was conducted in Vietnam to inform a media campaign aimed at improving infant and young child feeding (IYCF) (see Case Study 13). The research objectives were to identify: (1) current IYCF practices; (2) barriers and facilitators to optimal practices, such as exclusive breastfeeding through 6 months; and (3) strategies to improve feeding practices. With these objectives clearly in mind, the researchers began to read and code the data. They noted a number of barriers to breastfeeding. Returning to the study objectives, they focused the analysis on these factors and were able eventually to prioritize strategies for the media campaign. Internal barriers such as mothers' concerns about sufficient breast milk led to their recommendation for more effective counseling. External barriers, such as lack of prenatal and perinatal counseling, clearly pointed to certain policy changes.

Basic Steps in Qualitative Data Analysis

Qualitative analysis emphasizes how data fit together as a whole, bringing together context and meaning. There are many analytic approaches, and one way is simply to group data by each research question or theme within the topic guide and then look for similarities and differences. This approach may be particularly appropriate when time and resources are limited or when the research is a smaller component of a larger quantitative study and is conducted to provide further depth in predefined areas of interest.

In this book, we have chosen to describe a more in-depth, inductive analysis. We have organized analysis in five interrelated steps. Step 1 includes careful reading of the raw data, noting quality and identifying patterns. Step 2 moves on to coding, with details on what to code, how to create a codebook, and how to apply codes to the data. We also discuss coding as a team with implications for consistency and reliability. In Step 3, we offer advice on how to examine the data for finer distinctions within and among the themes, using data display memos and notes to track discoveries and begin to develop hypotheses. Step 4 we call "getting the big picture." It discusses how to reduce a large data-set to a manageable size, using matrices and other summary devices to arrive at central themes. Step 5 covers interpretation of the data, how to find essential meanings, ensure trustworthiness, and interpret data from mixed-method studies. The diagram in Box 6.1 shows the five steps and their relationships.

To illustrate the classic qualitative analysis procedure, we use a mixed-method study that was conducted among young women in India and Tanzania, also presented in Case Study 5 (Tolley, Kaaya, and others, 2014). The goal of the study was to assess the feasibility of recruiting adolescent women younger than age 18 into HIV prevention clinical trials. The qualitative component explored sexual and reproductive health (SRH) risk among adolescent and young adult women in two countries in different sociocultural and epidemiologic contexts. We take the reader step by step through our analysis to illustrate how to turn raw data into credible, publishable results.

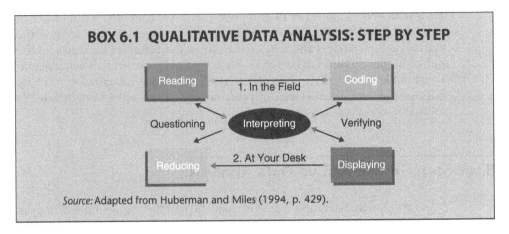

BOX 6.1 QUALITATIVE DATA ANALYSIS: STEP BY STEP

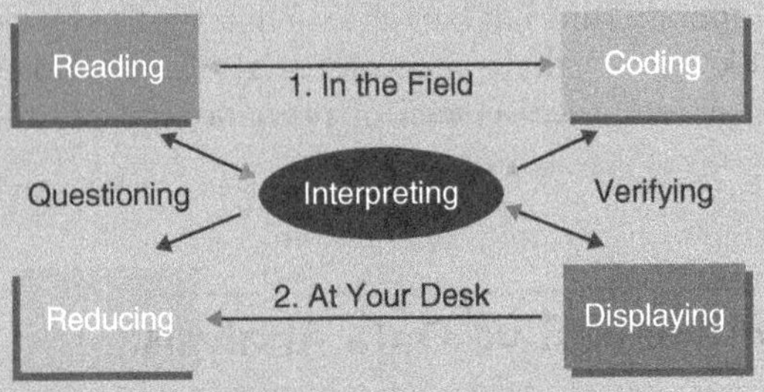

Source: Adapted from Huberman and Miles (1994, p. 429).

Step 1. Reading: Developing an Intimate Relationship with the Data

Most qualitative researchers would agree that qualitative analysis begins with data immersion. This means reading and rereading each set of notes or transcripts until you are intimately familiar with the content, noting content and quality and identifying patterns. As we have emphasized, the researcher does not wait for all the data to be collected, but starts a gradual immersion in a progressive review even as data are collected. The process is analogous to wading into a lake instead of diving in head first.

Reading for Content

What do you look for as you read? First, content. Are you obtaining the kinds of information that you intended to collect? Are responses full and detailed, or superficial? Perhaps the questions are not adequately framed or sequenced. Maybe the interviewers are not following up important leads with appropriate probes (see Chapter 4 for discussion of common errors in moderation of focus group discussions). Other aspects of the interview process may be inhibiting data collection, such as setting, composition of groups, or interviewer style or characteristics. As indicated in Chapter 5, it is helpful to note on transcripts where discussion might have been more thoroughly explored. Further questions can then be incorporated into future interviews.

In the study to examine adolescent barriers to participation in HIV prevention clinical trials, we wanted to understand the circumstances in which young women use health care services. The text shown in Box 6.2 is a verbatim excerpt from an interview with a young married woman who worked both as a peer educator and a clandestine sex worker in India. Interviewer questions are shown in italics, and sex worker's responses are in standard text. This segment suggests that nongovernmental organizations and peer educators may play an important role in young women's access to health care services. However, as noted in bold by one of the analysts, the interviewer could have explored this clue further before moving on to other topics. It is important to discuss these issues with data collectors or, if you are the one gathering the data, make note of them before moving on.

BOX 6.2 NOTING CONTENT IN TRANSCRIPTS: AN EXCERPT FROM AN INTERVIEW WITH A PEER EDUCATOR AND SEX WORKER

Q. What is a peer educator's work?

A peer educator's work means giving information to girls, taking their blood samples for HIV testing. Sirs [program officials] come and arrange meetings. We have to call these girls for meetings. We give them information about the meeting date and timing. We have to visit the lodges [where sex work happens]. We have to give information to the girls [sex workers] who work there. They tell us about their problems. We try to help them as much as possible.

[Analyst note: **This clue can be explored more. Probe on what kinds of problems the girls discuss, and in what ways you help them.**]

Q. How many girls are here?

There are many girls. We have different divisions. This friend and me, we work for [name of area]. Others are working in different areas.

Q. So is this your daily routine?

Yes, every day. If some of them [sex workers] are unwell, then we take them to the hospital in that area. We give them medicine. These girls do not go [into the city]. That is why we take them here.

[Analyst note: **Ask why these girls do not normally go to the hospital. What kinds of services are these girls provided? How are they treated by staff? Understanding barriers to health services will help us understand possible barriers to participation in HIV clinical research.**]

Excerpt from the transcript of an interview with a 21-year-old peer educator and clandestine sex worker in India.

While reading through the data, it is not too soon to begin identifying emergent themes and developing tentative explanations. Look for topics that the research may not have adequately addressed or that have emerged unexpectedly in the transcripts. You may find undeveloped or surprising new ideas to explore as fieldwork continues. As recommended in Chapter 5, these ideas could be directly typed into your transcripts, taking care to put them in brackets or italics to distinguish them from original text and coding them accordingly. Or record your ideas in a field journal or type them in separate memos. Some qualitative software programs allow you to link memos to specific text and then to print them together; doing so makes it easier to separate interpretations from observations and other field data.

Noting Quality

How were data obtained? If you are reviewing a set of field observations, how soon after the field activity ended were notes recorded? How vivid and detailed is the description? If the data report reflects an informal interaction in the field, how spontaneously was the conversation initiated, and do the notes explain the interaction? Were interview questions asked in a neutral way, or did the researcher suggest that some responses would be more valuable than others?

These methodological issues affect credibility. Responses should seem plausible and there should be enough contextual detail to add understanding. By including bracketed or italicized notes where problems arise it will be easier to differentiate responses obtained through open-ended questions from those obtained from less reliable, leading questions. You will also begin to develop a system, or audit trail, by which others can review your analytical work. (See Chapter 5 for more on audit trails.) Ultimately, it is the researcher's skill that will determine the quality of study findings.

Identifying Patterns

Look for patterns in the textual data. Patterns may occur in all or some of the data, revealing possible relationships between themes, contradictory responses, or gaps in understanding. In the adolescent participation in HIV prevention trials study, we set out to determine whether young women's sexual and reproductive health risks and potential clinical trial behavior differed by age (adolescents versus young adult women), by country (India versus Tanzania), or by specific contexts (i.e., marital, educational, or sex worker status). From these data we began to identify some interesting emergent themes. For example, a number of participants described precarious home lives and loss of parents through divorce or death. Our questions: Was this a common theme? And did missing parents lead some girls and young women to early marriage or sex work? Returning to the data, we discovered that indeed this was the case. Careful scrutiny of initial findings will almost always lead the researcher to discover new leads, new questions, and perhaps implications for further research.

Step 2. Coding: Identifying the Emerging Themes

After reading and becoming familiar with the initial texts, it is time to start coding themes. Codes are like street signs inserted into the margins of hand-written notes or typed after segments of text to remind you where you are and what you see. In qualitative analysis, using words or parts of words to flag ideas in the transcript can make analysis of a large data file easier and more accurate. Key themes coded in this way can later be searched and retrieved in a separate file. Having all the pieces of the text that relate to a common theme together in one place also enables you to discover and explore new subthemes.

Researchers differ on how to derive codes, when to start and stop the coding of a text segment, and how broadly or finely to code their text. Nevertheless, there are some common pitfalls to avoid. One is starting out with a coding scheme that is too complex or with too many fine distinctions among concepts. A complicated scheme can be difficult to apply and a diversion when attention should be solely on the data themselves. Another common pitfall is failure to refine the coding scheme as new ideas and clues emerge. When more than one person is involved in coding, develop a process to negotiate or reconcile coding decisions. Be guided by what is most useful as you organize and make sense of the text, and remember to document coding decisions as you make them.

> Common pitfalls include: (1) coding too finely (too many distinctions) so that important unifying concepts are missed, and (2) forcing new findings into existing codes instead of adding codes that could extend analysis in new directions.

What Aspects of the Text Are Coded?

Qualitative researchers develop their coding schemes in a variety of ways. Some begin their analysis by developing a set of **structural codes** that align with the research objectives or specific questions from the data collection instruments. For example, in the breastfeeding study discussed earlier, some structural codes might include: exclusive breastfeeding, complementary foods, and prelacteals (foods given to newborns before breastfeeding has been established). When the sequence of questions guiding a set of interviews or observations is similar, codes may represent each question number or topic domain. In this case, the application of structural coding allows the researcher more quickly to organize and bundle information on each topic for further exploration.

Other researchers develop their coding scheme prospectively in response to newly discovered themes. In that case, the codes may be emergent, theoretical, pragmatic, or a combination. **Emergent codes** closely match the ideas or language found in the textual data. For example, in both India and Tanzania, the term *trust* emerged frequently during discussions about perceived risk of HIV.

Some researchers may use emergent codes to avoid imposing words or concepts that might prevent them from seeing their data in a new way. Others borrow terms from the social science literature—for example, HIV risk perception or self-efficacy—that represent more abstract concepts important to their fields. These have the advantage of being clear to a wider audience. Others apply codes more pragmatically, for example, to identify particularly well-articulated ideas (i.e., "good quotes") or to highlight participant responses that were the result of special leading questions. Whether borrowed from theory or emergent from the unfolding data, codes allow you to assemble under one concept many seemingly disparate pieces of text and search for connections among them.

Consider the text in Box 6.3, excerpted from an interview with a single, out-of-school young woman from Tanzania, aged 18. She currently lives with a girlfriend in an area of town where alcohol shops and brothels are common. The analyst's initial thoughts about potential codes appear in boxes to the right of the text and are linked to specific lines of text.

Several important themes emerge from the excerpt presented in Box 6.3. They help us understand the relationship between this young woman's family and work situation, her sexual and reproductive health risks, and potentially her attitudes toward HIV prevention clinical trial participation. They include the following:

- Her living circumstances
- Family conflict
- Economic dependency
- The role of the social networks
- HIV risk behaviors—or, "big bars and brothels"

BOX 6.3 TRANSCRIPT EXCERPT AND EMERGENT CODES

I: HOW DID YOU GET IN *UWANJA WA FISI*? (a neighbourhood in Dar es Salaam)

I was staying in Ilonga with my aunt, but (she) found bus fare for me to come and look for my aunt who stays (in Dar es Salaam). When I first came here and was staying with my aunt, **I didn't expect that I will (end up) doing this job**. One day after two weeks, she was inside with her children. I was outside the window but they didn't notice (me). They started talking about me - **'Why doesn't she go and stay with her mother? Her mother has enough wealth** - why is she here?' I was angry about that, I was planning to go home to live with my aunt… but I didn't have money for bus fare. That thing hurt me and it was lunch time, they prepared it and called me to eat, but I refused and told them that I was full.

One day my aunt's son threw out my bag and told me 'Go back to your mother.' I was confused because… I didn't know any place - only the market and butcher. A lady passed outside to see what was going on; she decided to take me to stay with her. She was working at Kariakoo in the Indian shop. She used to leave me home and go to work. I was not comfortable that I was depending on her for everything. In the neighbourhood, there are ladies who used to go to big bars looking for men to have sex with in order to get money. They (told me) 'Your friend is saying bad things about you, she is tired of you. Don't wait until she chases you away.' So I started going out at night with those ladies, **we went to big bars like, Kili Time bar, Kona barSinza, where we look for men…**

Work situation

About parents

Conflict

Big bars (and brothels)

Excerpt from Transcript of Tanzanian Single Out-of-School Youth.

Many of these same themes appeared in different ways in interview transcripts from other young women. Developing and systematically applying a set of codes to each transcript enabled us to examine how they relate to sexual risk for different categories participant.

Developing a Codebook

How do you code your text to help identify all these themes? How many codes should be used, and how should they be labelled?

There are no clear guidelines on how finely to code the data. It may depend as much on personal preference as it does on research aims or preference for emergent- versus theory-informed approaches. Nevertheless, we suggest several strategies to facilitate codebook development:

- Limit the first round of coding to a small number of fairly broad labels that correspond to the study's main research questions.
- Avoid using coding labels that suggest interpretation or premature judgments about the meaning of text.
- Draft a preliminary codebook that documents agreed-upon codes and explanation of how they should be applied.
- If possible, work as a team. Team-based coding can increase the "dependability" of the research findings. Team-based coding is discussed below in sections on team-based coding and intercoder reliability.

The team involved in the study on adolescent participation in HIV prevention trials identified 42 preliminary codes that captured the basic themes emerging from repeated in-depth interviews with young women in India and Tanzania. Structured codes were drawn largely from the study objectives and topic guides, enabling the team to group information around specific themes like living circumstances (e.g., household description, parents, other family members); risk behaviors (e.g., sexual debut, concurrency, pregnancy, abortion, HIV/STIs); or access to health care (e.g., health care setting, health care provider, HIV testing behavior, HIV treatment). Others were drawn from theory (e.g., risk perception, self-efficacy). Some codes were more emergent, drawing on words used by different participants—including *trust* and *secrecy*. Box 6.4 shows examples of initial codes developed for this study.

Applying Codes

Whether working alone or in a team, consistency is critical. Have a well-developed codebook that is easy to navigate and provides sufficient description of what to include or not to include in a given code. Consult the codebook often. It is common during initial stages of coding to identify additional themes you wish to capture with a new coding label. Before adding a new code, however, verify that it is not already in the codebook or cannot be included with minor adjustments to existing codes. Multiple coding options that require decisions among similar codes make the task more complicated.

Coding is also made easier with guidelines on how to apply the codes. For example, in verbatim transcripts that include both questions and responses, apply one code to both. Whenever possible, apply a code to the whole paragraph. (Note: When a small text segment is embedded in a larger paragraph, a single code for the whole paragraph may obscure the meaning.) Guidelines help ensure that there will be sufficient context within which to interpret the text segments later. A coding guide also contributes to consistency in team-based coding.

Sometimes, multiple codes are applied to the same piece of text. It may be helpful first to apply the code or codes that are most central to the text and then to examine the text for other codes as well. It is better to over-code than not to apply relevant codes to text segments.

Team-Based Coding and Intercoder Reliability

Coding in a team can speed up the process. However, before launching into team-based coding, it is important that everyone have the same understanding about how to apply codes. Of course, coders may disagree on coding decisions or may apply the same code to text segments of different lengths (as shown in Box 6.5), but such differences usually can be negotiated and resolved early in team meetings.

"Lumpers," like coder 1 in Box 6.5, tend to apply their codes to larger text segments in order to keep more context. Whereas coder 1 applied the code "conflict" to the full two paragraphs, coder 2 was much narrower in how he applied the code; as a "splitter," he coded just the specific sentences that appeared to convey the idea of conflict. There are trade-offs in each approach. Applying codes too broadly means more text to reread and reduce in the next stage of data analysis. On the other hand, if you code too narrowly, it may be difficult to figure out how coded text from one transcript relates to coded text in others. Other points of disagreement might arise when applying a code to a text segment that does not express that code well or neglecting to apply a code to a relevant text segment.

BOX 6.4 PRELIMINARY CODEBOOK

Interview Context: Description of physical venue or social interactions that might influence the content of the interview.

Household Description: Description of house construction, number of rooms, size, cleanliness or content. Include composition—who lives in house, who shares a room?

Parents: Characteristics and/or interactions with parents or guardians.

Friends: Description of nonsexual friendships that may influence participant's attitudes and behaviors. Also code those who act as the opposite—adversaries.

Sexual Partner: Any partner, current or past, with whom the participant had sexual relations.

Conflict: Any description of verbal, physical, or sexual abuse; tension; and disagreements. Also code lack of conflict (e.g., when a participant says her partner never forces her to have sex, or never hits her).

Trust: Perceptions about whether a partner is faithful; signs of faithfulness or lack of it. Faithfulness of self or others. General thoughts on faithfulness and fidelity.

Risk Perception: Personal perception of risk for pregnancy or HIV, or more general attitudes and experiences that affect risk perception.

Meeting Places: Places where adolescents meet friends, sexual partners, or others.

Health Care Setting: Any description of health care services/settings, whether HIV-related or contraceptive or general health. Includes any general discussion about services provided, location, hours, access, and so forth.

HIV Testing Behavior: Own, partners', or general discussion on testing behavior or their lack of testing. Includes perceptions and attitudes toward testing behavior as well as description of getting tested.

BOX 6.5 APPLICATION OF THE CODE "CONFLICT" BY TWO CODERS

CODER

1 2

I: HOW DID YOU GET IN *UWANJA WA FISI*? (a neighbourhood in Dar es Salaam)
I was staying in Ilonga with my aunt, but (she) found bus fare for me to come and look for my aunt who stays (in Dar es Salaam). When I first came here and was staying with my aunt, I didn't expect that I will (end up) doing this job. **One day after two weeks, she was inside with her children. I was outside the window but they didn't notice (me). They started talking about me - 'Why doesn't she go and stay with her mother? Her mother has enough wealth - why is she here?' I was angry about that, I was planning to go home to live with my aunt... but I didn't have money for bus fare. That thing hurt me and it was lunch time, they prepared it and called me to eat, but I refused and told them that I was full.**
One day my aunt's son threw out my bag and told me 'Go back to your mother.' I was confused because... I didn't know any place - only the market and butcher. A lady passed outside to see what was going on; she decided to take me to stay with her. She was working at Kariakoo in the Indian shop. She used to leave me home and go to work. I was not comfortable that I was depending on her for everything. In the neighbourhood, there are ladies who used to go to big bars **They (told me) 'Your friend is saying bad things about you, she is tired of you. Don't wait until she chases you away.'** So I started going out at night with those ladies, we went to big bars like, Kili Time bar, Kona barSinza, where we look for men... looking for men to have sex with in order to get money.

How can you ensure that a team of different coders is applying codes in a consistent manner? Once the preliminary codebook is developed (as shown in Box 6.4), the following steps can be followed:

- Using a fresh transcript, ask each team member to code it independently, using the common codebook.

- Team members can highlight their coding in the margins (as shown previously), or with a software program, if one is being used.
- As a team, examine each paragraph and compare how individual coders applied the codes. (A team member may choose to fill out a **matrix** to compare how individuals applied their codes to the selected transcript, as shown in Box 6.6.)
- Notice which codes are being applied by all team members in a similar way. This means that the team has a common understanding of how to apply these codes.
- Also notice when team members use different codes for the same text segment. This may indicate that team members are unclear about the kinds of information that fit within a code, or that some members are forgetting to use some codes.
- Discuss and clarify how to apply codes that were used inconsistently.
- If needed, revise codebook definitions or document examples of when to use, or when not to use, codes that were applied inconsistently.
- Thorough coder training will better ensure consistency across numerous transcripts and a more efficient and accurate analysis in the long run.

There are several approaches to assessing **intercoder reliability** (ICR). Some researchers calculate a kappa statistic to assess the number of observed agreements as a proportion of total agreements possible or as a proportion of observed agreements plus observed disagreements (Hruschka et al., 2004). Some software packages will calculate such statistics for you. But there are limitations to quantifying ICR. First, such statistics generally are run for each code separately and examine agreements only between two coders at a time. Furthermore, codebook complexity—for example, having many codes or codes with multiple levels, or intercoder variations in how codes are applied—may skew the scores toward lower reliability.

It is possible to examine intercoder agreement more qualitatively by developing a matrix (as shown in Box 6.6) that summarizes whether an individual coder has applied a specific code to more text, less text, or the same text as others on the team, or whether the individual did not apply the code at all. In the example shown in Box 6.5, both coders have captured the essential text associated with "conflict." Spending time up front to ensure all team members are applying codes consistently will enhance the dependability of your findings. It may take several rounds of intercoder checks to achieve agreement in the group.

BOX 6.6 QUALITATIVE INTERCODER RELIABILITY MATRIX

Code	AKM	AM	DB	BT	Notes
Adolescent decision-making power		✓	+,–	+	DB: Broaden the amount of text that you code. Avoid coding phrases and short sentences, but select the entire response and question asked for better context.
Condom use: personal	–	✓	–	+	AKM: Missed a mention of condom use. DB: You coded a smaller portion of text re: condoms than the others and ended up cutting out an interesting paragraph on why they don't use condoms. This code is not just about use or nonuse, but also why they are used or not.
Conflict	✓	✓	+	+/–	BT didn't code lack of fear or forcing; others didn't code his constant visits and her refusal to come home.
Contraceptive use: personal	–	✓	✓	–	Whole team: If condom use is mentioned as a way to prevent pregnancy, code under "contraceptive use: personal" and "condom use: personal." Also, AKM and DB: Do not use this code when condom use is described as HIV prevention.
Faithfulness	–	–	–	+	AM, DB: Look at AKM's coding on faithfulness to see some sections of text that you missed coding. Also, no one coded text about not using condoms because of HIV testing or trust in partner.
Friends	0	0	+/–	+/–	Mention of nonsexual friendships should be coded here. That includes things like "My friends were drinking and I went out with them that night to the bars." Also, the start of a new sexual relationship as friends first.

(Continued)

BOX 6.6 QUALITATIVE INTERCODER RELIABILITY MATRIX (Continued)

Code	AKM	AM	DB	BT	Notes
Future dreams	0	0	0	+	Some of the text coded under fertility intentions for this participant should also be coded under "future dreams" because she obviously has hopes and desires of becoming a mother—wants children "faster faster."
Health care setting	+	✓	+	+	AM, HK, RE: This code includes info about clinic hours, days open, as well as the quality of services. See the coded text of DB and AKM for text examples that should be coded as health care setting.
HIV testing behavior	✓	✓	✓	0	All match. BT missed this.

✓ = All essential text coded
\+ = Coded some text segments that others did not code
– = Some text not coded that others coded
0 = Did not use a specific code

Advantages of Continuous Coding

Continuous coding as data collection proceeds has many advantages. First, it imposes a systematic approach, assisting the analyst in identifying gaps or questions while it is still possible to return to the field for more data. Continuously reviewing the coding structure in light of new texts may also reveal early biases and help you move beyond them, allowing you to redefine concepts without imposing unnecessary structure. As MacQueen notes in Box 6.7, some software packages make it easier to code texts and revise coding schemes as you go.

We suggest coding your first several texts using fairly broad, freestanding codes. However, as you continue to read and code texts, you may find that such broad headings give you little sense of the main ideas emerging from your data. You may want to refine further your coding scheme to include subcodes (e.g., the code, conflict, might include verbal, physical, or sexual) or to further divide a broad category into levels (low and high conflict).

To track changes in the coding scheme, keep a notebook or computer file in which each code is listed with its definition and an example of how it is used; record revisions and dates. Be sure that everyone is clear on who has authority to alter the master file with the most updated version of the coding scheme. (See Chapter 5 for more on training staff for data analysis.)

For practical reasons, researchers sometimes wait until all the data have been collected before starting to code. A transcription service may require submission of all transcripts at one time. However, coding cannot begin until you have text, whether handwritten or typed into a computer. Waiting too long to add notes could preclude later revising and refining the questions, thereby missing information related to the research topic. In this situation, good field notes and regular reviews of notes as a team are critically important.

TIP

Concentrate on one coding report at a time, selecting the most central themes to begin with and then working your way out to related themes as they appear important. If you work in this fashion, you will begin to see how certain themes connect.

Computer Software

It is possible to conduct qualitative analysis without a computer. For many decades, qualitative researchers have used handwritten notes or have transcribed verbatim interviews by hand. They have underlined text, written codes into page margins, or otherwise highlighted segments of print to distinguish ideas and messages. They have cut and pasted, sorted, and piled, organizing data around central themes. In fact, some researchers still worry that relying too much on computer shortcuts will distance them from the text.

However, modern computer software programs can ease the burden of cutting and pasting by hand while at the same time producing a vastly more powerful analysis by performing a number of basic data manipulation procedures. Such procedures include creation and insertion of codes into text files, indexing, construction of hyperlinks, and selective retrieval of text segments (Kelle, 1997).

Most software packages make the coding process quicker and more consistent. For example, instead of typing every code into computer-stored text files, some software applications keep a record of codes as you create them and allow you to select existing codes from drop-down menus. This feature protects against inadvertently altering the coding scheme and helps later to assemble related text segments for further analysis. It also makes it easier to automatically revise a particular coding label or set of codes across all previously coded text. For example, you might be able to merge two codes or move a code from a stand-alone position to a subordinate position as a subtheme of a larger code; one change in the master list changes all occurrences of the code.

Another function that most software packages offer is the means to search and retrieve text surrounding a specific word or combinations of words or move to the next occurrence of the word or phrase. For example, you may be able to:

- Find all words with a similar root: decide, decision (deci*)
- Specify a range of synonyms: money, salary, or shillings
- Join two concepts together: deci* or choice and health
- Restrict the search of one word or phrase to its proximity to another located within a specified number of words: e.g., the code, deci* (decision) located within five words of the code, health.

Hyperlinks enable you to cross-reference or link a piece of text in one file with another in the same or a different file. For example, you can write memos about a text segment or identify text from another source that relates to your original segment and then link them. If in separate interviews, for example, a husband and wife talk about how household decisions are made, you can link text segments from the two interviews for comparison. Hyperlinks also are used to link codes and their related text segments to one another.

A number of software programs permit hierarchical ordering of codes. That is, you can identify a general code, such as <decision making>, and link subcategories of codes, such as <joint, husband-controlled, wife-controlled>, under the main heading. Depending on the data, each of the three approaches to decision making might occur; no visible pattern exists. Or, you may find that women in the study tend to describe decision making as husband-controlled, whereas husbands were more likely to describe joint or wife-controlled patterns. Some packages allow text segments to be linked to each other without using codes, or they enable you to build nonhierarchical networks of codes or text segments (Kelle 1997). See Box 6.7 for more information on how to choose a software package. Also, for a complete discussion of selecting and using qualitative analysis software, see Chapter 9 in Guest, MacQueen, and Namey (2012).

BOX 6.7 WHAT TO LOOK FOR IN SOFTWARE FOR QUALITATIVE DATA ANALYSIS

Kathleen M. MacQueen, PhD

FHI 360

Software options available for qualitative data analysis (QDA) have been steadily increasing in recent years. This is both good news and bad news. Good, because it means it is getting easier to match the best tool to the task. Bad, because it means there are more opportunities to choose a tool that works poorly or not at all for the task at hand. How to make the best choice?

Concerns in choosing QDA software include the following:

- How complex are the data?
- How complex is the analysis?
- What resources—staff, time, and technology—are available?

As these questions suggest, QDA software decisions are an important part of the research design process. When researchers put aside those decisions until after collecting the data, they often find that they have collected more data than they can manage or analyze in a systematic way.

HOW COMPLEX ARE THE DATA?

Qualitative data present organization and management challenges that are different from those of quantitative data. Data such as field notes, recorded and transcribed interviews, video recordings, written responses to questions, and photographs can contain many layers of information that will need to be carefully peeled apart during analysis. The greater the amount of data, the greater will be the complexity of organizing and managing it.

Choose software that helps you organize the computer files containing your data. Particularly when working with large, complex qualitative data sets, you should look for software that lets you decide where to store your data files, rather than requiring you to place data files in a particular directory on your computer. For example, if you are conducting a two-stage multisite research project with three different data collection instruments per stage, you need to be able to organize

(Continued)

BOX 6.7 WHAT TO LOOK FOR IN SOFTWARE FOR QUALITATIVE DATA ANALYSIS (Continued)

the resulting data in folders or by using file tags or other file properties that reflect the underlying logic of the data collection design.

HOW COMPLEX IS THE ANALYSIS?

The more complex the analysis goal, the more important it is to choose software that is up to the task. Analytic goals can range from simple summaries of responses to complex theoretical modeling or hypothesis testing.

- At the simpler end, the goal of summarizing responses about individual topics may be fully met using a word processor to insert topical codes in the text, conduct word searches on those codes, and copy text excerpts to summary tables. Depending on the volume of text, this goal could also be achieved using paper, highlighters, scissors, and tape.
- A somewhat more complex goal would be a description of the way different topics are related to each other. For example, you might want to code issues from discussions on multiple topics. Software that produces reports on the co-occurrence of codes would be helpful. If the data are rich with layers of information, the software should also let you organize your codes into hierarchical trees and networks so that you can easily go from a broad overview to a detailed view of content. Look for software that will generate summary tables that show which codes occur together and how often, as well as text sorted by the codes assigned to it.
- If complex modeling or hypothesis testing is the goal, then you may need several software programs so that you can go beyond text analysis to decisional analysis, cluster analysis, and multidimensional scaling. A key issue here is the ability to import and export data. Of course, such complex approaches also require equally sophisticated research design and data collection strategies. Unless you already have at least some formal training in or experience with most of these methods, you probably should not choose this as your goal.
- Another issue is the amount of sociodemographic data that will be used as part of the qualitative analysis. For example, for a single analysis you may want to contrast responses for men and women, for different age groups, for different ethnic groups, and for different research locations. The more kinds of groupings you want in the analysis, the more important it will be to choose software

(Continued)

that lets you link this type of information to the qualitative data so that it will automatically sort the data in different ways.

WHAT STAFF, TIME, AND COMPUTER RESOURCES ARE AVAILABLE?

The number of staff who will be working on an analysis will affect your choice of software. As staff increases, so does the need for organization. This includes tracking who is doing what, ensuring that everyone is using the same standards, and merging the results of each team member's analysis task. If there is a lot of data or the analysis goal is fairly complex, you should choose software that helps with these tasks.

Many QDA packages require a significant amount of time to learn, and the packages may cost hundreds of dollars. Therefore, if you are familiar with a particular software package, continuing to use that package may be worthwhile if it meets most of the needs for a new project. But if you are attempting a project that is more complicated than your previous work, you should make a detailed outline of the data management and analysis steps that it will require. Then test them out using the software you intend to use to make certain it will work and determine the requirements in terms of time and effort. Also, you will want to make certain that you have enough memory to store the data and run the program without crashing (or straining your patience). If you plan to use cloud-based storage of data, check the compatibility of the QDA package and whether you can automate back-ups to the cloud, especially if you plan to have people working on multiple computers. For long-term projects you may want to reach out to the software developers to see what plans they have for future upgrades or plans to discontinue support for older versions you may be using.

SOFTWARE NEEDS BASED ON STUDY COMPLEXITY

Simple Qualitative Study

Such a study would have most of the following characteristics:

- A limited descriptive goal, for example, to summarize the range of responses on five or fewer major topics
- Limited data needed to achieve that goal, for example, less than 250 pages of text, no more than 20 in-depth interviews, or no more than 10 focus group discussions

(Continued)

BOX 6.7 WHAT TO LOOK FOR IN SOFTWARE FOR QUALITATIVE DATA ANALYSIS (Continued)

- Analysis to be done by one or two people
- Little or no sociodemographic data to be used during the analysis, for example, only sex and ethnicity differences to be noted

For example: In preparation for a larger community-based intervention trial to enhance access to prenatal care, a qualitative researcher conducts 12 in-depth interviews with women who gave birth at the local hospital without previously receiving care. The goal is to describe some of the experiences of women in this situation to enhance the training of the staff who will implement the intervention. The interviews elicit information on each woman's home environment, her access to transportation, the extent to which she relies on traditional healers, her perceptions of the value of prenatal care, and her experience with the hospital during her recent birth. Two focus groups are also held with hospital staff to determine what they perceive as the major barriers for women seeking prenatal care. The interviews are audiotaped and transcribed. A research assistant helps with data analysis. The software requirements are minimal; the objectives can be met by using a word processor with search, copy, and paste tools.

Moderately Complex

This type of study would have two or more of the following characteristics:

- An explanatory goal, for example, why a particular outcome is observed
- A moderate amount of data, for example, 250 to 1,000 pages of text, 20 to 50 in-depth interviews, or 10 to 20 focus groups
- Analysis team to have two to four people
- More than five major topics to cover in the study, with overlapping issues within at least some of the topics
- Limited sociodemographic information to be used during the analysis, for example, no more than 20 variables

For example: Once the intervention trial described here is under way, it becomes clear that first-time mothers are not being effectively targeted. The researchers implement a substudy to find out why. They begin by conducting five

(Continued)

focus groups with a variety of women to find out how to locate and enroll women who are pregnant for the first time or are likely to become pregnant for the first time. They initially use the interview guide developed for the simple study; but after conducting eight such interviews, they identify a new set of issues that have not been previously addressed. They modify the interview guide accordingly. In addition, they note that income, education, employment, and housing appear to influence access; so they develop a set of standardized questions on these factors. They conduct another 20 interviews. All focus groups and interviews are audiotaped and transcribed. Another research assistant joins the analysis team. This type of study works best with the help of software specifically designed for QDA. Almost any QDA software package will work.

Complex Study

This study would have two or more of the following characteristics:

- A major scientific goal, for example, theoretical modeling or hypothesis testing
- Data collection on a large set of topics organized into hierarchies or networks of information
- Very large volumes of text, for example, more than 1,000 pages or more than 100 text files
- Detailed quantitative measures or descriptors that will be linked to the qualitative results
- Coordination of one large analysis team (five or more people) or multiple small teams with discrete analytic tasks

For example: The community intervention trial to enhance access to prenatal care is successful, but a follow-up study two years later shows a subsequent decline in access, especially for first-time mothers. The researchers hypothesize that this is related to a combination of local cultural values that tend to isolate childless women, in combination with economic factors that increase the dependency of young women. They suspect that long-term, sustainable improvements in first-time mothers' accessing prenatal care will require greater involvement of their spouses or partners. They design an ethnographic study that will collect information on all of these issues (gender roles, age roles, family roles, socioeconomic status, pregnancy, motherhood) through a series of interviews with men

(Continued)

BOX 6.7 WHAT TO LOOK FOR IN SOFTWARE FOR QUALITATIVE DATA ANALYSIS (Continued)

and women aged 15 to 45. Data collection strategies include structured interviews that are audiotaped and transcribed, informal interviews for which notes are taken and then compiled, and field notes describing observed interactions in a variety of settings. Two senior researchers and four research assistants conduct data analysis in stages. Several structured interview guides are developed, based on interim data analysis.

A project of this magnitude requires systematic file and data management, the ability to link text and quantitative data, the ability to export summary data for use in other software programs, and the ability to track and replicate analysis decisions. Most QDA software packages will support some of these tasks but not all of them. In this situation it is important to carefully evaluate the options included in a software program to determine whether it will meet your needs.

INFORMATION ON QDA SOFTWARE

A number of qualitative software programs exist. Some common ones include:

ATLAS.ti	www.atlasti.com
MAXQDA	www.maxqda.com
NVivo	www.qsrinternational.com
QDA Miner	www.provalisresearch.com
Dedoose	www.dedoose.com

Chapter 9 in *Applied Thematic Analysis* (Guest, Namey et al., 2013) provides a good summary and discussion of the features available in a range of qualitative software packages that are currently available.

Coding Reports: Building Theme-Related Files

Familiarity with the data based on reading, re-reading, and coding text leads into a more formal analysis, examining separately and fully each important theme as it emerges from the data. One starting point is to generate **coding reports** for each of these broader codes and to begin working through each coding report, one after the other, for a finer understanding of each. (See Appendix 7 for an example of a coding report.)

A coding report is a new file that aggregates similarly coded segments of text from a set of original transcripts or field notes. Coding reports can be compiled manually using highlighting or cut-and-paste techniques, with simple word processing or with qualitative text analysis software. In fact, most qualitative software packages enable the user to generate different kinds of coding reports, from a report on an individual code that includes all relevant text segments to reports with summary information about the frequency with which codes appear in the dataset.

Box 6.7 shows an excerpt from a coding report on a code named <conflict>. The coding report was generated in NVivo 10 from the adolescent participation in HIV prevention trials study. The bolded lines in the coding report show the location where the text segments originated. For example, the first several text segments come from a transcript named INMTN004_2, which is located in a folder named MTN and is among a set of documents that are within (or internal to) the NVivo project. Our naming conventions helped us easily to identify the source of the information in the coding report:

- MTN denotes the folder of transcripts for "married teens"
- The file name INMTN004 denotes an Indian married teen, number 004
- The number 2 denotes the second of up to three repeated interviews with this participant

In addition to the name and location of each file from which text segments were extracted, the number of text segments (or references) within the document is indicated, as well as the percentage of the full transcript that each excerpt represents. In our example, three different segments from two transcripts are shown: both interviews with married teens, one each from India and Tanzania. If you do not use a software package to aggregate similarly coded pieces of text, you will need to enter identifiers that indicate the original source files for each block of text in the new, sorted file.

In most qualitative studies, coding reports consist of numerous text segments for each theme. The full coding report on <conflict> in the adolescent study includes 420 text segments extracted from 112 different transcripts. The three segments in our example in Box 6.8 come from two different transcripts—the second interview with a young married teen from India (INMTN004_2) and the second interview with a married Tanzanian teen (TZMTN011_2). These text references were selected to illustrate how comments on one theme, conflict, can be identified in different transcripts and clustered in a single file.

BOX 6.8 CODING REPORT ON CONFLICT

<Internals\MTN\INMTN004_2> - § 5 references coded (24.89% coverage)

Reference 1—0.84% coverage

Which things don't you like about him?

What else? It's an everyday thing. He wants to have sex every day. I do not like that.

Why don't you like it?

Once in a while it is okay. But he wants it often. I do not like it every day.

Reference 2—1.58% coverage

Okay. Do you feel pressured or scared of anyone—either at your mother's house or in your own house?

At my grandmother's house, I am afraid of my uncles. I feel they may get angry with me if I make some mistake. In the same way, I am afraid of my mother and father. They will scold me if I do something wrong. This is the only kind of fear I have. I am not afraid when I am in my own house.

So you aren't afraid of your husband?

I am not afraid of him.

<Internals\MTN\TZMTN001_N_2> - § 3 references coded (6.32% coverage)

Reference 1—3.01% coverage

During the first interview, i asked you if there is someone you are scared of and you said no one. And you told me that your husband used to beat you. Do the beatings make you scared of him in any way?

I was scared of him, because he used to beat me.

Could you speak a bit louder?

I mean I was afraid of him. Whenever he started talking, you become frightened, because you know he can beat you at any time.

Okay, and how is your relationship with your husband right now?

He wants me to come back to him, but I tell him to let me rest at home for the moment. He says he was wrong; he wants me to forgive him and come back to him.

And how do you take that?

I tell him I will come back but not now, for the moment I want to rest at home.

Step 3. Displaying Data: Distinguishing Nuances of a Topic

Having extracted and combined all the information on a specific theme in a coding report, you are ready to examine the theme more closely. Displaying data means laying out or taking an inventory of what you know related to a theme; capturing the variation, or richness, of each theme; and noting differences between individuals or among subgroups. One way to approach the data-display phase is to develop detailed memos related to each main code in the coding scheme. Similar to the coding phase, the first step of data display is to identify the principal subthemes that emerge from the data, working within a single coding report instead of the whole text.

In our illustration of the coding report in Box 6.8, participants describe sources of tension or conflict in their households. Even in these three short segments, several subthemes arise. The young Indian woman alludes to conflict with her husband over the frequency of sexual relations. Although she professes not being afraid of her husband, she is fearful of other family members, including her parents and uncles, who may verbally abuse her for behaving improperly. In contrast, the young Tanzanian woman is afraid of her husband, having suffered physical abuse in the past. Her fear has led her, at least temporarily, to seek refuge with her parents.

As analysis continues, subthemes emerge to reflect ever finer distinctions. For example, further review of the conflict coding report reveals additional information on the types of and reasons for conflict and how various people deal with conflict. It also sheds light on factors that give rise to conflict or help women avoid it.

Writing Data Display Memos

Qualitative researchers write memos for a variety of reasons. As described previously, developing a separate memo further detailing information from each of the larger codes helps the researcher develop a deeper understanding of important themes. The example in Box 6.9 shows a brief excerpt from a memo on a code, "sexual behavior." A number of subthemes emerged from the coding report, including young women's experiences of sexual debut and thoughts about whether the timing of debut was too early or not; types and frequency of sexual behavior; circumstances around multiple sexual partners; and communication with partners or others about sex.

Memos may also be used to document insights into study participants or social relationships. In the study on adolescent participation in HIV prevention trials, the investigator and her team (Tolley et al., 2014) wrote memos that

BOX 6.9 MEMO ON SEXUAL BEHAVIOR

Date completed: 4/6/2012
Relevant code (s): Sexual behavior
Analyst: BT

Adolescents and young women in both Tanzania and India experience sexual debut early (in our sample, female teens aged 15-17 reported sexual debuts on average below 15 and young women aged 18-21 reported sexual debuts earlier than age 17); in many other ways, however, patterns of adolescent sexual behavior are quite different. In India, early sexual debut happens primarily within marriage, although many of our key informants did suggest that Indian adolescents were increasingly sexually active prior to marriage, especially boys. In our India cohort, 7 of 23 young women had been married at or before age 15 (despite legal restrictions on marriage before 18). All other married participants were married by the age of 18. Whether married early or slightly later, almost none had been informed about sexual relations until after marriage. For many/most girls in our India sample, their first sexual encounter was terrifying, painful, and even humiliating, and often followed by signs/symptoms of reproductive tract infections/STIs. In Tanzania, some key informants and community groups suggested that adolescents were engaged in sexual relations as early as 9 to 10 years old; several mothers' groups suggested adolescents knew more about sexual and reproductive information than they, as adults, did. Several of our female participants described learning about sex through traditional practices aimed at transitioning them to adulthood. In most cases, sexual debut in Tanzania occurred prior to or outside of marriage. Though many Tanzanian girls described being pursued or persuaded to have sex by their partners, very few described being coerced or forced. They maintained some autonomy in decision making. Such autonomy was rarely described in the India context.

SEXUAL DEBUT:

1. Timing—too early (India: 7 key informants, 18 adolescent/young women; Tanzania: 5 key informants, 3 FGDs, 13 adolescent/young women)
   - Participant 07, India, married young woman: *How does a woman have to behave with a husband?* Family members teach us how to behave after marriage. You have to be quiet, don't get irritated, don't quarrel, and mingle with family members. Stay in a joint family. Don't insist on a divided family. Share the household work. Don't instigate quarrels. This is the kind of preaching given by family members.

(Continued)

- Participant 016, Tanzania, single out-of-school youth: Nowadays we are having sex when we are too young. *How old were you?* When I had sex for the first time I was like 16 years old [. . .] even if we wanted to be older we couldn't do it; girls of this generation couldn't wait to be older to start having sex—we couldn't do it.

2. Timing—appropriate (India: 3 married young women; Tanzania: 9 adolescents and young women, single and married)
   - Participant 015, Tanzania, single out-of-school youth: *In what circumstance did you have sex for the first time?* As I told you, I was scared of pregnancy and diseases but I happened to fall in love with a certain man. That man had been my friend; then he approached me and we had sex. I did not refuse nor hesitate [she was 18] [. . .] it made me feel like I am just like any other girl. It made me feel like I am an adult. *Did you feel like you were the right age to have sex?* I was at the right age because if you reach 18 years old you are an adult and you know what you are doing, you cannot be easily seduced by men.

focused on individual participants, summarizing information across several interviews about the participant's family circumstances, life aspirations, and partner relationships. Some researchers also use memos to reflect on how their own personal or professional experiences might be influencing the data collection process or their interpretation of the data (see Chapter 2 on reflexivity).

There are no hard and fast rules about how to write memos. However, if they are well structured, memos will be a useful resource in the later stages of analysis and when writing up your results. (See Appendix 8 for an example of a data analysis memo.) Consider including some of the following features:

- Header, including date and subject of the memo and who produced it
- Summary statement that provides an overview of the code
- Subthemes and brief summary of main findings
- Specific text segments representing each subtheme

Developing Hypotheses, Questioning, and Verifying

We have shown how, by clustering text segments around a theme, such as <conflict> or <sexual behavior>, you can extract meaning from data. As you continue organizing information associated with each theme, you will start to form hypotheses—hunches about the data that you want to investigate further. In fact, throughout the entire process of collecting, reading, coding, and displaying data, the qualitative researcher is formulating questions, interpreting responses, developing theoretical explanations, and trying to validate or reject emerging conclusions.

- Do the categories that I have developed make sense?
- What pieces of information contradict my emerging ideas?
- What pieces of information are missing or underdeveloped?
- What other opinions should I take into account?
- How do my own biases influence the data collection and analysis process?

Attention to Data Credibility

How do you determine whether a research participant is giving you a credible response to a question? How do you make sense from the jumble of responses from different groups or individuals? Not all responses should be treated equally. It is important to examine how information was elicited and how it was delivered. Information is likely to be more credible when the following apply:

- The participant is responding to open-ended questions rather than highly leading or suggestive ones.
- The participant is talking about his or her own beliefs, motivations, or experiences rather than someone else's.
- The participant does not contradict him- or herself in subsequent dialogue.
- The participant speaks in detail rather than generalities.

In the adolescent participation in HIV prevention trials study, discussions about the theme <faithfulness> contained numerous contradictions that required further investigation. In both India and Tanzania, young women commonly described both trusting and not trusting their partners, often within the same paragraph. For example, a 21-year-old Indian college student responded this way when asked:

Do you ever feel worried about him having contact with some other girl when you are not around?

Yes, I do feel worried sometimes. He had an affair with a girl, but he did not have an intimate relationship with her. They did not have sex. Although her marriage was fixed she agreed to go around with him. When he mentions her, I get angry. Now, when he wants to make me angry, he talks about her.

In spite of this, would you say you trust him?

I trust him. I trust him immensely. . . . He takes me with him for outings. He cares for my expectations and desires and behaves accordingly.

Confronting these frequent contradictions around the topic of <faithfulness>, we began to develop some hypotheses and ask additional questions to check our hunches. For example, in India it seemed that young women generally assumed a partner's faithfulness and only believed differently if she had sufficient evidence. Was this the same among young Tanzanian women? What kind or amount of evidence was required before a woman would become concerned about possible risk of sexually transmitted infection or HIV? Some young women, including the one in the previous example, appeared more persuaded by positive evidence, such as a partner's attentiveness or gifts, or by absence of negative evidence, such as not seeing him on the street with other women or not finding another woman's emails or text messages on his mobile device, than they were by negative evidence. We wondered whether young women's tendencies to trust their partners or not differed by their own age, their sexual context (i.e., married, single in- or out-of-school, or involved in sex work), and whether perceived faithfulness was consistent with how they described their partner's behavior.

It is important to weigh the credibility of your data as you interpret what you hear and attempt to confirm early conclusions. From a tactical perspective, it is helpful to question your data at every stage of the analysis. Some researchers enter questions, uncertainties, and misgivings directly into their transcripts, distinguishing commentary from raw data with brackets or parentheses or setting them in italic or bold type. Others link interpretive information as separate memos. As you review transcripts, if you are still collecting data, you can integrate new or revised questions into the interview or discussion process. On the other hand, if data collection is complete and you are now working from the coding reports, you may want to enter separate memos about emerging conclusions, reminding yourself to return to your raw data for evidence to validate or reject your ideas.

Step 4. Data Reduction: Getting the Big Picture

Data reduction is the process of distilling the information to make visible the most essential concepts and relationships. Along the way you have read through transcripts, identified important themes, and developed a coding system to mark these themes. You have sorted data from your original transcripts into new files (or coding reports) organized by theme. You have explored the rich variation of each thematic file, identifying key concepts and discovering the perspectives of different subgroups in your study.

It is time to step back from the data. The reduction process usually happens once all the data are in and you have become familiar with their content. The goal now is to get an overall sense of the data and distinguish central and secondary themes, separating the essential from the nonessential. To get this wider perspective on the data, visual devices such as matrices, diagrams, or taxonomies is often helpful (Ryan & Bernard, 2000; Maxwell, 2010; Namey, Guest, Thairu, & Johnson, 2007).

A matrix may contain numeric or textual data, or both. It enables the researcher to further reduce information from a complicated data set to a manageable size. In Box 6.10, we show a matrix summarizing information from a coding report on <sexual behavior>. When constructing the matrix, the researchers decided to:

- Include the participants' IDs to be able to trace information back to original transcripts
- Leave matrix cells empty if a topic was not discussed by a participant
- Develop a numeric scale to summarize whether participants described their sexual debut as being voluntary (0), persuaded (1), or coerced (2)

The use of an Excel matrix enabled the researchers to better visualize potential differences in the data. For example, originally, the matrix was organized by adolescent (aged 15–17) and young adult women (aged 18–21) categories. However, there appeared to be few differences in subthemes by age group. Both age groups reported similar numbers of past sex partners; descriptions of first and current sexual partners included a similar range of positive and negative characterizations. Once the data were sorted by sexual context rather than age, several important differences emerged. For example, in-school youth reported slightly later sexual debut that young women in other categories. The sexual debut of young married women was more likely to have been coerced than for other women. Additionally, women were more likely to describe their first partner (most often the current or ex-husband) as abusive.

BOX 6.10 DATA REDUCTION MATRIX BASED ON SEXUAL BEHAVIOR CODING REPORT

Participant ID	Age	Age at Sexual Debut	First Sex Persuaded (=1) or Forced (=2)	Total Number of Partners	Description of First Partner		
Female Sex Workers					*Who*	*Age*	*Personality*
SOS011	19	15	1	2+	First boyfriend		Generous, calm, but became abusive
SOS012	18	15					
SOS018	15	15	0	>3	First partner	17	Civilized, not hooligan
SOS019	18	16	1	3	Current part	24.5	Likes his walk, sexy
Average	**17.2**	**15.5**		**3**		**20.7**	
Married Adolescent and Young Women					*Who*	*Age*	*Personality*
MTN001	17	15	0	2	Husband		Humiliates her
MTN002	17	16	0	1	Husband	20	Calm
MTN003	16	14.5	0	2	Husband	29.5	Can be harsh
MTN004	17	15	1	3	Husband	27	Doesn't like questions, can be harsh
MYW011	20	16	2	3	Husband		Quiet, likes sex with him
MYW012	20			2	Husband		Jealous, but loves him
MYW013	20	15	0	3	First husband		Cruel when angry
MYW014	20	17	2	1	Boyfriend	34	Humiliates, insults her
Average	**18.3**	**15.5**		**2.13**		**27.6**	

(Continued)

BOX 6.10 DATA REDUCTION MATRIX BASED ON SEXUAL BEHAVIOR CODING REPORT (Continued)

Participant ID	Age	Age at Sexual Debut	First Sex Persuaded (=1) or Forced (=2)	Total Number of Partners	Description of First Partner		
Single Out-of-School Youth					*Who*	*Age*	*Personality*
SOS013	16	14	0	2	Boyfriend	20	Womanizer
SOS014	17	15	0	4	Boyfriend	21	Womanizer
SOS015	20	18	0	2+	Friend	22	
SOS016	20	16	0	5	Child's father		Would force sex, doesn't like him
SOS020	17	15	1	2	Casual		
Average	**18.0**	**15.6**		**3.25**		**21.0**	
Single In-School Youth					*Who*	*Age*	*Personality*
SIS012	18	17	0	2	Boyfriend Zanzibar	19	Thin, black, likes his dimples
SIS014	16	14	0	3+	Boyfriend	22	Smart, financially good
SIS015	16	13	0	5	Boyfriend		Cheated on his friend
SIS013	20	18	0	2	Boyfriend		
SIS011	22	18		4	Boyfriend		Not her fiancé
Average	**18.4**	**16.0**		**3.25**		**20.5**	

Other matrices that were developed for this study included summary information on participant characteristics, partner characteristics, knowledge and experiences using condoms and/or contraceptive methods, attitudes toward microbicide use, and understanding of clinical trial concepts. Some software makes it easy to develop such matrices, but they can also be developed by hand. Although the process can be time-consuming, data reduction helps the researcher establish the boundaries of important themes. In fact, when multiple researchers are involved in the analysis process, each can pursue different themes and present findings to the group. Lively discussion may ensue as the group explores how themes connect, overlap, or contradict each other.

While it makes sense to develop matrices to capture the essence of some themes, different mechanisms may be more appropriate for other themes. Some data might be better visualized by developing a decision tree, taxonomy, graph, or other device. (See Part 2 of Miles, Huberman, and Saldana [2014] for more methods of data display and reduction.) For example, in the breast-feeding example presented at the beginning of this chapter, a decision tree might identify categories or specific conditions within which a mother might decide to give water or other food or drink to her newborn.

Data reduction may not be necessary for all codes; some may be discrete enough that further refinement is not needed. The code <good quotes> used in the adolescent study would be one such example. Other codes may contain multiple ideas and necessitate development of several different matrices, diagrams, or taxonomies in order to reduce complex constructs to main themes and subthemes.

Step 5. Interpretation

In Step 5, we focus on three issues: (1) how to arrive at the essential meanings of qualitative data, (2) how to ensure that interpretation is trustworthy, and (3) how to interpret data in a study that uses both qualitative and quantitative methods.

Interpretation is the act of identifying and explaining the data's core meaning. It involves communicating the study's essential ideas to a wider audience while remaining faithful to participants' perspectives. The purpose of interpretation is not simply to list a handful (or pages full) of interesting themes and their examples, leaving readers to draw their own conclusions; rather, it is to identify ways that the many different pieces of the research puzzle (emerging themes and subthemes, connections, and contradictions) fit and what they all mean. Meaning should reflect the intent of study participants' responses, but it must also have relevance to a larger population and provide answers to questions of social and theoretical significance.

Developing credible, or trustworthy, interpretations of qualitative research includes understandings that would make sense to the men and women who have agreed to be observed, answer questions, or participate in other ways in the study. Of course, some comments may reveal that some or all study participants do not want certain information acknowledged and will publicly deny or suppress it. Such might be the case, for example, if release of findings could undermine the relatively more powerful or privileged positions that certain individuals hold over others. Conversely, participants might deny or want to suppress information if they fear it will put less-advantaged individuals or groups at greater physical or social risk. In such situations, checking the trustworthiness of your interpretations against community understandings may be difficult. In addition, credibility of qualitative results does not necessarily mean that the findings are reproducible. Other researchers might examine the same data and interpret them differently. Contradiction in this case is similar to arriving at different quantitative conclusions when researchers have used different statistical analysis techniques. In both qualitative and quantitative scenarios, the researcher must reevaluate the first analysis, looking for factors that contribute to different results, using his or her best judgment to decide which procedure to favor, and present the process for external scrutiny. This convention is inherent to scientific method and the generation of knowledge.

When both qualitative and quantitative data have been collected and analyzed, the interpretive process must include integration of the two types of data. Qualitative and quantitative researchers working together identify where different approaches produce similar or complementary findings and where they are contradictory. When findings are contradictory, the researchers must decide how or whether to reconcile or prioritize them to arrive at an overall interpretation of study findings.

Synthesizing Findings: Gaps and Connections

Once you have read and reread your texts, developed and refined codes, and extracted central ideas, you may be tempted to conclude your analysis. But as experienced researchers know, the task now is to search for relationships among themes or concepts identified from the analysis. Doing so may be particularly difficult if there is a large number of themes and subthemes. As shown in Box 6.11, diagrams or other visual representations that highlight the relationships can help.

In the study on adolescent participation in HIV prevention trials, the researchers struggled to make sense of so many different themes, wondering how to present them in a way that a larger audience could understand them and find them useful. They drew on their memos and matrices in order to describe the similarities and differences in young women's sexual and reproductive health risks by cultural context.

Box 6.11 illustrates this point. It shows how to synthesize information distilled from the **coding memos** and data matrices, including the following:

- In both countries, sexual debut occurred early—between 13 and 18 years of age, and often around 15 years old.
- Whereas first sex was most often experienced within marriage in India, it usually preceded marriage in Tanzania.

BOX 6.11 USING A DIAGRAM TO ORGANIZE FINDINGS

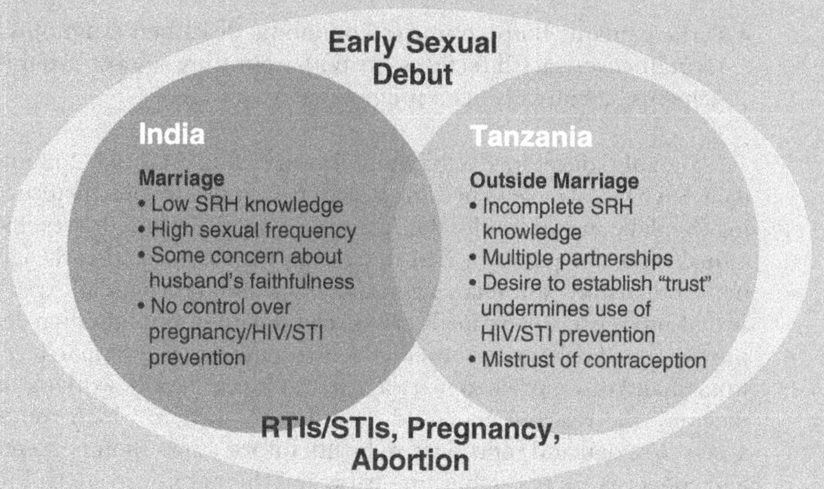
Early Sexual Debut
India
Marriage
• Low SRH knowledge
• High sexual frequency
• Some concern about husband's faithfulness
• No control over pregnancy/HIV/STI prevention
Tanzania
Outside Marriage
• Incomplete SRH knowledge
• Multiple partnerships
• Desire to establish "trust" undermines use of HIV/STI prevention
• Mistrust of contraception
RTIs/STIs, Pregnancy, Abortion

- Indian participants had quite low levels of knowledge about sexual and reproductive health issues. In Tanzania, participants were at least partially informed about HIV, but their knowledge was often incomplete.
- Few Indian participants reported more than one partner unless they acknowledged being engaged in sex work, whereas serial or concurrent sexual partners were common in Tanzania.
- In both settings, having "trust" in one's partner was important. Some Indian participants expressed concern about their husband's faithfulness, but they most often felt there was little they could do about it. In Tanzania, young women sought to establish "trust" even when they believed their partners might not be faithful. In other words, trust was more about emotional connection than about sexual fidelity.
- Young Indian women appeared to have little or no control over decision making about pregnancy or HIV/STI prevention. In contrast, young Tanzanian women could negotiate condom use, at least in the initial stages of a relationship. However, once trust was established, they discontinued such prevention behaviors, which were perceived as in contradiction to a trusting relationship.

- Contraception was rarely used by participants in either setting. In Tanzania, while condom use appeared acceptable in some circumstances, other hormonal methods of contraception were mistrusted.
- Participants in both countries commonly described symptoms indicating reproductive tract infections. In both countries, almost two-thirds of participants had already been pregnant at least once.

They also developed a diagram, shown in Box 6.11, to help summarize the data. Such visual devices provide a central organizational structure for presenting the data. For example, the researchers might frame the results section of a final report or paper by first describing the similar and early ages at which both Indian and Tanzanian girls initiate sex and their similar experiences with sexual and reproductive health risks. The researchers might then describe how the context of risk varies between the two countries, within marriage for Indian women and often prior to marriage in Tanzania. Finally, working through the diagram, the researchers could describe the ways in which young women's access to sexual and reproductive health information, their perceptions of risk and concerns about establishing trust, and their ability to control (or not) the use of preventive methods create vulnerability in each context, noting both similarities and differences across the two settings.

Interpretation of Qualitative Data in a Mixed-Method Design

Before linking the findings from qualitative and quantitative data analysis in a mixed-method study, it makes sense first to analyze each data set separately according to procedures associated with its paradigm (see Chapter 2). How to integrate these findings is guided by the purpose of each component in the study design. Their respective purposes influence whether qualitative and quantitative components will have equal weight in the study design, whether one is primary and the other secondary, and whether qualitative and quantitative components are conducted sequentially or at the same time (see A Practical Strategy for Mixed-Method Design section in Chapter 3).

The components of a mixed-method design may be conducted sequentially, but usually only one—the qualitative or the quantitative—is considered the principal approach of the study (see Box 3.5). If, for example, qualitative data were first collected to inform development of structured data collection instruments for a quantitative survey on teenage drug use, qualitative analysis would focus on identifying those issues that lead young people to consider, try, continue using, or reject drugs. It would investigate the ways adolescents obtain drugs, as well as the language they use to talk about such issues. Qualitative analysis would then be completed first, resulting in a list of topics and perhaps even specific questions with a range of structured responses—words or phrases, examples, or metaphors that the intended audience could easily understand. Quantitative analysis would be conducted separately, after the survey was completed. On the other hand, if the results of a regional stratified random sample survey among middle and high school students suggested that drug use was particularly high within several school districts, qualitative research might be conducted after the survey to help explain district-level differences in drug use, focusing on school- and community-based drug policies, the availability of extracurricular activities for adolescents, the characteristics of adolescent peer networks, and other emergent issues.

When qualitative and quantitative analyses are conducted sequentially, or when one set of analyses clearly dominates the study design, linking findings from the two research approaches can be fairly straightforward. However, linking qualitative and quantitative findings may prove more challenging when both methods in the study design have equal status (Tashakkori & Teddlie, 1998) or when they are conducted in parallel. In these more truly integrated studies, a combination of methods may be used to confirm research findings or to increase their explanatory power.

Difficulty arises when qualitative and quantitative methods uncover dissimilar or even contradictory conclusions. What should a researcher do when the data do not agree? A first step is to look for explanations that reconcile initially contradictory explanations.

Reconciling the findings may require additional analyses of either or both types of data. In a study in South Africa, qualitative findings on women's feelings of vulnerability and the difficulty of negotiating condom use conflicted with the quantitative finding that protection from STIs was within most respondents' control. After returning to the qualitative data and examining the language that women used to express their understanding of control, the researcher concluded that most women were giving hypothetical answers to the structured (quantitative) questions on control of STI prevention methods. They also appeared to have answered these questions from the standpoint of desired, rather than actual, decision-making responsibility. Another way to resolve contradictions is to stratify or regroup quantitative data for further analysis on the basis of the qualitative results. Or you can stratify the qualitative results by significant predictive variables in the quantitative analysis.

But despite all attempts to reconcile contradiction, different findings are sometimes irreconcilable. In such cases, we advise researchers to present the divergent interpretations and allow readers to draw their own conclusions. It is especially important in this situation to provide sufficient information on the data collection and analysis strategies to allow readers to evaluate for themselves the credibility of your interpretations and perhaps to arrive at different conclusions. Following are ways to maximize the credibility of your qualitative findings.

Establishing Trustworthiness

Analyzing qualitative data is intense. Having immersed yourself in a process of reading and rereading, labeling, dissecting, questioning, and synthesizing, you may find it difficult to step back from your emerging interpretations to determine their ultimate trustworthiness.

In Chapter 2 we introduced four criteria—credibility, dependability, confirmability, and transferability—by which to assess the truth value of qualitative findings. We now return to these four criteria and show how to incorporate them into the analysis.

Credibility

Credible interpretations of qualitative data offer explanations that are consistent with the data collected and are understandable to people in the study population. Such interpretations are contextually rich. They are sensitive to differing perspectives in the study sample—perspectives that sometimes diverge or even clash. Credible interpretations develop explanations that somehow reconcile or show how divergent findings relate to the context under study.

There are three techniques that help ensure that interpretation is credible: (1) looking for negative cases for emerging hypotheses; (2) testing rival explanations; and (3) seeking explanations for inconsistencies arising from triangulation of respondents, methods, theories, or researchers (Kidder, 1981; Krueger, 1998; Patton, 1999).

In a study to assess the quality of contraceptive implant services in Senegal (Tolley & Nare, 2001), the data yielded some apparently contradictory findings. Women in the study expressed different experiences with implant removal than researchers had anticipated. To ensure that their results would be credible, researchers probed the unexpected differences with both women users and providers. Closer analysis revealed that seemingly contradictory results did, in fact, reflect real issues for users and shed light on how women negotiate the decision to remove the device.

Showing that you have moved beyond your initial understanding of a research question to gain a more in-depth perspective also builds credibility. One way to show this progression is to consciously compare your final interpretation with what you first expected to find. By identifying and documenting your motivations, interests, and perspectives initially and throughout the research process, you will be better able to navigate around those biases to represent the study respondents more fully and credibly. Some researchers write down what they expect to find before implementing the study. If you find no surprises in the data, no contradictions or revisions to theories, then you may not have dug deeply enough but instead discovered only what you originally set out to discover (Lincoln & Guba, 1985).

Dependability

In quantitative research, an important test of reliability is the extent to which findings can be replicated. The goal is to replicate the results of a study. Given intervening time and change, replication of results may not be possible, but it is important nevertheless to be able to replicate the processes used to obtain those results (King, Keohane, & Verba, 1994).

To increase the dependability of qualitative findings, you might incorporate a team approach or use multiple independent coders or analysts. This tactic helps to offset the subjective bias of any one researcher. The process of resolving differences in interpretation can be a check against individual bias to some degree, but differences in individual power or status might still influence process. Or you may have a second independent investigator analyze data. This allows you to reduce the potential for individual influence over interpretation, but there is no way to rectify differences in independent interpretations. If two significantly different interpretations of the data emerge, you might need to resort to a third independent investigator or present both interpretations of the results, allowing the reader to draw conclusions from both perspectives.

Confirmability

By definition, qualitative research recognizes the researcher's central role in defining issues for study, interpreting information, and guiding the research process. Qualitative researchers do not claim to be detached and neutral scientists, unencumbered by their own experiences and values. They do believe, however, that by being conscious of their own subjectivity, they can better understand and limit its effects on their research activities (from data collection to analysis), thereby allowing participants to express their experiences, values, and expectations without constraint. Qualitative researchers can check whether they have sufficiently maintained the distinction between their own and their subjects' ideas by opening the study process to outside inspection and verification.

One such approach is the audit trail (Lincoln & Guba, 1985). An audit trail is a record that enables you and others to track the process that has led to your conclusions. It is created from notes and other field materials collected and stored along the way. Six categories of information contribute to a good audit trail:

1. Raw data: uncoded transcripts, audio recordings, field observation notes
2. Data reduction and analysis products: list of codes, theoretical notes about working hypotheses, matrices
3. Data reconstruction and synthesis products: diagrams and notes showing how different themes relate, a final report
4. Process notes; methodological notes, notes about trustworthiness, audit notes
5. Materials relating to intentions and dispositions: study protocol, personal notes about motives and expectations of the study
6. Instrument development information: interview guides, data collection protocols

An audit trail also enables other researchers who review analysis decisions to decide for themselves if interpretations are well grounded in the data.

Transferability

Because qualitative analyses are so firmly rooted in specific contexts, some researchers believe it is not possible to make inferences to other populations. Others appear to draw general conclusions from their research too casually. Although the first approach limits the usefulness of qualitative research, the second limits its potency or effectiveness. The middle ground is to apply lessons learned in one context to similar contexts. But how can we do this?

First, as qualitative researchers, we should draw our conclusions carefully, ensuring that the data support them. Second, we can describe enough of the research context, the characteristics of the study participants, the nature of their interactions with the researcher, and the physical environment that others may decide how transferable the findings are to other contexts. Finally, the results are more likely to be transferable if one objective of the original research design was to test a model or build a theory. Such designs will have identified theoretical constructs or components of a conceptual model to be tested in or adapted to a new study population. We can then expect that the study outcome will lead to support or refinement of a model, clearer limits on generalizability, or an alternative model or theory. Thus, the analysis process will have moved discrete fragments (segments) of data to a credible conclusion that is based on evidence and is capable of advancing our understanding of a complex behavioral health phenomenon.

Summary

The power of qualitative research lies in its ability to explore new and relatively unknown topics, examining how individual, social, and cultural contexts shape reality and acknowledging the potential for multiple and at times contradictory perspectives. Attention both to context and multiple perspectives, however, can make qualitative analysis a daunting task. How does one make sense of hundreds of pages of text, identifying relevant themes while paying close attention to subtle meanings in the data? How do you ensure that the findings you extract from the data reflect local, "on-the-ground" realities and are not influenced by your own predisposed ideas?

In this chapter, we have described a set of five interrelated steps that can help you move from pages and pages of raw data to a cohesive set of findings that explain the study topic from the perspectives of those who influence or are influenced by it. When beginning the analysis process, we emphasize the need to revisit the research purpose. This means reviewing the theoretical or conceptual framework basis and returning again to the research objectives and questions. We then suggest engaging in a process of (1) reading, (2) coding, (3) displaying, (4) reducing, and (5) interpreting the data, providing detailed explanations and some specific examples for each step. While most qualitative researchers use some or all of these steps when synthesizing their data, they may move between them in a different order or incorporate different ways to memo, display, or reduce their data. We encourage flexibility and creativity, while at the same time documenting the process and double-checking how and/or why you have arrived at the meanings you extract from the data.

Fittingly, we end this chapter with a discussion on trustworthiness. As discussed in Chapter 2, qualitative researchers acknowledge that subjectivity is an important element of the qualitative process. Our aim is to understand the subjective experiences and understandings of our research participants. And, in doing so, our own backgrounds, values, and experiences will influence the questions we ask and how the responses are interpreted. Attention to the subjective nature of experience (both the participants' and our own) can be a real strength as long as we pay close attention to how we generate our findings. By following a systematic process that helps us remain close to the data and by documenting each step in our analysis process, our study findings will be more credible and have greater impact.

Key Terms

1. **Coding:** The process of attaching labels, or codes, to lines of text so that the researcher can group and compare similar or related pieces of information.
2. **Data display:** The process of deconstructing or taking an inventory of the types of information captured in a larger concept or theme in order to understand how the theme is produced and/or varies across contexts or research participants.
3. **Data reduction:** Using matrices, diagrams, or other visual devices to identify the most pertinent components or outcomes from data analysis.
4. **Structural codes:** Codes that correspond to the basic structure of the topic guide or conceptual model of your research. They allow you to quickly group and begin coding your text.
5. **Emergent codes:** Codes that arise from the textual data and may be expressed by words or phrases that frequently appear in the transcripts or capture more concrete or context-specific information than was specified prior to data collection.
6. **Matrix:** A table that tallies analyzed data across relevant structural or emergent codes among the items contained in the data set (e.g., cases, participants).
7. **Intercoder reliability:** Level of agreement between two or more data analysts. This can be calculated by percentage of agreement or Cohen's kappa coefficient, or it can be assessed more qualitatively.
8. **Coding reports**: Compilation of similarly coded sections of text from different sources into a single file or report. Coding reports can be generated automatically, if using a qualitative software program, but they can also be assembled through cut-and-paste methods.
9. **Coding memo:** A written summary produced by the researcher that describes information contained in a coding report, including key questions or sources for the data, pertinent results, and a brief of the analysis process. It may contain representative quotes/text and quantitative results if applicable (i.e., frequencies or percentages). Memos may also be used to document a researcher's insights about the social or physical environment or the way that the researcher's own background and experiences influence the data collection and analysis process.

Review Questions

1. What are five basic steps that are often included in qualitative data analysis? What kinds of qualitative analysis activities would be conducted within each step?
2. Qualitative research is often described as an iterative process. What is meant by this?
3. What kinds of decisions does a researcher need to make when beginning to code qualitative data?
4. What kinds of information might be included in a memo?
5. Describe some ways that a researcher might "visualize" his or her data.
6. What are some ways that you can increase the credibility of your analysis?
7. Identify several qualitative research papers published in the peer-reviewed literature and read the research methods sections. What analysis steps are described in each? Which papers provide the clearest description of their analysis process?
8. Read through the study findings of one published paper. In your opinion, how credible are the findings? What elements of the methods and/or findings sections make you feel this way?

Recommended Readings

Miles, M. B., Huberman, A. M., & Saldana, J. (2014). *Qualitative data analysis: A methods sourcebook*. Thousand Oaks, CA: Sage.

Ryan, G. W., & Bernard, H. R. (2000). Data management and analysis methods. In N. K. Denzin & Y. S. Lincoln (Eds.), *Handbook of qualitative research* (2nd ed., pp. 769–802). Thousand Oaks, CA: Sage.

Tashakkori, A., & Teddlie, C. (1998). *Mixed methodology: Combining qualitative and quantitative approaches*. Thousand Oaks, CA: Sage.

References

Guest, G., MacQueen, K. M., & Namey, E. E. (2012). *Applied thematic analysis*. Thousand Oaks, CA: Sage.

Guest, G. S., Namey, E. E., & Mitchell, M. L. (2013). *Collecting Qualitative Data: A Field Manual for Applied Research*. Thousand Oaks, CA: Sage.

Hruschka, D. J., Schwartz, D., St. John, D. C., Picone-Decaro, E., Jenkins, R. A., & Carey, J. W. (2004). Reliability in coding open-ended data: Lessons learned from HIV behavioral research. *Field Methods*, *16*(3), 307–331. doi:10.1177/1525822X04266540

Huberman, A. M., & Miles, M. B. (1994). Data management and analysis methods. In N. K. Denzin & Y. S. Lincoln, *Handbook of qualitative research* (pp. 428–444). Thousand Oaks, CA: Sage.

Kelle, U. (1997). Theory building in qualitative research and computer programs for the management of textual data. *Sociological Research Online*, *2*(2), U1–U13. doi:10.5153/sro.86

Kidder, L. H. (1981). Qualitative research and quasi-experimental frameworks. In M. B. Brewer & B. E. Collins (Eds.), *Scientific inquiry and the social sciences* (pp. 226–256). San Francisco, CA: Jossey-Bass.

King, G., Keohane, R. O., & Verba, S. (1994). *Designing social inquiry: Scientific inference in qualitative research*. Princeton, NJ: Princeton University Press.

Krueger, R. A. (1998). Analyzing and reporting focus group results. In D. L. Morgan & R. A. Krueger (Eds.), *The focus group kit* (Vol. 6). Thousand Oaks, CA: Sage.

Lincoln, Y. S., & Guba, E. G. (1985). Establishing trustworthiness. In Y. S. Lincoln & E. G. Guba (Eds.), *Naturalistic inquiry* (pp. 289–331). Beverly Hills, CA: Sage.

Maxwell, J. A. (2010). Using numbers in qualitative research. *Qualitative Inquiry*, *16*(6), 475–482. doi:10.1177/1077800410364740

Miles, M. B, Huberman, A. M., & Saldana, J. (2014). *Qualitative data analysis: A methods sourcebook*. Thousand Oaks, CA: Sage.

Namey, E., Guest, G., Thairu, L., & Johnson L. (2007). Data reduction techniques for large qualitative data sets. In G. Guest & K. MacQueen (Eds.), *Handbook for team-based qualitative research* (pp. 137–161). Lanham, MD: AltaMira Press.

Patton, M. Q. (1999). Enhancing the quality and credibility of qualitative analysis. *Health Services Research*, *34*(5 Pt 2), 1189–1208.

Ryan, G. W., & Bernard, H. R. (2000). Data management and analysis methods. In N. K. Denzin & Y. S. Lincoln (Eds.), *Handbook of qualitative research* (2nd ed., pp. 769–802). Thousand Oaks, CA: Sage.

Tashakkori, A., & Teddlie, C. (1998). *Mixed methodology: Combining qualitative and quantitative approaches*. Thousand Oaks, CA: Sage.

Tolley, E., & Nare, C. (2001). Access to norplant removal: An issue of informed choice. *African Journal of Reproductive Health/La Revue Africaine de la Santé Reproductive*, *5*(1), 90–99. doi:10.2307/3583202

Tolley, E. E., Kaaya, S., Kaale, A., Minja, A., Bangapi, D., Kalungura, H., . . . , & Baumgartner, J. N. (2014). Comparing patterns of sexual risk among adolescent and young women in a mixed-method study in Tanzania: Implications for adolescent participation in HIV prevention trials. *Journal of the International AIDS Society*, *17*(3, Suppl 2), 19149. doi:10.7448/IAS.17.3.19149

CHAPTER 7

DISSEMINATING QUALITATIVE RESEARCH

OBJECTIVES:

- To discuss the rationale for dissemination of research results
- To describe how to develop a dissemination strategy and implement dissemination activities
- To describe dissemination approaches appropriate for different audiences, including:
  - Communities
  - Research participants
  - Policymakers and other health decision makers
  - Funders
  - Other researchers and technical experts

> **Knowledge translation strategies can harness the power of scientific evidence and leadership to inform and transform policy and practice.**
>
> ***(World Health Organization, 2006)***

WHEN WE WRITE about people's notions of health risk or quality of care, we are fulfilling a practical and social mandate common to applied research: to create information for use by programs to improve services or by decision makers to inform policies. The end product of applied qualitative research on public health should be to give public voice or visibility to private or hidden issues, cast new light on puzzling questions, make invisible problems clear (allowing solutions), and make health problems more understandable (allowing better solutions) (Rubin & Rubin, 1995).

> **The ultimate goal of qualitative research is to transform data into information that can be used.**
>
> *(Rossman & Rallis, 1998, p. 11)*

Because applied research generates information for a purpose, it must have a projected audience and a plan for reaching the stakeholders, or end users. Therefore, the **dissemination** of study findings—what, why, by whom, to whom, and how—needs to be considered from the beginning. If you want your results to be used, start planning for dissemination even when you are designing the study and developing a budget. Your specific purposes for dissemination can vary and may include the following processes:

- Strengthening and increasing the frequency of communication between the researcher and study participants
- Providing tools or materials for researchers and health advocates to communicate in support of policy change
- Helping other researchers, scientists, or decision makers understand the social, cultural, political, or economic factors that influence public health
- Empowering marginalized, silenced groups (such as victims of sexual violence)
- Providing practical information to solve programmatic problems
- Developing awareness of a particular issue within a stakeholder group or audience (Barwick, 2011)
- Keeping health issues alive in the media, donor, and public health communities

Dissemination activities may include individual or group discussions before, during, or after study completion; professional meetings and conferences; publication in peer-reviewed journals; reports presented to public health stakeholders and funders; distribution of fact sheets and infographics; use of entertainment and print media (e.g., songs, posters, puppet theater); coverage by news media; engagement via social media; audiovisual presentations or webinars; or training workshops. It is never too early to ask a stakeholder the simple question, "What do you need to know?"

Contrary to the popular notion that dissemination implies only end-of-study activities, such as a seminar to brief senior health administrators, research dissemination is a communications process, not a one-time event. You do not have to wait until you have analytic saturation before you start to disseminate. From the first day you introduce your study to department of health officials or community leaders, you are actively disseminating information on the purpose, scope, and potential impact of the study. This act of inclusion helps to create a sense of community ownership for the study. Engaging with stakeholders about their questions and reactions can also help you understand how to shape future dissemination activities. Later, when you return to key informants to say "This is what I'm hearing in the research. Does it make sense to you? Why or why not?" you are sharing preliminary findings and opening a collaborative dialogue on their meaning.

In short, dissemination is an ongoing part of the dialogue with stakeholders that characterizes applied qualitative research. The methods used in qualitative research bring you into repeated contact with opinion leaders, community members, and other stakeholders; these interactions serve both to gather and to share information. Having unearthed in-depth, often deeply personal information on what people think about health issues, you must share study insights as widely as possible, whether such dissemination is formal or informal, direct, or indirect.

As you develop a research dissemination strategy appropriate to your study, you will likely encounter obstacles. These can range from resource constraints or skepticism about the validity of findings on the part of policymakers and scientists unfamiliar with qualitative methods to personal reservations regarding your interpretive role or resistance on the part of health bureaucracies to information suggesting new practices. You also may have underestimated the often considerable amount of time and effort needed to prepare for dissemination activities. Many researchers believe either that research dissemination—and more broadly, "knowledge translation"—is outside their professional capacity or simply not their responsibility. Others think they are responsible for dissemination only to the research community. It is important to consider from the outset where your research responsibilities will end and whom to involve in order to promote effective use of results.

Although many of the strategies and activities used to disseminate qualitative research are identical to those used to disseminate other types of studies, a few issues are specific to qualitative work. For example, a frequent complaint among both scientists and policymakers who have little previous experience with qualitative studies is this: "Why should we believe that these results mean anything? This information is anecdotal!" To accomplish the ultimate purpose of applied research—to produce new and useful information—you will need a strategy for presenting your results effectively and persuading audiences that your findings are credible. We recommend at the very least disseminating your findings to study participants, health advocates, and the local or international research community. Incorporating participatory dissemination from the beginning, a process to which qualitative methods lend themselves, will generate better data and give your research results a better chance of being used.

Research Ethics Require Dissemination

> **Neither academic nor medical and health research institutions . . . regard it as their responsibility to communicate their research findings to local policymakers, practicing health professionals, or the public.**
>
> *(Kitua, Mashalla, & Shija, 2000, p. 821)*

The obligation to disseminate information back to study participants has been part of the professional code of applied sociologists, anthropologists, and other social scientists for decades, as has been the public disclosure of findings. The Association of Social Anthropologists of the UK and Commonwealth (1999), for example, states that a researcher's "obligations to the participants or the host community may not end (indeed should not end, many would argue) with the completion of their fieldwork or research project.... [Researchers should] communicate their findings, for the benefit of the widest possible community."

Qualitative researchers are ethically bound to disseminate findings for several reasons. First, we share the fruits of research—namely, information on study findings—because it is unethical to collect data and then not disseminate the main findings. Second, the use of qualitative research methods—whether focus group discussions with seniors at risk of depression or structured interviews with health educators—is based on creating trust. We reciprocate that trust by sharing information, returning the benefits of research to the individuals and communities that have contributed their insights. This ethical commitment to reciprocity has been formalized in guidelines for the informed consent process for international research involving human subjects, including qualitative research. In large part because community members in countries where research on HIV is being conducted have demanded that the benefits of research accrue to them more directly, international guidance documents are increasingly recommending that communities as well as study participants be informed of study findings after research is finished (Heise, McGrory, & Wood, 1998; Joint United Nations Programme on HIV/AIDS, 2000).

An Inclusive Dissemination Process Promotes Use

Ideally, qualitative study designs include a component in which study participants are contacted and asked whether the preliminary findings appear valid to them. For logistical and financial reasons, this phase is not always possible. Nevertheless, do what you can to check that your findings would make sense to your conversational partners or others in the same population. You might, for example, conduct exit interviews with stakeholders before leaving the study site. Every time you ask your participants how they understand the meaning of the data you are generating, you are inviting them to contribute to shaping the messages that will emerge from the research, while at the same time disseminating information on the study. Such interactive dissemination leads to more grounded and therefore more credible study findings. Experts in diffusion of information agree that an inclusive and ongoing approach to research dissemination also leads to a greater likelihood that findings will be used (Cernada, 1982; Havelock, 1971; Rogers & Storey, 1987). "Sustained interactivity" between researchers and practitioners promotes research utilization (Huberman, 1992), with results having a stronger influence on practitioners if interactions with researchers occur before, during, and on completion of the study, especially face-to-face interactions (Huberman, 1990, p. 365). To foster a climate in which research is seen as relevant, involve stakeholders in as many research dissemination activities as possible.

Stakeholder participation can mean very straightforward, simple activities. Maintaining frequent communication with key groups through visits, telephone calls, email correspondence, or technical support is a powerful way to promote interest in and use of study findings. A study on the dissemination of research-based HIV prevention models to community service providers in the United States found that dissemination efforts are more successful when they "occur in the context of ongoing relationships between researchers and service providers, and when staff-training technical assistance is followed by opportunities to plan and problem-solve how to implement the research-based intervention" (Kelly et al., 2000, p. 1087). The authors of this randomized control trial concluded that the frequency of outside contact reinforcing and supporting initial dissemination messages to health administrators and providers had a significant impact on adoption of new research-based HIV service delivery approaches. Box 7.1 outlines ways to encourage this kind of two-way communication between researchers and stakeholders.

Communication and participation are actually two words sharing the same concept. Etymologically the Latin *communio* relates to participation and sharing.

(Dagron, 2001, p. 33)

BOX 7.1 WAYS TO FOSTER TWO-WAY COMMUNICATION IN RESEARCH

Research stakeholders are more likely to use study findings if they feel they have participated in creating the results and are consulted and kept informed throughout the research process (Rothman, 1980). To promote use of study findings, plan to include two-way communication steps such as the following:

- Collaborative development of subprojects
- Regular two-way communication and consultation with stakeholders
- Regular written feedback to stakeholders on study purposes, progress, and findings
- Substantial face-to-face dialogue about progress, preliminary study results, and implications of results for programs or policies
- Field trips with managers and stakeholders to view activities in order to create understanding, enthusiasm, and ownership of study results
- Collaborative seminars to interpret findings
- Joint development of a family of related print materials written at appropriate levels for different audiences
- Follow-up visits to ministry of health officials or other key parties to personally deliver and review the study report
- One-on-one discussions with stakeholders for informal discussion of results, with written communication regarding next steps
- A facilitated series of conversations ("multistakeholder consultations") to deepen understanding or encourage action (World Bank Institute 2013a, p. 119)

Source: Adapted from Population Council (1994).

How to Develop a Communication and Dissemination Strategy

A **communication strategy** consists of planning for all forms of communication with stakeholders throughout the life cycle of the study, and it may include planning for how to deal with crises. It implies reciprocity, a two-way exchange of information. It is broader than a **dissemination strategy** (a plan for communicating information about a study, typically study results), which may be limited to dissemination of research findings at the end of your study. Some researchers develop overarching communication strategies, whereas others choose to develop only a results dissemination strategy; that is, they may focus only on communication related to dissemination of research results. (See Box 7.2 for a checklist that can be used to develop either strategy.) A strategic communication planning template that may double as a template for a dissemination strategy appears in Figure 7.1 and also may be found at http://communications4clintrials.org/wp-content/uploads/2013/10/Appendix-3-1.pdf.

No matter how modest or ambitious your dissemination goals are, develop a written strategy based on audience needs, your needs and resources, current and emerging opportunities, timing, and the power of your study findings.

(Rogers & Storey, 1987)

A simple version of the communications planning template shown in Figure 7.1 can be downloaded as a Word document at http://designlab360.org/commhandbook/wp-content/uploads/2013/10/Box-6-1_Dissemination_plan_template.doc. It covers the following:

- Background and environmental analysis (also called a needs assessment)
- Goals and objectives
- Identification of key stakeholders
- Strategy for ongoing communication with stakeholders
- Strategy for managing controversy related to research
- Dissemination plan for study results
- Materials to support the study (Robinson, Baron, Heise, Moffett, & Harlan, 2010, pp. 90–91)

To develop a strategy for disseminating study findings and promoting their use, you will need to make decisions on what to say, to whom, and through which means, and you need to make sure you have the staff and financial resources to implement your plan. In practical terms, a modest but effective package of dissemination activities might include determining appropriate modes for dissemination, publishing a newsletter with research results, collaborating on country-specific research reports, contributing the study report

BOX 7.2 CHECKLIST: ELEMENTS OF AN EFFECTIVE COMMUNICATION AND DISSEMINATION PLAN

This checklist can be used when planning for the dissemination phase, even at the start of the research project. Ask yourself the following questions:

Objectives: What do I hope to accomplish in disseminating the results?

Users: Who are my audiences?

Content: What will I need to share with each of the audience groups?

Sources: What sources of information will each audience most respect (e.g., government statistics, photographs taken by community members)?

Media/channels: What media, interpersonal, or other channels of information will be most effective for delivering the message to intended audiences? (See Box 7.3 on working with the media, and Box 7.4 on using social media.) Which messengers will be most trusted?

Evaluation: How will I know if the proposed dissemination activities have been successful?

Access: How can I ensure that the information my research generates will be accessible, both now and in the future? (See Box 7.5 on making research results accessible.)

Availability: How can I make intended audiences aware of the availability of research-based information from this study?

Barriers: What possible barriers can I predict now that later might interfere with access to or use of the information? What can I do to offset possible interference?

Source: Adapted from Westbrook and Boethel (2006).

FIGURE 7.1 Strategic Communications Plan

Below is a sample plan developed by Family Health International to guide trial communications in one country. It has been left partially filled out to show what a written plan contains.

Strategic Communications Plan for X Trial

Below we describe the study's major vulnerabilities (issues, groups, individuals, or community concerns that could limit the success of the study) and our plans to address these issues before they become problems (what we will do, why, with whom, and how). The key elements in the plan include:

- Environmental scans
- Partnering and networking
- Ongoing communication with stakeholders
- Engagement with activists
- Public information and research dissemination
- Selective outreach to news media
- Good internal communications
- Research dissemination

Introduction/background

[Fill in here]

Team/roles

[Fill in here]

Environmental scan and analysis of vulnerabilities

[Fill in here]

Objectives (internal/external)

[Specify objectives clearly, as shown in examples below.]

1. *Improve how scientific information is disseminated within the network.*
2. *Improve dissemination of scientific information to the community where trials are conducted.*
3. *Improve the utility, accessibility, functionality of the Web site.*
4. *Increase visibility of the network among interested stakeholders internationally and locally to facilitate community and stakeholder engagement.*

FIGURE 7.1 Strategic Communications Plan (Continued)

Existing relations and outreach to key research partners and stakeholders
The study team will continue making contact with researchers and community members at various levels. The two PIs are well recognized in their areas and will be quite useful in keeping contact with the network of researchers in their site. Existing communication with partners and stakeholders includes the following: [List as appropriate for your trial.]

1. *Relations with government officials and other decision makers*
2. *Relations with the local study communities*
3. *Relations with local, national, or regional advocacy groups*
4. *Donors active in supporting HIV programs: USAID, DFID, WHO, Gates Foundation, Clinton Foundation, EG-PAF, UNAIDS*
5. *Health professionals*

Strategy for rapid response to controversy
As a controversy emerges, the communications team will work with appropriate individuals from the groups listed above to identify: [Write down what is relevant for your trial.]

1. *Possible steps to change the course of the issue's progression: This may include communication intended to inform, advise, demonstrate due diligence, demonstrate caring, etc.*
2. *Other communications activities will be implemented to build consensus or support among opinion leaders and key stakeholders, such as meetings, press briefings, and the placement of op-ed pieces by prominent colleagues with credibility in health and human rights.*
3. *Site-specific communications: In all network sites, we will depend very heavily on local CABs to acquire information and to respond to community concerns, rumors, and other misinformation within the sites. CAB members will be trained on the importance of their role. The PIs will be the project's spokespeople at the sites, and the network can assist them to prepare responses to issues as they emerge.*

Ongoing communications that target specific audiences

[Write down key groups you will need to inform on an ongoing basis, and how you will do that.]

1. *News media: The network can stay in touch with a small group of journalists through whom communications about the network will be made. These journalists will be identified through their previous work on covering research and HIV/AIDS and through their media affiliation.*
2. *Local community: Community education forums will be conducted by site teams.*
3. *Government or ministry officials: Quarterly briefing sessions will be organized for Ministry of Health officials to keep them up to date with the site-level activities. They will also receive regular information through the newsletter.*
4. *Public health professionals will receive updates through the newsletter.*
5. *Study staff/research teams: Staff members will be trained in the area of research literacy and will learn how to answer tough questions that may be asked by community members during community education forums.*
6. *Activists or other civil society groups.*

FIGURE 7.1 Strategic Communications Plan (Continued)

Materials needed to support communication and dissemination plans

We will identify the communications materials that will need to be written and distributed (including language and target audience) and determine who is responsible for each of these materials. These will include: [List materials you need to support your plan.]

1. *A statement about the network*
2. *A list describing other HIV prevention studies being conducted in each country and key events for these*
3. *Annotated lists of activists in each country*
4. *Calendar of relevant meetings and conferences, nationally and globally*
5. *Q&A*
6. *Contact list of site staff*
7. *Media guidelines governing coordination and procedures for media inquiries*
8. *Materials to include in training of study team: presentation on communications, research literacy issues (including research concepts and study procedures as well as issues pertaining to prevention trials) and how to answer difficult questions*
9. *Rapid response plan*
10. *List of key resources*
11. *Internal Web portal/Basecamp site with network materials*
    - *Protocol*
    - *Community assessments*
    - *News clips*
    - *Photographs*
    - *Backgrounders and Q&As*
    - *Contact lists*

Source: Reprinted with permission from Robinson, Baron, Heise, Moffett, & Harlan (2010, pp. 192–194).

BOX 7.3 WORKING WITH THE MEDIA

The media play a key role in conveying health information on important topics such as Zika virus to researchers, clinicians, and the general public (Grimes, 1999; Kaiser Family Foundation, 2001).

Mass communication using news media, advertising, and marketing channels works particularly well to publicize new information and influence social norms. Media coverage of public health issues can demonstrate the benefits of particular policies, articulate obstacles to health services, or model behaviors such as responsible parenthood (Smith, 1995). If your study purpose involves communicating results to a wide group of people and you have sufficient resources to do so, seek out a media professional or health advocate who can help you plan effective activities, keeping these guidelines in mind:

- Establish your message.
- Consider your audiences and direct your messages to them. Your audiences are mostly interested in how they are affected by what you say.
- Know your facts.
- Use human language. Everyone relates best to human experiences, so use stories drawn from your research to make your key points easier to absorb. Try to avoid technical terms. Use quotes from research participants to illustrate your message.
- State your conclusions clearly, from the beginning (Seidel, 1993). For example, you might say, "This study showed that prophylactic use of aspirin prevents recurrent heart attacks, and let me tell you why."
- When interviewed, stick to a couple of key points; practice articulating a very brief message that broadcast journalists can use as a sound bite.

and relevant materials to a local library or resource center, holding a meeting with members of civil society to discuss the results, publishing journal articles, defining messages or talking points of importance to stakeholders, or translating results for policy audiences.

At a minimum, aim to do the following:

- Plan a half- to full-day presentation meeting for key decision makers, health professionals, and advocacy groups.

BOX 7.4 USING SOCIAL MEDIA TO SHARE RESEARCH

Use of social media, especially blogging, represents an expanding channel for researchers to communicate study results and narrow the research-to-policy communication gap (Grande et al., 2014).

At the 2014 International AIDS Society (IAS) Conference, Futures Group (now Palladium), an organization that focuses on global health policy, developed a social media campaign to share study and program results with funders, partner organizations, governmental officials, influential social media figures and bloggers, and the broader international AIDS community. Three websites served as the primary communication channels and repositories for all content to be shared, while social media outreach was used to drive audiences to materials posted on the websites. Twitter, in particular, was used to engage audiences at the conference and those following proceedings from afar. The group also sent announcements about new findings shared at the conference using email, always directing recipients to the official event portal, which included links to summaries of oral presentations, PowerPoint slide presentations, YouTube videos of presentations, and posters on policy-related studies, including on geomapping of HIV "hotspots" and HIV-related stigma and discrimination. Researchers then wrote daily blogs and submitted them to the official conference blog site, *Science Speaks*, which posted them. Facebook was also used to post photos, whose captions linked readers back to materials on the websites.

One tactic that proved useful was to write "canned" tweets prior to the conference and then modify them as needed when live tweeting. This approach can be especially helpful if key messages need to undergo review by funding agencies before being broadcast publicly.

- Return information to the community through community discussions, a brochure on findings (see Figure 7.2, which shows a brochure designed to share study findings with the communities that participated in the research), or other means.
- Distribute copies of your report to local universities, libraries, and key local and international organizations.

To increase the likelihood that your study results will be used, keep in mind that the information must be communicated to the appropriate potential users of the findings (primary and secondary users). Study findings must address issues that your research stakeholders perceive to be important, and

BOX 7.5 HOW TO MAKE STUDY FINDINGS ACCESSIBLE

- Obtain an International Standard Book Number (ISBN) number or other standard cataloging information for each substantial document you produce. It will help promote correct cataloging and easy retrieval by local and international library reference staff and users.
- Submit your citation to bibliographic indexing databases such as POPLINE, if it is related to population or reproductive health, and to relevant Wikipedia pages to ensure that researchers will have worldwide access to your article or abstract through libraries, commercial information services, and the Internet. Most databases automatically get citations from journal publishers (PubMed, Web of Science, Social Sciences Index, etc.), so if you publish in a journal that is included in these databases your study will be indexed.
- Post study reports for which you hold the copyright on the Internet, either on your institution's website or that of a sister agency interested in disseminating health information. You can also post citations and abstracts to large clearinghouses on international development, such as Zunia (http://zunia.org).
- For tips in retaining your copyright when you publish with traditional publishers, or if you self-publish, check Creative Commons License for license options and other tips and tricks regarding copyright at http://creativecommons.org.

Appendix 9 also contains information on how to make findings accessible.

reports must be presented in a form that users of the findings will understand and consider credible. There is evidence that "readers processed new scientific information more rigorously when articles provided analogies" (Shapiro, 1994, p. 435). Other characteristics of effective dissemination efforts include "brevity, repetition, and reinforcement" (Sechrest, Backer, & Rogers, 1994, p. 193). Box 7.6 summarizes strategies for utilization of findings.

Information must be delivered to each audience in time to be useful, such as during revision of national guidelines on health service delivery practices (Morris, Fitz-Gibbon, & Freeman, 1987). Special events such as World AIDS Day, International Women's Day, or World Day Against Trafficking in Persons may offer an opportunity to focus attention on your study. Also, try to make your communications activities as pleasant as possible; consider serving lunch at your dissemination seminar or combining tea and an informal talk with government officials to whom you hand the report.

FIGURE 7.2 Flyer Disseminating Results from the LinCS 2 Durham Study to the Community

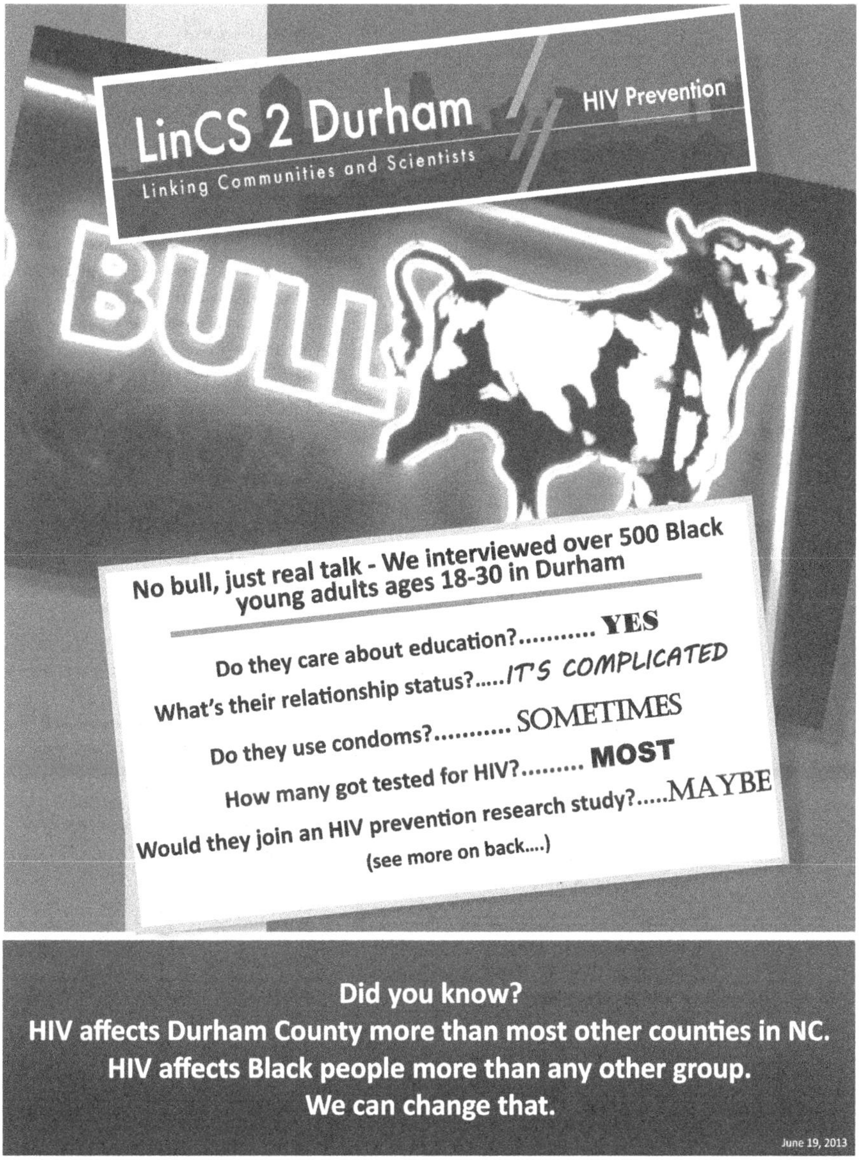
LinCS 2 Durham
Linking Communities and Scientists
HIV Prevention
BULL
No bull, just real talk - We interviewed over 500 Black young adults ages 18-30 in Durham
Do they care about education?........... YES
What's their relationship status?.....IT'S COMPLICATED
Do they use condoms?........... SOMETIMES
How many got tested for HIV?......... MOST
Would they join an HIV prevention research study?.....MAYBE
(see more on back....)
Did you know?
HIV affects Durham County more than most other counties in NC.
HIV affects Black people more than any other group.
We can change that.
June 19, 2013

FIGURE 7.2 Flyer Disseminating Results from the LinCS 2 Durham Study to the Community (Continued)

Who did we talk to?

Half of the survey participants reported living in Durham County since childhood

More than 4 out of 5 were single - not married or in a domestic partner relationship.

They care about education: more than 4 out of 5 had at least a high school diploma or GED.

Most wanted more education. About 3 out of 5 wanted at least a bachelors degree.

About one quarter were enrolled as students.

Of those not enrolled as students, 2 out of 5 were unemployed.

Some have been incarcerated.

About 2 out of 5 men

About 1 out of 5 women

About 1 in 5 did not have health insurance.

About 1 in 5 **men** did not know if they had health insurance

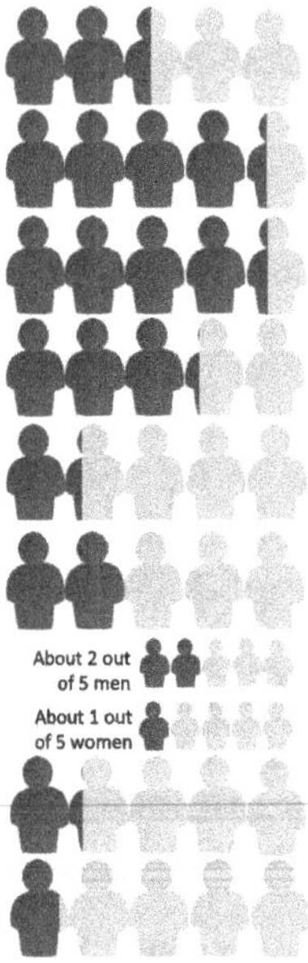

Let's talk about sex:

To join the study, the Black young adults had to be sexually active in the previous 6 months. More than 4 out of 5 people said they had a steady person in their life. But, several people (1 out of 4 women and even more men) also said they went back and forth between sex partners (had concurrent relationships) in the previous 6 months.

Only about 1 out of 4 women and slightly more men reported using condoms consistently with their steady partner. Men in concurrent relationships were less likely than other men to use condoms with any of their partners.

Did you know that:

- sex transmits HIV
- Concurrency increases your risk of HIV (going back and forth between sex partners)
- Condoms help stop the spread of HIV - but they need to be used, even with a steady partner

HIV Testing:

3 out of 4 men and even more women (9 out of 10 women) had been tested for HIV. 1 out of 5 said they and their partner decided to get tested together.

Here is where you and your partner can get tested:

- Durham County Department of Health
- Lincoln Community Health Center
- CAARE, Inc.
- Alliance for AIDS Services
- Ask your doctor or at any clinic - many offer testing for free.

Why would they participate in HIV prevention research?

- Because they believe in the importance of helping others.
- Because they think others would participate.
- Because they don't feel stigma toward HIV (they don't have negative feelings for or actions against people with HIV).

Without participants, we won't find what works. You can participate in many ways, including advising researchers on how to work in your community.

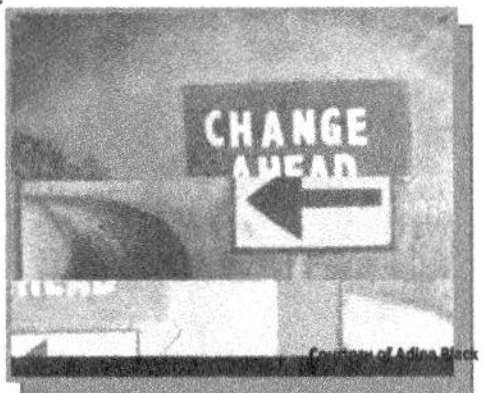

June 19, 2013

Visit our website (www.lincs2durham.org); Follow us on Facebook (www.facebook.com/LinCS2DurhamFan) or Twitter (@LinCS_2_Durham)

BOX 7.6 DISSEMINATION FACTORS THAT PROMOTE UTILIZATION

- The information needs of specific audiences are considered when designing the study.
- The credibility and reliability of the research findings are accepted by users of the study.
- Findings are disseminated to multiple audiences using a variety of proactive and reactive channels and formats, including person-to-person contact, written information, and electronic media.
- Presentation of findings emphasizes the important lessons learned, especially from the point of view of the intended audience, rather than the need for more research.

Source: Adapted from Sharma (1996).

Taking into consideration dissemination factors that promote utilization of research results, as shown in Box 7.6, to be most effective as a communications or dissemination strategy would include the following 12 components.

1. **Conduct a needs assessment to help shape the dissemination of findings.** One of the most important elements in dissemination to promote use of research findings is adequate understanding of what the users of findings need (Havelock, 1971). Determine the degree of interest among researchers, health professionals, stakeholders, women's groups, and others who work to improve the public's health.
2. **Develop a list of what various people or groups want to know and why they want to know it** (Morris et al., 1987). Consider the decision-making process and the most influential people working on this issue in the setting you are studying. Your stakeholders, including any local study staff and key informants, should also help create this list; do not assume you know all the groups that could benefit from the information. Also, be aware that sometimes stakeholders may not want to disseminate information to certain groups; try to ascertain whom they do not want you to talk to and why. Remember that different groups of people need different kinds of information in different forms and at different times (Morris et al., 1987). Ask who

might be influential in action to improve health conditions, attitudes, programs, or policies suggested by research findings or recommendations and whether such individuals or groups have an explicit advocacy agenda.

Audiences that may be appropriate to involve in dissemination, either as creators or recipients of information related to your study findings, may include other researchers or technical experts, health program directors, planning and finance ministries, donor agencies, news media (see Box 7.5), or nongovernmental or civil society organizations that focus on women's health, human rights, adolescent health, or health policy.

3. **Have a clear idea of the importance (or lack of importance) of your findings to your audiences.** Be realistic. Ask whether the information in your report provides the level of contextual information needed (given current issues and competing knowledge), and ask whether it is:
   - Relevant to the user's real and compelling problems
   - Practical from the user's perspective
   - Useful and applicable to their situation
   - Understandable to potential users
   - Timely (Morris et al., 1987; Westbrook & Boethel, 2006)

4. **Determine whether the findings may have a negative impact or be controversial.** When you originally designed your study, you should have considered the potentially disadvantageous uses of the data you planned to collect. In planning your dissemination strategy, be sure to revisit these issues. Anticipate whether your study results might be embarrassing to program administrators, parliamentarians, or other community leaders accountable for decisions and oversight of health programs and policies (Hess, 1989). Consider whether news media or citizen groups may take the findings out of context. Be aware that "the study will be used, one way or another, and sometimes those uses are different from the ones [the researcher] intends" (Rossman & Rallis, 1998, p. 11).

   Sometimes study findings lend themselves to misinterpretation and therefore need special consideration in dissemination planning. For example, in a combined qualitative and quantitative study of the social and economic consequences of family planning use in the southern Philippines, researchers found that one-fourth of all women, rural and urban, reported ever having been physically harmed by a spouse (Cabaraban & Morales, 1998). The study found that among the significant correlates of violence were the wife working for pay and the husband sharing household chores. When initially presenting these results in the community, some audiences mistakenly concluded that male involvement in cleaning and washing leads to violence. One man commented, "Therefore, in order to avoid violence, we must not do household chores." To correct further misinterpretation of the results, the research team met with stakeholders to develop a dissemination strategy (M. Cabaraban, personal communication, August 2001). Jointly, they developed an approach to serve the community interest while avoiding potential distortion of the data. They recommended that churches use the research results in developing guidelines for marriage counseling, that local institutions be encouraged to provide safe haven and legal services for battered women, and that health providers—including traditional midwives and healers—be trained to provide assistance and referrals for women experiencing violence.

How your study results will be used may be outside your control, but you are responsible for anticipating the potential negative uses of the information. By planning ahead, you can assist stakeholders and members of your research team in preparing for findings that may be controversial or lend themselves to distortion.

5. **Gain an understanding of the criteria the audiences use to assess the information they get.** To promote effective communication, determine which sources of information different groups consider to be credible, useful, or timely (Goldstein, Wrubel, Faifeles, & DeCarlo, 1998). Note the style of dissemination that best meets each group's needs. Some may prefer brief or graphically interesting materials, whereas others do better with a more comprehensive or academically oriented presentation. Spatially referenced results, presented through maps or infographics, are increasingly used to convey information to policy audiences (Moise, Cunningham, & Inglis, 2015). Sometimes written dissemination is not culturally appropriate, whereas a series of community discussions would be. Different groups need different information, in different languages, using different terminology, delivered in formats that respect cultural or other norms. Timing and opportunities for dissemination will also differ by group (Moise et al., 2015).

6. **Identify people to work with.** If you have determined that you have time to disseminate your findings only through written reports or journal articles, consider working with local groups that could plan and implement broader dissemination of the findings. These might include professional associations, librarians, broadcast journalists, NGOs, advocacy groups, or folk media committed to disseminating health messages.

7. **Identify the best people to deliver the information back to key groups interested in the findings.** The knowledge dissemination and use literature shows that information produced internally—in contrast to information imported from outside an organization or a country—is often more acceptable and more credible. Consider various options, including co-presenting

the information with local study staff or a local health program manager who intends to use the findings. Find out if existing consortia, such as a national health task force, can either integrate their dissemination efforts with yours or reinforce your efforts with supporting messages. Offer a local health website the opportunity to post your study report's executive summary, or share your findings with an influential blogger who understands health issues well.

8. **Identify opportunities for dissemination and the possibility of controversy.** Identify other relevant activities going on in the setting (e.g., conferences, events, or media coverage of a related issue) that could either support or conflict with your dissemination plan.

All information is subject to misuse; and no information is devoid of possible harm to one interest or another. Researchers are usually not in a position to prevent action based on their findings; but they should, however, attempt to pre-empt any likely misinterpretations and to counteract them when they occur.

(Association of Social Anthropologists of the UK and Commonwealth, 1999)

In short, plan specific ways to reach out to each important audience through channels that have appropriate "reach, frequency, and cultural impact" (Seidel, 1993, p. 2). One channel that is increasingly used to share research results is social media, described in Box 7.4. If time and financial resources allow you to collaborate with a communications consultant or a local NGO skilled in dissemination, ask them to develop and pretest materials and messages for various intended audiences.

9. **Collaborate with individuals who can help your strategy.** Perhaps you work at a major university and have conducted in-depth interviews on approaches to prevent fall injuries among the elderly in collaboration with research partners in several locations. You might decide—and your study participants might tell you—that health professionals, advocates for senior citizens, and policymakers all could benefit from the findings. In this case your strategic priorities, developed with appropriate input, might be to do the following:

   - Widely disseminate technical data on risk of falling among the elderly and the specific study results (locally, nationally, internationally).

- Help local experts or other partners understand that how they translate findings and technical information into political or programmatic terms is key to gaining support for policy or program changes.
- Build local capacity for ongoing dissemination and policy reform related to injury prevention among the elderly.
- Work with the media to encourage accurate reporting on key findings to audiences concerned with the elderly (see Box 7.3).
- Leverage existing resources, relationships, and professional and social networks (Community Alliance for Research and Engagement [CARE] and Yale Center for Clinical Investigation, 2003) to reach allies and ensure that technical experts in your field understand and can explain your findings to others.

If you intend to influence an audience, know its motivations and its idiosyncrasies.

(Morris et al., 1987, p. 15)

As a researcher, you likely will not implement a comprehensive dissemination strategy without assistance. You may be too busy, may not consider it appropriate, or may not have the needed resources or skills. But your role in identifying dissemination priorities is crucial: You have sifted through the data and articulated what they mean.

10. **Begin disseminating from the outset.** From the first day of your contact with stakeholders, inform them of your study's purpose, its limitations, and its potential outcomes. A participatory approach increases the likelihood that the eventual results will be discussed and used. Where feasible, inviting policymakers to contribute questions of importance to them encourages interest among leaders in a position to initiate change.

11. **Help study participants play an active role in informing others.** Simple early dissemination activities, such as handing out a short letter describing your study's goals, may help to create a climate conducive to research and empower research stakeholders to support your work. Prior to distributing written materials to participants, find out if you will need ethics committees to approve the materials. Be cautious to present such material in a way that avoids implicating individuals as participants in the study, as this would be a breach of confidentiality and could result in social harms. Consider also that once you have provided written materials to individuals or groups, your materials may be inappropriately used or printed in a local newspaper.

12. **Help your readers identify the most important information.** If you are developing printed materials, use headings, write topic sentences, and pay attention to spacing, margins, and graphic design. In short, do what you can to improve the readability of your material (Morris, Fitz-Gibbon, and Freeman, 1987).

Choosing a Format for Dissemination

Qualitative research is primarily about text, although in some research, images, body maps, and photos are used and analyzed as forms of visual language. Like modern scientific writing, which reflects conventions first developed in the late 19th century, qualitative research writing has its own traditions and conventions regarding presentation of data and the visibility or invisibility of the author-researcher in the writing itself. However, these conventions are still evolving as qualitative research expands in its use and application.

An array of stylistic conventions can be used for presentation of qualitative data on public health. Not all qualitative researchers choose conventional scientific formats for presenting findings; many experiment with form, format, voice, shape, and style. Reporting people's insights can be accomplished through genres such as fiction, poetry, performance, graphic arts, photographs, videotapes, and multimedia presentations (Gergen & Gergen, 2000). Other approaches range from testimonials, such as first-person accounts by hospital obstetric patients regarding the quality of labor and delivery services, to scientific papers (covered in Chapter 8), which might include selected quotes from study respondents.

Determining how to write—that is, which presentation style to choose—requires first determining your purpose. Are you writing to influence community opinion leaders, to inform policymakers, or to promote changes in health provider practices? Is your purpose to further academic discussion with scientific colleagues, to satisfy your faculty tenure committee, or to fulfill an obligation to share findings with study participants? Being clear about your purpose and identifying secondary objectives will help you determine what audiences to write for. At the same time, balance your aims with available resources by undertaking a frank assessment of your time and resource constraints.

Writing intended for lay readers or the public typically presents the human face of a persistent public health problem, for example, post-traumatic stress disorder among people exposed to conflict settings. Such writing should either suggest reform of current practices or policies or give guidelines for how to alleviate a problem or improve practices (Denzin & Lincoln, 2000).

Choosing a **dissemination format** requires determining the basic story you are going to tell, who is to do the telling, and what type of narrative format you plan to use to weave your data. Your choice of presentation style will depend on your audience, purpose, and obligation to the study participants. The format you select may also depend on your study's characteristics. For example, a narrowly focused ethnographic study of commercial sex workers in one establishment may lend itself to a narrative style, but a more widely focused study may not. Your selection of a format may be influenced by various other factors as well, including availability of staff time or financial resources for writing, upcoming opportunities for presentation at conferences, or a tradition in your organization to write reports instead of publishing in journals. Once you have ascertained which primary and secondary audiences you intend to reach with your dissemination, you will be able to assess which writing practices would be appropriate for a presentation of methods and findings.

How to Disseminate to Community Stakeholders

When preparing to disseminate study results to members of the local community at large, it is important to use formats that ensure accessibility so that people with various levels of familiarity with scientific research or the study topic will be able to fully understand the results and their significance. Avoid using technical terminology or expressing statistical approaches that lay audiences may not be familiar with or might find confusing, and avoid presentation formats that are better suited to scientists or technical experts. Brainstorm with key informants and other community liaisons about communication formats that will enable you to engage with community audiences and vice versa.

Such formats might involve traditional media like printed materials (e.g., flyers, posters, and newspaper articles) and radio or television programs or announcements, or they could include artistic performances such as theater performed in public gathering spaces. Community meetings are another option and could involve oral or visual presentations and question-and-answer sessions. More formal approaches appropriate for meetings in academic or business settings might consist of presentations in which you use slides summarizing the main findings and their significance. These audiences may also appreciate one- to two-page research briefs or factsheets in which results are summarized. (See Appendix 10 for examples of communication materials distributed to community stakeholders and Case Study 14 in Appendix 1 for an example of developing communication materials in collaboration with community stakeholders.) What you say and how you say it all depends on who your audience is.

In the LinCS 2 Durham HIV prevention study conducted among 18- to 30-year-old African-Americans in Durham, North Carolina, researchers teamed up with community members in the "Collaborative Council" to brainstorm about how to disseminate preliminary study results to different subsets of the community (see Case Study 3 in Appendix 1). The Collaborative Council came up with a diverse set of activities tailored to each audience (Table 7.1). Of note was the group's work with local artists to interpret

Table 7.1 Community Dissemination Formats and Audiences for the LinCS 2 Durham HIV Prevention Study

Presentation Format	Event/Location	Audience
Art exhibition of visual works interpreting study results	Local café	General public
Public service announcement on television	Local public access television stations	General public
Display of flyers briefly describing key points	University campus	University students and faculty
Newspaper article featuring perspective of collaborative council community member	Local African-American newspaper	General African-American public
Posting of summary results	Popular social media site	General public, social media site community
Oral presentations with slides	Local, NC-based professional meeting	Undergraduates, graduate students, and health educators representing a variety of institutions throughout North Carolina
	Multiple university lecture series	Undergraduates, graduate students, and faculty
	Featured topic at regular joint meeting of local health department and community members	Human services practitioners and community members
	Local university community advisory board	Community advisers, including researchers, students, health care professionals; people living with HIV; leaders of area HIV organizations, historically black colleges and universities, and faith-based organizations; and community members
Oral presentations with distribution of flyers briefly describing key points	Meeting with local housing community	Housing community residents

study results in a way that would be visually engaging for the general public, particularly the local African-American community. The resulting artwork was exhibited at a local café, and the art opening featured live music and other artistic performances. Researchers and the Collaborative Council also developed flyers for display on local college campuses and distribution in community meetings, such as in a meeting with members of a local public housing community who were interested in HIV prevention. The flyers briefly summarized key points and used visual representations of statistics rather than numbers alone, as shown in the "Who did we talk to" section of the flyer (Figure 7.2). In addition, the project produced public service announcements that were broadcast on public television stations, posted results on social media sites, and held presentations at academic meetings.

How to Disseminate to Research Participants

Communicating study results to research participants can be a challenging endeavor because of the potential for inadvertent disclosure of participants' identities and social harms resulting from others finding out about an individual's participation in a study. For example, family members unaware of the person's participation may feel that she or he has gone behind their backs; they may also misinterpret participation in a study about prevention of a particular health condition as indication that the person suffers from that condition, or a person's actual health condition might be disclosed. When disseminating study results to participants, therefore, it may be inappropriate to call them to a joint dissemination meeting, contact them in person or by phone, or distribute paper copies of study results to them. More appropriate efforts might be to post or publicize key study results in a public venue where participants, as well as members of the public, can see or hear them. This could include posting flyers in public places, using media such as radio and television to disseminate the results more generally, using artistic performances open to the study community, or using social media or email, being careful not to implicate any individual involved in the study.

How to Disseminate to Policy Audiences

Health policy reform is a process composed of several dynamic, interactive activities: defining a problem, generating solutions, building political consensus (Porter & Hicks, 1995), and advocating for and monitoring implementation (Health Policy Initiative, 2010). If shared effectively, your research findings can influence policy in defining health problems and shedding light on possible solutions. (See Box 7.7 for tips on disseminating to policy audiences.) Translating research findings into terms that address the interests and concerns of decision makers and other groups active in public policy is not

BOX 7.7 POLICY DISSEMINATION TIPS

- Keep reports brief.
- Provide actionable messages for decision makers who may either use or disseminate your study results (Lavis, Robertson, Woodside, McLeod, & Abelson, 2003).
- Recognize that research results may have larger political implications that require the consensus of many stakeholders before action can occur.
- Encourage policymakers to weigh data from different sources.
- In planning for use of information for policy purposes, consider the availability of resources, the institutional capacity to change practices, and political risk (Rist, 2000, pp. 1013–1014).

easy, but it is vital (Porter & Prysor-Jones, 1997). As Rist (2000, p. 1005) notes, "Qualitative research can be highly influential... with respect to problem definition, understanding of prior initiatives, community and organizational receptivity to particular programmatic approaches, and the kinds of impacts (both anticipated and unanticipated) that might emerge from different intervention strategies." Make use of the power of your participants' words and stories to engage those who influence policy. Select the "face" or aspect of the problem that is most relevant to the interests of your particular audience; a simplified understanding of the problem is crucial in generating support for solutions (Porter & Hicks, 1995). (See Appendix 11 for examples of research briefs distributed to policy audiences. Appendix 12 shows a pocket card that was developed as an advocacy tool.)

Identify locally credible champions—not necessarily experts, but respected individuals able to convey research-based information—to make the case for change with those who can actually influence health policies and their implementation. Working to influence policy is a form of behavior change intervention, a field in which both theory and data point to the importance of participative decision making and face-to-face interactions that lead to commitments to change (Stevens & Tornatzky, 1980). Never underestimate the importance of personal contact in your policy dissemination efforts.

When planning for dissemination to policymakers and other local public health stakeholders, consider hosting a half- or full-day meeting in which you invite decision makers or their representatives from key national and local organizations—such as government, private, and nonprofit institutions—to learn the findings. If you worked with local partners, it may be a good idea for them to present some or all of the findings to promote local ownership of the research (see Case Study 8 in Appendix 1).

Develop your list of invitees for the dissemination meeting with local research staff, key informants, or others with an understanding of the politics of dissemination in the local context. It will be important for the people who are most likely to use your research results to attend the meeting. You will want to write a letter inviting the identified individuals or their representatives to attend. In the letter, include the date of the meeting, the location, the name or topic of the meeting, and a short description of the study on which you will be reporting. If possible, include a draft agenda.

When developing the agenda, be sure to balance time for presentations with question-and-answer periods. Provide time for periodic breaks, as well as lunch. In many settings, working lunch meetings are not customary and should be avoided. After the introductory remarks, it may be wise to follow with a general presentation on the health topic in order to ensure that all attendees have the background information necessary to interpret the results of the research. Describe the research, including the participant categories, recruitment methods, when data were collected, the data collection methods, and the quantities of each type of data collected. If you use slides, include a maximum of five bullet points per slide. You might want to prepare discussion questions to stimulate discussion on, for example, the significance of the results and the next steps. Consider ending with a wrap-up session of closing remarks and distribution of an evaluation form.

How to Disseminate to Other Researchers

Many researchers may find dissemination to other researchers to be the most comfortable in terms of knowing the language and style to use. Although we advocate for avoiding technical jargon whenever possible, you can more safely employ technical language when presenting to colleagues, students, professors, or other research scientists than when presenting results to nonresearchers.

Dissemination to other researchers can take written or oral formats or some hybrid of the two. Presentations made at academic or professional meetings are often oral presentations with slides, or they may be poster presentations. Consider printing handouts of your slides or poster for people to take with them, and be sure to include your contact information in case someone has questions about your work. You may also want to use slide presentations during professional working group meetings, brown bag presentations, and of course class presentations.

Writing up your research results for publication in scientific peer-reviewed journals is the other most common form of dissemination to other researchers. We cover this in detail in Chapter 8.

How to Disseminate via Oral Presentations

Oral presentation of qualitative findings is very similar to presentation of quantitative study results, with the distinction that treatment of quotes from participants usually replaces statistical summaries of the data. As with all dissemination formats, be sensitive to audience needs and expectations (e.g., by determining the time your audience has to listen and speaking less than the maximum time allotted); know whether overhead slides or projection images will be better received and what contextual information will be important to provide; and focus on the main question, paying attention to the quality of what you say. Keep in mind who your audience is and what will be of interest to them.

When structuring your oral presentation, include the following four sections:

1. *Opening.* Set the scene by telling a story that will interest your audience.
2. *Introduction.* Tell your listeners what your presentation will cover.
   - What health issue did you study?
   - Why did you conduct the study (objectives), and why was it important?
   - What questions did you ask, and how did they evolve as you analyzed initial responses?
   - What methods did you use, and how close did you get to the participants in the study setting?
   - Which results will you discuss?
3. *Body of the talk.* Discuss your results sequentially, and relate them to your theoretical framework. Clarify each point by using examples and presenting selected short quotes from study participants to illustrate major findings. Offer your interpretation of how applicable the findings may be to other settings, and describe the limitations of your work.
4. *Summary.* Summarize for the audience the important points in your talk. Articulate any unanswered questions, and identify areas that need further study.

Two of the most important elements of successful presentations are (1) to keep overheads, slides, or other visuals short and simple; and (2) to practice giving your talk beforehand. To hold your audience's interest and to share ownership of the findings, consider inviting a key informant or other stakeholder to co-present the findings. Remember that you are sharing the words and experiences of people who entrusted their stories to you. Do not be afraid to try presentation formats that convey the drama and emotion of their lives.

How to Disseminate via Final Reports

At the outset of your project, ascertain any requirements funders might have for end-of-project reporting of study results. Some funders require detailed final reports with executive summaries, while others prefer summary documents, such as research briefs, or they may have their own reporting forms and requirements. Still others may be willing to wait for publications in peer-reviewed scientific journals (see Chapter 8).

If you want to prepare a final report for public health stakeholders such as decision makers or funders, you may choose to follow a fairly standard scientific format. Most final reports follow a general outline as shown in Chapter 8.

In addition, include an executive summary to accompany a more lengthy report if you want to capture the interest of busy policymakers and funders. An executive summary should state the following: (1) what you studied; (2) why you conducted the study; and (3) what major findings, conclusions, and recommendations you have generated. Some readers may not have the time or expertise to read through your report, but they will want to know what you found and how it applies to them.

Outcome Indicators for Dissemination

Outcome indicators for dissemination are measures that tell us whether we have achieved what we intended to accomplish (i.e., the outcomes or effects). Because you do not know precisely where the research will lead or to whom the findings will be important, you cannot define outcome indicators for effective dissemination at the outset of your qualitative study. Nevertheless, as you proceed with the study, do your best to identify appropriate indicators for use of the results. Defining possible ways to measure the effects of dissemination will help focus your efforts on activities with greater impact (Ohkubo, Sullivan, Harlan, Timmons, & Strachan, 2013).

To develop outcome indicators, try to visualize how different groups might use your study to address health care or service delivery problems; how the findings might influence relationships among individuals or groups concerned with your topic; and how your study findings might affect future research, public awareness, or community empowerment to improve health. These possible outcomes may become your outcome indicators for dissemination. They may include changes in the information resources available to stakeholders or changes in their knowledge base, information-seeking behavior, or decision-making processes (Menou, 1993, 1999a, 199b; Thorngate, 1995).

Process indicators for dissemination of study findings are data and indicators compiled at the program level. What might the application of your findings mean to program planning, allocation of resources, procedures, or functions (Buckner, Tsui, Hermalin, & McKaig, 1995)? Process indicators for the short-term or intermediate outcomes (or effects) of public health research dissemination may include the following:

- Publication of study findings in-country as well as internationally
- Presence of study reports in local, national, and international libraries
- News media coverage of study findings
- Number of individuals or groups who need the information reached with summaries of results
- Locally initiated translation of study findings into local languages or easier-to-read formats
- Increase in the number of ongoing opportunities for and instances of communication between community stakeholders and health researchers or policymakers
- Number of short courses or conferences at which study results are disseminated
- Funds allocated for additional communication of results
- Adoption by sister research agencies of future research priorities suggested by your study

The long-term or ultimate outcomes (or impacts) of qualitative research dissemination are harder to measure but nevertheless important (Beck & Stelcner, 1996, 1997). They may include the following:

- The number, variety, and mutuality of relationships between those interested in the health issues you studied and those who are in a position to help them (Cernada, 1982; Havelock, 1971; Human Interaction Research Institute, 1976)
- Enhanced mutual understanding of terminology or language used by different groups (researchers, politicians, community members) to describe health concepts
- Increased accuracy in the information that stakeholders share in dialogue or debate
- Growing respect among research stakeholders for each other's perspectives, manifested in changed attitudes, shared understanding, improved collaboration, and greater degree or regularity of consensus on action steps favoring improved health care delivery (World Bank Institute, 2013b, p. 21 and 68)

- The number, variety, frequency, and persistence of forces that can be mobilized to use the knowledge generated (Havelock, 1971)
- Changes in health services or policies attributable to your research
- A high level of citations of your report in scientific papers and international bibliographic indexing databases
- Increased long-term news media coverage of the topic you studied (as measured through content analyses over time)
- Allocation of funds or government support for further research on aspects of the topic you studied
- Systematic use of study findings in public health, educational, and training institution curricula
- The percentage of organizations that subsequently offered an evidence-based model of services in line with your research findings

Common sense tells us that if we know where we want to go, we are more likely to get there. Identifying outcome indicators for dissemination is one way to keep your sights on the potential use of your study findings by people who need them.

Summary

Researchers have both an ethical and a practical obligation to research participants and the study community to disseminate the results of studies conducted there, as well as to other audiences with a stake in the findings. When study results are shared with a variety of stakeholders at different points in the process, they are more likely to be seen as relevant and consequently to be used. Well-thought-out study communication and dissemination strategies—plans that may be one and the same—will go far to promote use of findings and avoid misinterpretation or inappropriate use. This chapter has presented a variety of communication formats and channels for different purposes and different audiences, including community members, research participants, policy audiences, program managers, or other researchers and technical experts. The effectiveness of these communications can be judged by outcome and process indicators, all of which are part of a comprehensive dissemination design.

By starting the dissemination process early and working methodically through the steps to the end, you can be assured that the results of your study will ultimately reach their goal of better health for the community.

Key Terms

1. **Dissemination:** The act of circulating information about a study to stakeholders, that is, people who share an interest in the research.
2. **Communication strategy:** A plan for two-way communication with stakeholders about a study, including study progress and results.
3. **Dissemination strategy:** A plan for communicating information about a study, typically study results.
4. **Dissemination format:** A stylistic convention for presenting information, including written, oral, and visual forms.
5. **Outcome indicators for dissemination:** Measures that tell researchers whether they have achieved the outcomes or effects they desired to achieve through dissemination.
6. **Process indicators for dissemination:** Measures for dissemination that are compiled at the program level.

Review Questions

1. Why is ongoing dissemination of research important for both researchers and research stakeholders?
2. Imagine that you are planning a study on child mortality and health care-seeking behaviors of mothers in Mozambique. What elements do you need to include in an overall study communication strategy? What specific steps need to be in place in a plan for dissemination of study results? How will you overcome skepticism about the validity or generalizability of qualitative results when addressing policy audiences who consider such research anecdotal?

Recommended Readings

Hovland, I. (2005). *Successful communication: A toolkit for researchers and civil society organisations.* London, UK: Overseas Development Institute.

Meredith, D. (2010). *Explaining research: How to reach key audiences to advance your work.* New York, NY: Oxford University Press.

National Center for the Dissemination of Disability Research. (2001). *Developing an effective dissemination plan.* Austin, TX. Available at http://www.researchutilization.org/matrix/resources/dedp/index.html#ten

Ohkubo, S., Sullivan, T. M., Harlan, S. V., Timmons, B. T., & Strachan, M. (2013). *Guide to monitoring and evaluating knowledge management in global health programs.* Baltimore, MD: Center for Communication Programs, Johns Hopkins Bloomberg School of Public Health. Available at http://www.globalhealthknowledge.org/sites/ghkc/files/km-monitoring-and-eval-guide.pdf

Robinson, E. T., Baron, D., Heise, L. L., Moffett, J., & Harlan, S. V. (2010). Preparing for and disseminating study results. In *Communications handbook for clinical trials: Strategies, tips, and tools to manage controversy, convey your message, and disseminate results* (pp. 86–113). Washington, DC: PATH and Research Triangle Park, NC: Family Health International.

World Bank Institute. (2013). *Art of knowledge exchange: A results-focused planning guide for development practitioners* (2nd ed.). Washington, DC: International Bank for Reconstruction and Development.

References

Association of Social Anthropologists of the Commonwealth. (1999). *Ethical guidelines for good research practice.* Available at http://www.theasa.org/ethics/guidelines.shtml

Barwick, M. (2011). *Making science stick: Developing the KT plan* (webcast #30). Available at http://www.ncddr.org/webcasts/webcast30.html

Beck, T., & Stelcner, M. (1996). *The why and how of gender-sensitive indicators: A project level handbook.* Quebec: Canadian International Development Agency.

Beck, T., & Stelcner, M. (1997). *Guide to gender-sensitive indicators.* Quebec: Canadian International Development Agency.

Buckner, B. C., Tsui, A. O., Hermalin, A. I., & McKaig, C. (1995). *A guide to methods of family planning program evaluation: 1965–1990: With selected bibliography.* Chapel Hill, NC: Evaluation Project.

Cabaraban, M., & Morales, B. (1998). *Social and economic consequences of family planning use in the southern Philippines.* Research Triangle Park, NC: Family Health International.

Cernada, G. P. (1982). *Knowledge into action: A guide to research utilization: Vol. 1. Community health education monographs.* Farmingdale, NY: Baywood.

Community Alliance for Research and Engagement & Yale Center for Clinical Investigation. (2003). *Beyond scientific publication: Strategies for disseminating research findings.* New Haven, CT.

Dagron, A. G. (2001). *Making waves: Stories of participatory communication for social change.* New York, NY: Rockefeller Foundation.

Denzin, N. K., & Lincoln, Y. S. (Eds.). (2000). *Handbook of qualitative research* (2nd ed.). Thousand Oaks, CA: Sage.

Gergen, M. M., & Gergen, K. J. (2000). Qualitative inquiry: Tensions and transformations. In N. K. Denzin & Y. S. Lincoln, *Handbook of qualitative research* (pp. 1025–1026). Thousand Oaks, CA: Sage.

Goldstein, E., Wrubel, J., Faigeles, B., & DeCarlo, P. (1998). Sources of information for HIV prevention program managers: A national survey. *AIDS Education and Prevention, 10*(1), 63–74.

Grande, D., Gollust, S. E., Pany, M., Seymour, J., Goss, A., Kilaru, A., & Meisel, Z. (2014). Translating research for health policy: Researchers' perceptions and use of social media. *Health Affairs, 33*(7), 1278–1285. doi:10.1377/hlthaff.2014.0300

Grimes, D. A. (1999). Communicating research. In P. M. O'Brien & F. B. Pipkin (Eds.), *Introduction to research methodology for specialists and trainees* (pp. 210–217). London, England: FCOG Press.

Havelock, R. G. (1971). *Planning for innovation through dissemination and utilization of knowledge.* Ann Arbor, MI: Center for Research on Utilization of Scientific Knowledge, Institute for Social Research.

Health Policy Initiative, Task Order 1. (2010). *The art of moving from policy to action: Lessons learned from the USAID: Health Policy Initiative (2005–2010).* Washington, DC: Futures Group and Health Policy Initiative.

Heise, L. L., McGrory, C. E., & Wood, S. Y. (1998). *Practical and ethical dilemmas in the clinical testing of microbicides.* New York, NY: International Women's Health Coalition.

Hess, D. J. (1989). Teaching ethnographic writing: A review essay. *Anthropology & Education Quarterly, 20*(3), 163–176. doi:10.1525/aeq.1989.20.3.04x0657g

Huberman, M. (1990). Linkage between researchers and practitioners: A qualitative study. *American Educational Research Journal, 27*(2), 363–391. doi:10.3102/00028312027002363

Huberman, M. (1992). *Linking the practitioner and researcher communities for school improvement.* Keynote address: International Congress for School Effectiveness and Improvement, Victoria, British Columbia.

Human Interaction Research Institute. (1976). *Putting knowledge to use: A distillation of the literature regarding knowledge transfer and change.* Los Angeles, CA: Human Interaction Research Institute.

Joint United Nations Programme on HIV/AIDS. (2000). *Report on the global HIV/AIDS epidemic June 2000.* Geneva, Switzerland.

Kaiser Family Foundation. (2001). *September/October 2001 health news index.* Menlo Park, CA: Harvard School of Public Health.

Kelly, J. A., Somlai, A. M., DiFranceisco, W. J., Otto-Salaj, L. L., McAuliffe, T. L., Hackl, K. L., . . . & Rompa, D. (2000). Bridging the gap between the science and service of HIV prevention: Transferring effective research-based HIV prevention interventions to community AIDS service providers. *American Journal of Public Health, 90*(7), 1082–1088. doi:10.2105/AJPH.90.7.1082

Kitua, A. Y., Mashalla, Y. J. S., & Shija, J. K. (2000). Coordinating health research to promote action: The Tanzanian experience. *British Medical Journal, 321*(7264), 821–823. doi:10.1136/bmj.321.7264.821

Lavis, J. N., Robertson, D., Woodside, J. M., McLeod, C. B., & Abelson, J. (2003). How can research organizations more effectively transfer research knowledge to decision makers? *Milbank Quarterly, 81*(2), 221–248. doi:10.1111/1468-0009.t01-1-00052

Menou, M. J. (1993). *Measuring the impact of information on development*. Ottawa, Canada: International Development Research Centre.

Menou, M. J. (1999a). Electronic communications in African development: Tracking their impact. In S. Macdonald & J. Nightingale (Eds.), *Information and organization: A tribute to the work of Don Lamberton* (pp. 371–392). New York, NY: North-Holland.

Menou, M. J. (1999b). Impact of the Internet: Some conceptual and methodological issues, or how to hit a moving target behind a smoke screen. In D. Nicholas & I. Rowlands (Eds.), *The Internet: Its impact and evaluation*. London, England: ASLIB.

Moise, I. K., Cunningham, M., & Inglis, A. (2015). *Geospatial analysis in global health M&E: A process guide to monitoring and evaluation for informed decision making*. Chapel Hill MEASURE Evaluation, University of North Carolina at Chapel Hill.

Morris, L. L., Fitz-Gibbon, C. T., & Freeman, M. E. (1987). *How to communicate evaluation findings*. Newbury Park, CA: Sage.

Ohkubo, S., Sullivan, T. M., Harlan, S. V., Timmons, B. K., & Strachan, M. (2013). *Guide to monitoring and evaluating knowledge management in global health programs*. Baltimore, MD: Center for Communication Programs, Johns Hopkins Bloomberg School of Public Health.

Population Council. (1994). *Communication strategy: The Africa operations research and technical assistance project II*. [Unpublished manuscript]. New York, NY.

Porter, R. W., & Hicks, I. (1995). *Knowledge utilization and the process of policy formation: Toward a framework for Africa*. Washington, DC: Academy for Educational Development.

Porter, R. W., & Prysor-Jones, S. (1997). *Making a difference to policies and programs: A guide for researchers*. Washington, DC: Academy for Educational Development.

Rist, R. C. (2000). Influencing the policy process with qualitative research. In N. K. Denzin & Y. S. Lincoln (Eds.), *Handbook of qualitative research* (2nd ed., pp. 1001–1017). Thousand Oaks, CA: Sage.

Robinson, E. T., Baron, D., Heise, L. L., Moffett, J., & Harlan, S. V. (2010). *Communications handbook for clinical trials: Strategies, tips, and tools to manage controversy, convey your message, and disseminate results.* Washington, DC/Research Triangle Park, NC: Path and Family Health International.

Rogers, E. M., & Storey, J. D. (1987). Communication campaigns. In C. R. Berger & S. H. Chafee, *Handbook of communication science* (pp. 817–846). Beverly Hills, CA: Sage.

Rossman, G. B., & Rallis, F. R. (1998). *Learning in the field: An introduction to qualitative research.* Thousand Oaks, CA: Sage.

Rothman, J. (1980). *Using research in organizations: A guide to successful application.* Beverly Hills, CA: Sage.

Rubin, H. J., & Rubin, I. S. (1995). *Qualitative interviewing: The art of hearing data.* Thousand Oaks, CA: Sage.

Sechrest, L., Backer, T. E., & Rogers, E. M. (1994). *Synthesis of ideas for effective dissemination. Effective dissemination of clinical and health information: Conference summary* (pp. 187–196). Rockville, MD: Agency for Health Care Policy and Research.

Seidel, R. (1993). *Notes from the field in communication for child survival.* Washington, DC: Academy for Educational Development.

Shapiro, B. (1994). *What children bring to light: A constructivist perspective on children's learning in science.* New York, NY: Teachers College Press.

Sharma, R. R. (1996). *An introduction to advocacy: Training guide.* Washington, DC: Academy for Educational Development.

Smith, W. A. (1995, January 25). *Mass communication for health: A behavioral perspective.* Presentation at the National Academy of Sciences Expert Meeting on Reproductive Health, Washington, DC.

Stevens, W. F., & Tornatzky, L. G. (1980). The dissemination of evaluation: An experiment. *Evaluation Review, 4*(3), 339–354. doi:10.1177/0193841X8000400304

Thorngate, W. (1995). Measuring the effect of information on development. In P. McConnell (Ed.), *Making a difference: Measuring the impact of information on development.* Ottawa, Canada: International Research Centre.

Westbrook, J. D., & Boethel, M. (2006). *General characteristics of effective dissemination and utilization.* Austin, TX: Southwest Educational Development Laboratory.

World Bank Institute. (2013a). *Art of knowledge exchange instrument—Multi-stakeholder dialogue/consultation.* Washington, DC: International Bank for Reconstruction and Development.

World Bank Institute. (2013b). *Art of knowledge exchange: A results-focused planning guide for development practitioners* (2nd ed.). Washington, DC: International Bank for Reconstruction and Development.

World Health Organization. (2006). *Bridging the "know-do" gap: Meeting on knowledge translation in global health.* Geneva, Switzerland.

CHAPTER 8

PUTTING IT INTO WORDS

REPORTING QUALITATIVE RESEARCH RESULTS IN SCIENTIFIC JOURNALS AND REPORTS

OBJECTIVES:

- To describe how to write up qualitative data for scientific audiences
- To frame the write-up of study results as part of responsible conduct of research
- To provide guidance on what to do before, during, and after writing
- To describe how to organize sections of journal articles and reports
- To advise on how to work with co-authors
- To discuss selection of a target journal
- To discuss the importance of distinguishing between presentation and interpretation of results
- To describe use of quotes in write-up of qualitative results
- To present techniques for combining quantitative and qualitative findings
- To provide guidance on submitting an article to a peer-reviewed journal
- To advise on how to respond to the comments of journal reviewers

APPLIED PUBLIC HEALTH RESEARCH frequently has the goals of influencing policy, strengthening programs, or changing health provider practices. The main product of qualitative research, however, is text—articles, reports, books, theses, and data archives.

As researchers, what can we do to make our writing matter and have an impact? What influence do we have over how people will interpret or use the text we have generated? How can we present results convincingly, especially to people who may be more accustomed to understanding issues in quantitative terms (including many journal editors and reviewers)?

Writing up qualitative data is a process that includes determining whom to address and why, revealing one's theoretical and methodological approaches in relation to the data, and dealing with special issues of trustworthiness. This chapter discusses publication of qualitative data in scientific publications. It discusses selecting a target scientific journal, how to organize Methods and Results sections of manuscripts, the importance of distinguishing between presentation and interpretation of results, treatment of quotes, techniques for combining quantitative and qualitative findings, appropriate length, working with co-authors, submission of your article to a journal, and responding to journal reviewers' comments. Most of these elements pertain equally to the writing of technical reports.

While the emphasis in this chapter is writing articles for submission to peer-reviewed journals, qualitative researchers have a variety of options for how to write up findings, depending on their purposes. We present our work in different ways to different audiences, depending on the purpose of the investigation. Applied research may speak to academics interested in the theoretical and methodological base, or the target audience may be health managers vested in solving practical problems in day-to-day work. And, as discussed in Chapter 7, we sometimes direct research results to lay audiences who have their own needs for information or to intermediaries, such as news media, who have a "knowledge translation" function. Whether presenting research results in scientific publications or in reports to donors, managers, or civil society advocates, the researcher must apply the same criteria of clarity, persuasiveness, and honesty to the needs of these different audiences.

Writing up qualitative research "convert[s] private problems into public issues, thereby making collective identity and collective solutions possible."

(Richardson, 1990, p. 28)

The Role of Writing in Responsible Conduct of Research

The very nature of qualitative research—the active generation of insights and meaning by study participants sharing their stories—has important practical and ethical implications for how researchers report study findings. Writing up your research results is a normative and important step in the responsible conduct of research, and it is an assumed element in research integrity (Northern Illinois University, 2004). Publishing is a key way to make your results accessible and known so that they can later be applied in valuable ways. Be aware of qualitative reporting conventions even before you begin your study, and use them to guide your work.

In general, the ethical norms that govern how we write about people's lives include "the four non-negotiable journalistic norms of accuracy, nonmaleficence, the right to know, and making one's moral position public" (Denzin & Lincoln, 2000, pp. 902–903). When you write up sensitive information on public health, keep four basic principles in mind:

1. *Aim for balance and accuracy, not neutrality.* Qualitative writing aims for balance and accuracy in reporting findings, not neutrality. It presents multiple sides of the particular public health issue being studied. It aims to elicit the knowledge, understandings, and insights of the research participants and to present their insights in context.
2. *Ensure that no harm comes to participants.* You must not only ensure that no harm comes to those interviewed as a result of their participation in a study, but you must also ensure that no harm comes to them as a result of the publication, presentation, or dissemination of their views or experiences. Even when the published work does not give names, some information could reveal the identity of some participants.
3. *Give public voice to findings by sharing participants' own words.* The aim of most social scientific inquiry is to generate knowledge and insights for the scientific community and ultimately to benefit society. The tradition in qualitative research of presenting study participants' insights in their own words is both a philosophical commitment and a qualitative writing norm. Try to include quotes or even brief phrases (if possible, in the participants' original language, along with translation). By presenting participants' perspectives in their own words, you both empower them and convey important contextual information to readers, such as depth, detail, emotionality, and nuance (Denzin & Lincoln, 2000).
4. *Describe the context of your interactions and disclose your role.* Generally, qualitative researchers learn about other people through interaction in specific roles such as interviewer/interviewee or participant-observer/persons observed (Richardson, 1990). If you are conducting team-based research, particularly in developing country settings where you may not know the local language(s), local members of the research team may be collecting the data and your role might be as lead investigator. In order to judge the quality of the research, readers must have adequate information about when and how you or your team gathered information, awareness of the nature

of the relationship of the data collector(s) and investigators with those studied (your conversational partners), and knowledge of your standpoint and motivation in carrying out the study.

Before You Write

Recognize When to Write

Many investigators new to qualitative methods ask when they should begin writing up research for publication. Because qualitative research generates rich information, determining where to focus one's attention, getting organized, and deciding on the level of detail to be shared is often difficult. How do you know when your research process has reached the writing stage? Do you have other considerations—time, money, donor interest, and so on—that may impose time frames of their own?

You do not need to have the entirety of the study data analyzed before writing up the results of a particular component or topic area, depending on the breadth of your study. You can also begin to work on some sections of your article or report even before completing the data analysis, such as conducting a literature review for eventual use in the Introduction or Discussion sections and for drafting the Methods section. However, once you have completed data analysis, we recommend turning your attention to writing up your results.

How do you know when you have completed data analysis? When you have come as close as possible to the point of saturation in your analysis of a given dataset (you may have multiple sets or categories of data in a single study)—that is, where additional data are not yielding new insights—you are ready to write up those results. At this point, if you have followed a systematic research process, you should have a full set of files that document your reflections on what you have learned. You will also have the following:

- A final list of codes
- Tables, matrices, or other summary devices that identify aspects of the public health concepts you have studied
- A clear understanding of the thematic structure: how your themes fit together and how they relate to your conceptual framework

In conducting your study, you have generated information in the form of text, photos or images, and perhaps numbers. As you interpreted and analyzed the information you gathered, you also began to write up your thinking. You may have made notes in the margins of your transcripts or used notes or memo functions in coding software (e.g., "most married women are reluctant to ask husbands to use condoms"), or you may have determined text headings to depict sort categories (e.g., "fear of pregnancy" or "fear of sterility"). Now your task is to put what you have learned from the study into a narrative: to produce text that weaves everything together and will make sense to your intended readers—text that members of the group you have studied would also consider accurate and complete.

Chronicle What You Have Learned

There is an intermediate step between data analysis and compiling a report, writing for scientific publication, or preparing a presentation: writing a chronicle of what you have learned. After completing data analysis and before beginning to write your article or report, take time to articulate how your data fit together with respect to particular objectives (i.e., of the study or of a particular analysis) or themes. Take the insights you have gathered and start writing what you have learned. Your task is to take all you know and make it concrete for yourself in a relatively concise summary. Later you will use this summary to organize your Results section.

Different qualitative researchers develop distinct processes for figuring out how their data weave together into a coherent picture. People who are more visually oriented may return to their visual or graphic diagram of how the key themes or concepts fit together, as described in Chapter 6. To then summarize these data in prose, they touch on each aspect of the diagram, writing a few sentences describing how the concepts are related.

Qualitative researchers who take a more verbal approach may use the process of writing itself to think through relationships in the data. This entails taking the data as summarized in tables, matrices, or memos and beginning to arrange and juxtapose themes within a word processing document to see how they relate to one another. Then think through these relationships by writing what is effectively a first iteration of the Results section of a scientific manuscript or report.

Another approach to sorting out the links between study themes is to convene a meeting of key informants and the research team, break into small groups to discuss how the themes fit, then reconvene as a larger group to work toward consensus on the meaning of the data and relationships among key ideas. Documenting conclusions drawn during the meeting will be an important starting point for developing a written account of the relationships among your data.

With any of these approaches, begin by clustering the fragments of thematic ideas and integrating them into a meaningful account of what is going on. Talk about linkages and interrelationships you see among ideas or themes. You may take different vantage points on the findings—a gender or economic perspective, for instance—but focusing on a clearly defined aspect of the material will help you organize your account. Your report will be more credible if it is organized around a conceptual framework, if the framework is elaborated throughout the report, and if it is supported with adequate qualitative evidence (Lofland, 1974).

Often there is more than one possible analysis for a study, and you will need to focus on a particular set of findings for a particular scientific article. (Reports may comprise more comprehensive accounts of what you found in your study.) One mistake qualitative researchers sometimes make is attempting to include too much data of too wide a scope in a given article, particularly for complex studies. Keep in mind that it may be possible to write more than one article for a given study, although journals discourage the practice of slicing up the data artificially simply to have multiple publications.

Having a clear understanding of how your concepts are linked is the most important signal that your analysis is finished. If you are getting ready to write your article or report and do not yet have a clear understanding of how key themes fit together, go back to your data before proceeding.

Choose an Audience and Format

Before you begin to write, consider whom you want your findings to reach. In general, those writing for academic audiences and public health researchers and practitioners commonly choose to submit their articles to social science, health, policy, or medical journals.

Such papers typically articulate conceptual frameworks or theories, describe methodologies used, present results, interpret the data, and relate findings to other published study findings. Papers published in journals for less academic audiences, including some health practitioners, may also provide theoretical frameworks for better understanding an issue, such as the gender dimensions of risk behavior and sexually transmitted infection (STI). Writing that targets an audience of health providers often includes concrete suggestions for better practices, as well as broad policy recommendations. See Box 8.1 for the standard format for scientific papers.

If you want to reach policymakers or funders, reports or briefs are commonly used. Reports are typically less theoretically oriented, start out with an executive summary for busy readers and may include recommendations. (In Chapter 7 we discuss other formats appropriate for disseminating research results to different types of stakeholders, including policymakers, research participants, and community members.)

Like modern scientific writing, which reflects conventions first developed in the late 19th century, qualitative research writing has its own traditions and conventions regarding presentation of data and the visibility or invisibility of

BOX 8.1 HOW TO ORGANIZE A STANDARD SCIENTIFIC ARTICLE OR REPORT

If you want to publish in a **peer-reviewed journal**, you may choose to follow a fairly standard scientific format. Most journals limit articles to 3,500 to 5,000 words, plus references and two to three tables. Many research organizations choose to write reports instead of publishing in journals, with reports following this same general outline:

I. Introduction
   A. Context
      1. The general state of your field (e.g., malaria-related mortality and existing prevention approaches)
      2. Relevant background
   B. Literature review
      1. Relevant facts about your focus from previous studies
      2. Questions unanswered by previous studies
         a. Specific knowledge gap that your study seeks to address; your specific focus (e.g., community perceptions of malaria prevention interventions)
         b. Brief description of the study
   C. Purpose of the study, including main research question and summary of basic approach used to answer it
   D. Brief description of the study
      1. Who did the study, where, and when
      2. Very brief description of the methods and participants, with some indication of the scale of the study
      3. Mention of relevant cultural or contextual information (e.g., religion or religiosity, socioeconomic context)
      4. Anticipated contribution of study results (potential implications)

(Continued)

BOX 8.1 HOW TO ORGANIZE A STANDARD SCIENTIFIC ARTICLE OR REPORT (Continued)

II. Methods

E. Study design

F. Sampling methods

G. Data collection methods (including how data collectors were trained)

H. Data analysis methods

I. Ethics statement (e.g., IRB approval or waiver)

III. Results

A. Presentation of the results, including any figures or tables. (Note that study reports tend to be longer than journal articles and often present more detailed results, whereas journal articles focus on key results and tend to not have more than five tables.)

IV. Discussion

A. Interpretation of the findings

B. How the results relate to earlier studies and your conceptual framework

C. Strengths of your study and what it contributes to the knowledge base

D. Limitations, including how methodological issues could have affected results

E. Recommendations for policy, service delivery, or community action (as applicable)

F. Logical next steps for research

V. Conclusion

A. Implications of findings for the specific purpose of the study

B. Importance of the results to others thinking about the problem

VI. Acknowledgments

VII. Bibliographic references and citations

the author-researcher in the writing itself. For example, the concepts of voice and reflexivity are of central importance in qualitative writing. Reflexivity in writing means letting readers see our individual insights as historically, culturally, and personally situated. Because qualitative research always explores the context in which phenomena occur, qualitative writing involves presenting relevant aspects of the larger historical, political, cultural, or scientific context of the issues we study and the findings we generate.

IMRAD Format

Writing scientific publications and reports constrains the types of accepted formats you might use to present your findings and interpretations. In this chapter, we present the most common organization of content used in both articles and reports: Introduction, Methods, Results, and Discussion (IMRAD) sections.

Variations in the Standard IMRAD Format for Reports However, for reports, depending on your study, purposes, and audience, you may need to modify the standard IMRAD structure to fit your material. The major sections of your report outline should reflect your audience's information needs and other factors, such as the importance you assign to discussion of theory. Other widely used approaches to organizing qualitative writing include much of the same material as presented in a standard scientific report, but with certain variations in the ordering of contents.

Problem-Solving Approach State the problem and describe the importance of the research topic and its implications for health policies or practices or its impact on theory. Briefly describe your methods. State what you have learned about individual public health themes or concepts. Offer your conclusions.

Narrative Approach Tell your story by way of a chronological narrative, illustrating a problem or process (such as barriers related to stigma that HIV-positive women experience as they attempt to access the cascade of prevention of mother-to-child transmission services) step-by-step or from multiple perspectives. A narrative approach can be very dramatic; see an example in Ronai (1995). In your conclusion, explain why and how the process occurs. For example, if your study examines community perspectives on female genital cutting and adherence to the practice varies from village to village, you might organize your findings by site.

Policy Approach Present a conclusion as to why a process or behavior occurs or fails. Walk through the evidence to show how you reached this conclusion. Journalistic and policy-oriented reports typically follow this pattern, which is ideal for busy readers who have little time for reading a lengthy article until they have grasped the relevance of the material. (See example of a policy brief on the female condom in Appendix 11.)

Analytic Approach Organize your findings in terms of the theoretical or conceptual framework you used to develop your study. Describe what you have learned and how it fits in the larger framework. (For an example, see Hardee, Irani, & Rodriguez, forthcoming). If you use a locus of control model (Rotter, 1966) to examine domestic violence, for example, explain how your findings support or differ from the model and related thinking. If you used a conceptual model to guide your study design, explain how the model may have changed as a result of your qualitative analysis. (See Appendix 1, Case Study 4 and supplementary case study materials on sustained acceptability of vaginal microbicides.)

Select a Target Journal for Your Scientific Article

If you have identified publication in a scientific journal as the most appropriate format for your audience, it is time to identify two to three potential journals to target. There are several factors to consider when deciding where to submit.

Consider the subject and geographical areas of your study. Some journals focus on a particular public health issue or disease, whereas others are broader in scope, focus on specific methodologies, or are domestically or internationally focused. It is also essential to identify journals that publish the kind of data that you have, that is, qualitative data or a combination of qualitative and quantitative data. A third factor to consider is which journals reach your intended audience(s). This involves thinking about issues of access: Do you want to submit your article to an open-access journal that anyone with an Internet connection can access (knowing that this will incur a fee on your part or the part of your funding mechanism or employer)? Or will your audience have access to journals requiring a subscription, perhaps through their institutions? Look into the types of articles the journals publish, for example, research articles, brief communications, case studies, review articles, research notes, commentaries, and so forth. Lastly, you will want to be aware of the word count limits for your article type. A complex qualitative study may be difficult to present in 3,500 words, but some journals, particularly open-access journals, have longer or no word limits. All of this information is typically found on the journal's website in the instructions for authors.

You may wish to consult your colleagues for suggestions about possible journals or to see whether your tentative target journals are realistic options. You can also query the editor of a journal to see whether your paper topic would be suitable for publication in the journal.

After you have narrowed down your list of potential journals to two or three, rank them in order of preference. The reason for having a ranked list is to expedite resubmission of your article to another journal, which you will have already identified, in the event that the article is not accepted by the first journal.

Once you have identified your target journals as well as determined your audience and the basic format you will follow, find and read examples of articles that address audiences and studies similar to yours. Your target journals are a good place to look for such articles. Analyzing styles and formats used by other researchers in your field can help you organize your data and insights effectively. In addition, these are *published* articles, and since your goal here is to publish your article, their style and format may be worth emulating.

For example, if you are writing about a series of focus group discussions on health decision making, try to find articles that describe research that uses comparable methodologies. Consider the following:

- How is the material organized?
- Does your material lend itself to this kind of format?
- How does the author describe his or her methods and analysis strategies?
- Where is the author in the text? How has the author dealt with reflexivity; that is, how has the author revealed his or her standpoint vis-à-vis the topic (Richardson, 1990)?

You will need to anticipate the approximate length of your manuscript, based on the target journal's word limits, so that you can balance detail with space considerations. Even for journals without word limits, it is important to provide enough description to convey meaning but without overwhelming the reader with length. The level of detail you provide about your study and the length of your writing will depend to a large extent on the audience you choose to address. (See Appendix 13 for information on where to publish qualitative studies on public health.)

Finally, if you are writing as a research team, determine from the outset who will be an author, agree on roles before you begin, and verify once done that the author order fairly reflects contributions.

Authorship Considerations for Scientific Articles

Who Qualifies as an Author?

Most journals specify who qualifies to be listed as an author. Typically, and according to the International Committee of Medical Journal Editors

(ICMJE) (see http://www.icmje.org/recommendations/browse/roles-and-responsibilities/defining-the-role-of-authors-and-contributors.html), one of the most widely accepted sources, co-authors need to meet all of the following four criteria:

1. Substantial contributions to the conception or design of the work or the acquisition, analysis, or interpretation of data for the work
2. Drafting the work or revising it critically for important intellectual content
3. Final approval of the version to be published
4. Agreement to be accountable for all aspects of the work in ensuring that questions related to the accuracy or integrity of any part of the work are appropriately investigated and resolved

Given these criteria, ghost writers do not qualify for authorship. Some journals also require that the contributions of each author be spelled out as part of the manuscript submission to ensure that each author listed indeed qualifies. People who contributed to the study but who do not meet the criteria should be thanked in the acknowledgments section.

One way of involving co-authors in the development of a manuscript is by having different people write particular sections. For example, someone who co-analyzed the data might write a paragraph on data analysis for the Methods section and write up a portion of the results. Or, collaborators in the field might draft the description of data collection and verify that the results have been represented accurately and interpreted in a way that makes sense locally. It is also often very worthwhile to tap your co-authors for their ideas about what to include in the Discussion section, including what they see as the significance of the research and its strengths and limitations. If you want your collaborators to appear as authors but they have not been involved in drafting the manuscript, it is imperative to include them in the review process so that they have the opportunity to make contributions to the intellectual content of the paper by providing critical feedback. (See Appendix 14 for more information.)

Authorship Agreements

You will quite likely have co-authors on your article or report. With scientific articles in particular, conflicts sometimes arise about who qualifies to be an author and in what order they will appear on the manuscript. To preempt such conflicts, it can be a good idea to draft an authorship agreement before you begin to write. The agreement should spell out the authorship requirements, such as the ones listed previously. You will also want to indicate who, specifically, will be listed in each position, as well as the conditions under which the order will be changed or a person removed from the list entirely. Lastly, the agreement should contain a description of the responsibilities of each author.

Author Order

There are no standard rules on the order in which to list the authors of the paper. However, in the field of public health, it is common for the lead author of the paper to be listed first. Often, if the principal investigator is a different person from the lead author, she or he will be listed in the last position. The positions in between first and last can vary and might be determined according to contributions to the drafting of the manuscript or by contributions to the research itself. Tentative author order should be determined at the beginning of the writing process; it can subsequently be adjusted to reflect the weight of each person's contributions.

Writing Your Article or Report

Each researcher's writing style and process are different. Here we present an approach that has helped many authors ensure that their writing is succinct and covers what they focused on, why they studied the topic, how they conducted the research, what they found, how they interpreted their findings, and the implications of their work. In addition, see Box 8.2 for a checklist of what to include in study write-ups.

Statement of Purpose

Before launching into the writing of your article or report, write a statement of purpose. This helps you find and maintain a focus (Wolcott, 1990). Here are two examples:

> Given the relative novelty of Option B+ [lifelong antiretroviral therapy to all pregnant women living with HIV] as a "treatment as prevention" programme, it is important to widely explore the risks and benefits of the intervention, as well as feasibility and costs, particularly for women living with HIV who are the end users of the programme.... [We] aimed to assess how Option B+ is understood and accepted by the population that will receive the programme [in Malawi and Uganda], and to ensure that their perceptions, values, and preferences are considered during the [WHO] guidelines development process.
>
> *(Global Network of People Living with HIV, 2013)*

> Access to health information in developing countries is key not only for designing sound health programs at the national level but also for implementing quality services at the facility and health post level. We conducted a qualitative study to document current systems and resources for managing and sharing health information; analyze the use of family planning and reproductive health information by health professionals, communicators, policymakers, and professional networks; identify obstacles to information sharing; and identify perceived needs and recommendations for strengthening knowledge management systems. The results from this study are intended to inform national efforts to strengthen access to and use of health information in Senegal.
>
> *(Sylla, Robinson, Raney, & Seck, 2012)*

Do not continue writing your article until you are satisfied that your brief statement of purpose captures the essential components of your study: what you looked at and where, and how and why you studied it.

Outline

Next, put together a detailed written outline or list of topics in the order you plan to present them. In addition, decide first how you are going to present your authorial voice (Wolcott, 1990). Your stance or voice should reflect the basic processes of data collection used in your study. Rubin and Rubin (1995, p. 268) recommend that "if the interviews were deeply interactional, with the parties exploring ideas together and coming up with a joint conclusion, then the researcher's voice and role should be apparent in the report."

Once you have identified your audience, chosen a presentation format, written a clear statement of purpose, and written an outline, you should be ready to begin your article or report. We discuss next what is typically included in the main report sections—Introduction, Methods, Results, Discussion, and Conclusion—and where that differs from scientific writing on quantitative studies.

Introduction Section

A good rule of thumb for the introduction of a scientific article is to go from broad to narrow. That is, start by presenting the broader context of the topic first. With each succeeding paragraph, narrow down the information you

BOX 8.2 CONTENT CHECKLIST: WHAT TO INCLUDE IN STUDY WRITE-UPS

Whether you write up your data as an oral history, final report, or a scientific journal article, your manuscript will need to answer the following questions:

- What was the research question, and in what context does the problem exist?
- How was the research designed?
- What techniques or methodologies did you use for data collection and analysis? What types of data were collected?
- Why were the research design, sampling strategies, data collection approaches, and analysis techniques appropriate to the question you posed in the particular context of your research?
- Was the research process iterative?
- Is the interpretive process used in the analysis clearly described?
- What did you find out, and what do you think it means?
- What was your relationship with informants, and how did you and they influence each other during the research process?
- Have you demonstrated an understanding of the world portrayed in your text in a way that readers will feel accurately represents the local perspective?
- Have you conveyed adequate levels of detail about the people and context you studied, including specialized or commonly used language regarding the aspect of public health you examined?
- Have you grounded your findings by systematically integrating negative cases and contrasting them with cases that are very different (Flick, 1998)?
- Have you explicitly shared with readers your own personal biases, perspectives, and motivations and how these might affect your research?
- What were the limitations in your study?

Sources: Adapted from Golden-Biddle and Locke (1999); Miller and Crabtree (2000).

present until you finally present your statement of purpose at the close of the introduction.

For example, if you studied maternal mortality in the Dominican Republic by interviewing husbands of women who died in childbirth, you could begin by citing the epidemiologic and ethnographic literature on maternal mortality in independent nations in the Caribbean region. A good starting point for your literature review is the background or introductory section of your study protocol, which should include information on the topic area and geographical context of your study, as well as the relevance of the study in relation to what is already known about the topic. After mining the study protocol, do a literature search to identify articles published since the study protocol was written.

This brief summary of existing knowledge would be followed by data specific to the Dominican Republic, including important aspects of the local context or culture, such as prevailing cultural or religious beliefs. Studies in sexual and reproductive health often include reproductive history of the study population, as well as number of pregnancies, age at first birth, and contraceptive use. You may also want to present literature on the methodology that you used—in this case, literature on the use of family members as key respondents for reporting reproductive health events. Describe how your topic and design fit in the existing body of literature on the topic you are studying.

The last paragraph of your introduction should state succinctly what you studied, where, and when; list the basic methodology used; and include the potential use of your results. For example:

> We conducted qualitative in-depth interviews with husbands of women who had died in childbirth in [city name], Dominican Republic, in 2016. Our objective was to learn husbands' perceptions of maternal mortality, including its causes and lived consequences, as well as whether and how it might be avoided. It is our hope that the results will be of interest to program planners working to reduce maternal mortality in the Dominican Republic and similar Caribbean contexts.

Methods Section

The Methods section is where you describe what you did to conduct the study and analyze the study data. Describe how you went about your study in as much detail as space allows, presenting those aspects that most affected the collection and analysis of data. This is the place to discuss any problems you encountered during data collection that may have had an impact on your ability to achieve the study objectives.

Because this section concerns what you *did*, in the past, it should be written in the past tense. Subheadings like those used for the sections that follow may help to organize your account (e.g., study context, data collection, data analysis, ethics statement), but they should be adapted to your particular case because they are not standard.

Study Context

Name the study site(s) and describe the geographical and cultural contexts of the study. In addition, provide the reader with information that conveys the scope of the public health problem in that context. For example, in a study of health beliefs related to diabetes among Bangladeshis in the United Kingdom (Greenhalgh, Helman, & Chowdhury, 1998), the authors provided important cultural, gender, and dietary contexts:

> In 1971 Bengal seceded from Pakistan and became the separate state of Bangladesh. The country is flat, with a monsoon climate, prone to flooding, and served mainly by inland waterways. The economy is pre-industrial, and most people live in scattered homesteads with an atomistic social organisation (that is, the family is the dominant unit with no effective social organisation or hierarchy beyond the family). The staple crop is rice, and the diet is largely fish, rice, and vegetables. Although about 95% of the population is Muslim, the society contains vestiges of its Buddhist and Hindu cultural roots. In the 1960s and '70s, large numbers of economic migrants came to Britain, particularly from certain villages in rural Sylhet. Men tended to emigrate several years before their wives followed.
>
> *(Greenhalgh et al., 1998)*

Data Collection

An important part of the Methods section is a detailed description of the data collection itself. If you collaborated with other organizations or institutions for any aspect of your study, name them and describe their overall roles. Did another group provide input on the development of the data collection materials? Conduct the data collection? Analyze the data? Note in the text that you (and your team, if applicable) were trained in research ethics and qualitative data collection methods (plus quantitative methods for a mixed-methods study). For example, orientation for interviewers would have included an introduction to ethical issues such as transparency, confidentiality, and treatment of sensitive topics (Barnett & Stein, 1998).

Also include the dates of data collection, what types of methods were used, and how many of each type of data (e.g., interviews, focus groups) were collected, and in what language(s). Note how the data were collected and documented. Were interviews recorded, transcribed, and translated? Was a checklist used for observations? Were field notes taken? It can also be useful to provide the objective(s) of each type of data collection, such as by listing broad topic domains from the interview guides. This helps the reader know what you intended to learn from each category of data collected. You will often have included this information in your study protocol.

Describe your participant sample. It may make sense to weave the broad description of your sample into the discussion of each type of data collection event. For example, you might say, "The local data collection staff conducted eight focus groups: four with married women ages 18 to 35 and four with married men 18 to 35." Also make sure to describe your final sample, including sociodemographic characteristics such as age, marital status, religion, sex, education, and other descriptive information related to the research problem. Presenting this information in a table format is often reassuring to audiences who are more familiar with quantitative methods.

A clear description of the sampling process, along with a brief explanation of how you recruited participants, will add credibility to your results. If space allows, many readers will be interested to know how you gained access to the interviewees and why they were willing to talk to you (Rubin & Rubin, 1995). How long were you in the field and what was your role? By presenting context and events related to the data collection, you are inviting the reader to be present in the study situation, which in turn will lead to better understanding of the findings.

Data Analysis

Last, discuss how you analyzed the field data. Who conducted the data analysis? What software was used? Describe the process for analyzing the data and its iterative steps. If multiple people coded the qualitative data, how was intercoder reliability assessed? Under what circumstances and how was information cross-checked? How were data reduced? Tell the reader what steps you took in the study to ensure that the study question and results were consistent with the participants' views of their world.

Ethics Statement

The Methods section should always include an ethics statement. This is a paragraph that describes the ethical approval(s) obtained prior to commencing the study, specifies that informed consent was obtained from research participants, and describes safeguards for ensuring the confidentiality of the participants' identities. This typically appears at the end of the Methods section, but there is no set rule for where this statement should be located; thus, use your judgment to identify the most logical placement. The statement often carries its own subheading, such as "Ethics" or "Ethics Statement."

Results Section

The Results section is where you present the findings from your study. It is essential to make a clear distinction between the presentation and interpretation of your results by locating them in the Results and Discussion sections, respectively. On the one hand, virtually every stage of your work at this point is simultaneous analysis and interpretation; your study findings in the Results are, in fact, interpreted data. However, interpretation in the sense of your reflections about what you believe the findings *mean* in relation to other data or other questions belongs in the Discussion section rather than in the Results section. Write this section in the past tense.

Presenting Your Findings

There are many ways to present qualitative data. A typical way is to move through themes sequentially as you follow the evolution of some issue. With this approach, how you order your presentation of themes is like constructing an argument. "Qualitative theory is developed by elaborating and interpreting the unexpected and the apparently contradictory. If you have evidence for both sides of an argument, then present it and explain it" (Rubin & Rubin, 1995, p. 263). For example, in a qualitative study in Haiti of women's roles in sexual decision making, the authors led the reader through five themes to illustrate how Haitian women's capacity to negotiate safe sexual behavior, including the use of condoms, may be related less to their knowledge of AIDS than to the powerlessness they feel as a result of economic dependency (Ulin, Cayemittes, & Metellus, 1995). Expanding on key thematic ideas, they present a range of study participant perceptions and descriptive information about participants who offer comments and quotes that illustrate both themes (e.g., beliefs about vulnerability to and consequences of AIDS) and subthemes (e.g., social rejection, destruction of family, uncertainty about a spouse's fidelity) that they determine to be important. Following this presentation of results, the authors offer a conclusion, which contains their analysis of the findings with regard to the eight specific study objectives posed at the outset of their investigation. They present the Conclusion section much like a series of distinct Discussion sections for a scientific journal article, each about a page long. Finally, the authors end with a Recommendations section, presenting their viewpoint on the study's implications for intervention.

You can also organize the presentation of your findings to reflect aspects of your research design, for instance, by presenting the results of each type of data collection and/or participant category. For multicountry qualitative studies, some investigators choose to present results by country, and then within each country by the main study questions or themes, with the synthesis of cross-country themes in the Discussion section (e.g., Global Network of People Living with HIV, 2013). In this approach, the order of presentation of results is parallel to the order in which study methods were described.

Whatever your approach, if your presentation of findings is logical and coherent, you increase the probability that readers will accept your work. Having a consistent structure for presenting results helps you organize the material more efficiently and will help those who read your article make sense of the information. This principle is valid even when dealing with multiple sources of data and presenting highly complex issues. The use of subheadings, for example, to indicate each theme is strongly recommended to help your reader follow your organizational structure.

One of the greatest challenges that qualitative researchers have in writing up findings is to remain focused on the research questions and objectives while linking the questions to the findings. In qualitative research, the study findings—which are the product of analysis—are the researcher's insights from sorting the data, identifying a small handful of key themes, describing how they fit together, and understanding how they fit in the larger sociocultural context. Quotes from participants, the raw data, should not be considered or presented as results but rather as illustrations of insights arrived at through your analysis. Just as a quantitative researcher would not provide raw line listings in the Results section of a paper, a qualitative researcher must do more than present strings of quotes. The results or findings represent a synthesis. The quotes provide richness and detail.

Tables, Figures, and Maps

Tables can be an effective way to summarize qualitative data in the Results section, especially when illustrating differences among subsamples or results yielded by different qualitative techniques (e.g., structured interviews vs. questionnaires).

Be sure to create a title for each table and figure and to reference each table and figure in the text. Note that it is customary not to present information in the text that is already presented in a table. Instead, simply refer the reader to the table. You may, however, summarize or highlight results presented in a large table in your text. For example:

> As Table 3 shows . . . at the health district level, most health centers and a few health posts have computers with Internet connections. In contrast, access to these technologies is virtually nonexistent at the community level.
>
> *(Sylla et al., 2012)*

Make use of numerical tables and other quantification where you can. It can help your readers learn, for example, that "individuals in all but one of the six focus groups believed in some way that the oral polio vaccine spreads HIV." Appropriate use of numbers gives readers an indication of the relative importance of an idea and allows them to weigh the evidence you present. (See Box 8.3 on writing results from mixed-methods studies.) But be careful! One of the most common mistakes in reporting qualitative research is to treat

BOX 8.3 HOW TO ORGANIZE AND REPORT FINDINGS FROM MIXED-METHOD STUDIES

A structure that works particularly well for studies using more than one methodological approach is to organize the presentation of all findings by key themes. You will need to be selective in your choice of themes; with so much data, it will be essential to leave some material out. As you write, guide the reader through findings from one methodological approach, present the findings from a different approach, and then tell the reader what you think the combined findings mean regarding that theme. After treating all your key themes sequentially in this way, write a conclusion that explains the linkages between themes, explains the findings in light of your theoretical framework, examines how applicable the findings would be in other contexts or with other groups, and discusses whether the findings are consistent with other studies.

Sometimes a study that uses both quantitative and qualitative methods gives different results when examining the same phenomenon. Reaching a unifying conclusion regarding discrepant findings is not your responsibility, but you should present these contradictions and offer supporting data for the reader to assess.

(Continued)

BOX 8.3 HOW TO ORGANIZE AND REPORT FINDINGS FROM MIXED-METHOD STUDIES (Continued)

In his combined-methods study of sexual cultures and sexual health among young people in Lima, Peru, one author (Cáceres, 1999) begins by presenting his study objectives and discussing the social theories or philosophies he employs. Second, he outlines the qualitative and quantitative phases of his study, describing the tools and processes used in data collection and analysis, stating ethical considerations, and providing sociodemographic information on the study population. Next, he leads the reader through each thematic topic, alternately presenting qualitative and quantitative findings, as available. He organizes the findings by thematic areas: gender images and norms, factors in sexual socialization, sexual experience, the process of sexual initiation, the structure of sexual risks, and special contexts for sexual experience (paid sex, coercive sex, and concomitant use of alcohol or drugs).

In writing on sexual risk, Cáceres presents quantitative data on the proportion of young women who report having experienced undesired pregnancy and on cofactors for undesired pregnancy. Without interrupting the narrative flow of his elaboration on this phenomenon, he shifts into qualitative findings regarding young people's thoughts on factors that lead to undesired pregnancy, factors such as the relative stability of the couple or the use of tricks by one partner to achieve pregnancy as a way of trapping the other in the relationship. In his analysis he provides selected quotes by adolescent study participants to illustrate key insights. Finally, once all relevant findings are presented on a given theme, he provides a unifying conclusion: his interpretation of what the findings mean, how variations in the findings can be understood, and what is important about what he learned.

Likewise, in a study of the determinants of underimmunization in urban Dili, Timor-Leste, the investigators presented their results not by study method but by theme, in order to enable triangulation of findings from different informants and situations. The study methods included directly observed immunization encounters and exit interviews at service delivery sites, focus group discussions (FGDs), and in-depth interviews with community leaders and health staff. The researchers organized their results by broad themes amenable to focused interventions—by caregivers' and health workers' knowledge, attitudes, and practices; the availability of service provision; and access to health information and education—citing data from the mix of methods that yielded results (Amin et al., 2013).

Like Cáceres and Amin, you can successfully alternate between or combine presentation of qualitative and quantitative data on specific points—even where themes break into subthemes—and still retain your focus.

data from qualitative samples as if they were quantitative. Since sampling for qualitative studies is not representative, overemphasizing numbers and distributions is erroneous and misleading. For this reason, it is preferable in most cases to use ordinal terms such as *most, some, about half, around a third, nearly all,* and the like rather than numbers on a metric scale, which would presuppose a large random sample and more precise quantitative data.

Finally, cartographic images or maps generated through use of geographic information system (GIS) technologies can be used to present relationships among variables explored in qualitative research as well as insights on the scale of those findings (Cope & Elwood, 2009).

How to Use Transcript Quotes in Narrative

Use quotes in the Results section to illustrate your findings and enrich the readers' understanding of the context of the themes in research participants' lives. As you select and present quotes, take care to represent participants' viewpoints fairly and respectfully. Some recommendations for using quotes are:

- Use representative quotes to illustrate norms or shared perceptions. These quotes should succinctly represent views that interviewees would recognize as their own. For example, in one West African study of service delivery for a contraceptive implant, the majority of respondents independently mentioned the phrase *va-et-vient* ("coming and going" or "being given the runaround"). Hearing so many women say that to get their implant removed they had to endure being given the runaround by service delivery personnel alerted the researcher that this service delivery phenomenon was entrenched. The women's shared phrase pointed to this phenomenon as a key theme to explore in future research.
- Use provocative quotes to highlight insights not generally held but that are perhaps innovative or pioneering. For example, if a focus group participant mentions that women like the female condom "because they can insert it before they leave work," you might explore whether potential users in that area perceive themselves to be at high risk of rape when commuting and whether they feel the female condom would offer disease protection. While we caution readers not to give undue importance to atypical positions, an unexpected response can be a clue to an aspect of the findings that might warrant further exploration.
- Draw on a variety of people's voices, not just the most articulate. Be sure to check whether the range of people you quote reflects the range of people

interviewed. One way to illustrate a range of perspectives and variations in language is to list short phrases related to your theme:

My wife and I decide together how many children we'll have.

It's up to the man to decide how many children he can afford, because he's the one who earns the money.

- Use quotes to show the importance not only of what people say, but also how they say it. The nature of language use, including tone, can indicate decision making, discord, ambivalence, underlying emotions, or social expectations. Things said with great emotion or powerful word choices may indicate provocative issues below the surface.

Identifying Quotes

Identifying quotes that illustrate a given theme ideally happens during analysis. You may want to identify key quotes associated with a theme as you create data reduction tables or memos summarizing types of responses. You can also mark key quotes to use in your results write up as you read through your transcripts during the coding process by designating a code for salient quotes. (See Chapter 6). Otherwise, trying to relocate a memorable quote when you need it can be a frustrating search.

Incorporating and Formatting Quotes in the Text

The usual approach for incorporating quotes into your results is to make the point in your narrative and follow it with an illustrative statement from a participant. You can wrap the quote into the narrative: "The lack of cohesion and communication between hospital managers of different districts resulted in difficulty in finding joint solutions in responding to regional shocks. As one hospital manager mentioned, '*access to resources is so limited that we compete with others to recruit a new ophthalmic nurse for example. Instead of finding solutions to common problems, we find solutions against each other*'" (Blanchet & James, 2013).

Or, you can set longer quotes off as indented paragraphs, usually with a slightly smaller font. Use quotation marks when the quote is embodied in the narrative, but not when it is set off in its own indented paragraph, as shown next.

A 42-year-old nonliterate mother of six volunteered the following illustration to explain how friends help each other:

When two women meet, they talk about the disease. I will say, "My dear, the AIDS disease is out there. Are you being careful?"

And my friend might say, "I have this man I've been sleeping with, but I don't know if he has other women. Do you think I should break off this relationship?"

And I say, "You can use a condom."

(Ulin, Cayemittes, & Metellus, 1995)

As a general rule, use verbatim quotes. However, minor changes may be needed to make a quote clearer, especially if it is a translation. Do not let clarification change some subtle meaning. If you need to shorten a quote or change some words, the convention is to put your substituted words in square brackets [ ] and replace omitted words with periods or ellipses in brackets. For example: "My boyfriend and I want to protect ourselves from these [sexually transmitted] diseases, but [. . .] we don't always have condoms when we need them."

Labeling Quotes

Remember to manage the marking of quotes within transcripts efficiently, and present them in ways that preserve the contextual information necessary for readers to understand them accurately. Note that quotes become more alive if they are labeled with descriptive information, for example, "a 16-year-old woman pregnant for the first time," or "a 40-year-old unemployed factory worker." Remember never to put the respondent's name in your article. You may have descriptive information in background data sheets (see Chapter 5). Your choice of descriptors will depend on the information you consider most relevant to the point you are making in your narrative. These descriptors can also follow the quote, for example:

I hide the pill packet in my clothes when my husband is home. I don't want him to find it, because he does not know I'm going to the family planning clinic.

—Market woman, primary schooling, 27 years old
(Ulin, Cayemittes, & Metellus, 1995)

You can also link several short, related quotes, indicating clearly that they are different speakers, for example:

> *I hide the pills in my clothes when my husband is home.*
> —27-year-old market woman
>
> *I take my pills before he comes to bed—I go to bed before he does.*
> —33-year-old teacher
>
> *When my husband asks, I just say I'm not using them.*
> —30-year-old farmer

Keep quotes short—enough to suggest the context and not so long that the reader loses the thread. Ask yourself whether the segment is a good reflection of the point you want to make. Because very long quotes tend to distract the reader from the narrative flow, make them just long enough to give some life to the text.

Managing Foreign Language Translations

Many words or expressions in other languages have no literal translation, or if translated, they lose the subtlety of the original statement. The best way to handle these is to use the word that the translator believes comes closest to the original but also to include the original word or phrase in italics within parentheses. For example: "An [informally] married (*placé*) woman agreed that 'life on the streets is hard [. . .]. A woman without employment can't stand up to her partner.'"

Include key foreign words or phrases to enable readers who do know the language to judge the validity of the translated data. For example:

Moderator: What kind of people can contract HIV?

First Haitian respondent: People who are fooling around (*viv deyo*), living promiscuously (*nan epav*), but if both people are not living like that, you will not get it.

Second Haitian respondent: What she says is right, [but] some women who live with men are not involved with other men (*li pa nan anyen*), while their men may be involved in everything (*nan tout afel*).

Like the choreographer, the researcher must find the most effective way to speak to the audience, to convince them of the meaning of the study. Staying close to the data is the most powerful means of telling the story, just as in dance the story is told through the body itself.

(Janesick, 2000, p. 389)

Discussion Section

The Discussion section is where you interpret your results, where you tell the reader what you think the results mean. It is also where you situate your results in the context of what is already known from other studies and describe why your study matters. (Box 8.4 offers suggestions for questions to ask yourself to help you determine this.) There is no one correct way to write the Discussion, but certain basic elements typically appear in this section.

BOX 8.4 DOES YOUR STUDY MATTER?

- Have you identified gaps in the literature and suggested ways your work offers new thinking in an area of importance?
- Are the results consistent with other studies? How applicable are the findings in other contexts or with other groups?
- Does your study provide new ways of thinking about the public health topic you addressed?
- Does your writing provoke readers to reexamine their assumptions underlying prevailing theories or lines of thought?

Sources: Adapted from Golden-Biddle and Locke (1999); Lincoln and Guba (1985).

Start out by restating the purpose of your research. Then state your main conclusion(s) based on your results in a concise, straightforward way. For example:

> Our study is the first to triangulate findings about stakeholders' perceptions of the effect of introducing the new MenA [meningococcal A] vaccine on health services with routine health facility data. The study found that many aspects of the health system were not affected by the MenA vaccine introduction, either positively or negatively, while some aspects improved and others—notably, continuity of routine services—suffered.
>
> *(Mounier-Jack, Burchett, Griffiths, Konaté, & Diarra, 2014, p. 125)*

Your next task is to interpret your key results, both from your own perspective as a researcher involved in the study, as well as in the context of the literature. One approach is to explain what you think the key results mean and why, perhaps providing several possible explanations. You might also compare and contrast key results from multiple sites or participant categories and offer reasons for why the findings are similar or different. Make clear the multiple and sometimes contradictory perspectives reflected in your data.

Also include here a discussion of whether your findings and interpretations are supported by or are different from the findings of similar studies, such as studies on your topic with the same populations in distinct geographical regions or studies that used similar methodology. If your findings conflict with other studies, explore the reasons why. You will also want to highlight interesting or unanticipated findings. Note that no new data—that is, data not presented in the Results section—should appear in the Discussion.

Another important point to cover is the strengths of your study, including what is new and different about it compared to previous studies. Did you use a data collection method in a new way? Was your study the first to explore that particular public health issue with a specific population? Note as well the gaps in the literature that your study fills. Readers (and editors) must understand how your study adds to the accumulation of knowledge in the field.

Just as every study has its strengths, every study will also have its limitations. These must be stated frankly. There is no need to be apologetic or self-deprecating; no one can think of everything when designing a study, for example, or get funded for a study of ideal duration. There are also unforeseen circumstances that can affect the conduct of a study or the quality of the data collected, for example, new legislation in the study country criminalizing the groups being studied, such as men who have sex with men. In addition, researchers must make choices at every turn, and each choice has its corresponding set of consequences. Limitations can include factors over which you both did or did not have control, such as methodological problems or drawbacks, recruitment obstacles, or a small sample size. Be sure to discuss any ways you tried to address the limitations—for instance, through other aspects of the study design—or to resolve obstacles you encountered. Also include mention of how the limitations had an impact on your study.

This paragraph (or two) on limitations may also flow logically into a discussion of recommendations for future research following from questions that your study was unable or not intended to answer. It is also the place to draw attention to unexpected findings that invite further exploration, perhaps using alternative methods in a new design. Implications for new research may refer to work that you intend to pursue or a more general recommendation for future research.

In addition, discuss the theoretical implications, relating your themes to your statement of purpose and original question(s) and describing how your data support your explanation of the question or your conceptual framework, if you used one. If you have created a visual diagram showing how your themes fit together, reflect on your original framework and its validity in the light of new findings. Practical implications can be discussed by stating the policy or programmatic implications of your findings, if applicable. If you elect to make recommendations, be sure that these are supported by your data; a less prescriptive way of stating what follows from your study findings might be "considerations" for policy or programs.

Lastly, journal editors, reviewers, and ultimately readers will also want to know what your findings mean in a broader context. How might these findings apply beyond the original study population? Be careful not to suggest that your findings can be generalized, but rather state or show why you believe they are extensible (meaningful to a wider public health community) or not. Sometimes it is possible to recommend use of your study's innovative methodological process in other contexts, such as different populations or geographical areas, even when your actual findings are not themselves generalizable.

Conclusion Section

Some journals do not require a separate Conclusion section, or they may combine the Discussion and Conclusion into one section. For journals that do require a Conclusion, we recommend a short, concise paragraph (or two) that communicates the take-home message of your article—the main conclusion and its significance in a broader context. Here is an example from a qualitative study on resilience after natural disasters:

> This study was an exploratory qualitative analysis giving voice to lay knowledge regarding the nature of interventions which aid resilience in people who have experienced a disaster in the Australian context. The findings have been synthesized within a model of ecological disaster resilience to describe a key outcome of getting on with rebuilding for the participants who experienced a bushfire or flood. The model facilitates the translation of scientific and lay understanding of resilience to provide direction for disaster management services aiming to address the consequences of psychological harm.
>
> *(van Kessel, Gibbs, & MacDougall, 2014)*

Acknowledgments Section

By the time your reach the Acknowledgments section, you may have run out of steam. However, this opportunity—obligation, even—to thank the people who contributed to your study is essential.

Whom should you thank? The answer will, of course, depend on your study. Some suggestions are the study participants (as a group); key members of the research team who are not authors on your article, for example, recruiters or data collectors; people who may have facilitated your access to the study population; and reviewers of the drafts. You will need to state clearly all sources of funding for your work. You may want to seek permission to acknowledge individuals who are named; some journals require this.

After You Write

Internal Review

An important step in writing for publication is to get the draft of your article reviewed by your colleagues, fellow students, professors, advisors, supervisors, or mentors, as applicable, and most definitely by your co-authors. Your department or organization may have protocols for review or signoff on manuscripts prior to their submission to a journal. However, even if they do not, review by **internal reviewers** is an essential step in the process of writing an article for publication. Your article will likely benefit, in fact, from several rounds of review.

You may want to solicit such reviews prior to completing the draft. Although not everyone feels comfortable showing others an unfinished draft, early review can be particularly helpful, for example, for getting feedback on your statement of purpose, the organization of your results, or certain points in the Discussion section.

At the least, you will want to get the paper reviewed once you have completed a draft of your manuscript. It is a good idea to identify internal reviewers earlier, however, and to let them know your timeline once you have a good idea of when your draft will be ready for review. Sometimes reviewers may request to see the article again once you have made the revisions they suggested. Or, you may simply want to get additional feedback in order to gauge how well you have addressed reviewers' concerns, or to solicit reactions to a certain section.

Submitting Your Article to a Journal

Plan to spend several hours, or even a whole day, preparing to submit your manuscript to a journal electronically. Pull up the "instructions for authors" on the journal's website and follow them closely. Some journals provide a manuscript template that shows exactly how they want manuscripts to be formatted.

Formatting

For the title page, be sure you have the full name of each author as she or he likes it to appear in professional contexts, and each author's academic degrees (for some journals), department, institution, city, country, and email address; you may also be required to enter this information electronically during the submission process.

Pay close attention to formatting requirements such as line spacing, font and font size, line numbering, heading and subheading styles, and reference styles. If you selected the journal before writing, as is recommended, you will not have to worry about the section headers (such as Introduction or Background, Methods, Results, Discussion, and Conclusions), but if you are resubmitting your manuscript to a different journal, ensure that your section headers match those required by the journal. Recheck the word count limits for the abstract and the body of the manuscript. References, tables, and figures typically do not count toward the word limits.

Cover Letter

When you submit your manuscript to a journal, you will also need to upload a cover letter. Write the cover letter on letterhead if you are affiliated with an institution. Consult the journal's instructions for authors to find out what to include in the letter. If you can identify the editor, address the letter to him or her by name. Typically, you will start out the body of the letter by requesting that the editor consider your article (provide the title) for publication in the journal (provide the name). Then, describe the paper topic in a sentence or two. Explain why the editor should consider your article for the journal by relating it back to the journal's topic areas of interest and mission statement. Also describe the main contributions and significance of the paper to the field, and consequently, its interest for readers.

Many journals request that authors suggest potential reviewers of the paper. These should be experts in the subject area but not people with whom you have published in the past five years or colleagues from the same organization. If the journal requires suggestions for reviewers and you do not have anyone in mind, consult your colleagues and advisor or supervisor. You can also look to the reference section of your paper for ideas; if you cited them, chances are they are well versed on the topic. Journals may or may not follow your suggestions; sometimes, they may pick one of your suggestions and choose a second person from their pool of reviewers. Typically two reviewers are used.

Some journals like you to specify that the paper is not being considered elsewhere and has not been published previously. Similarly, specify the conference name and date of any results included in a poster or oral presentation. Also declare that you and the other authors have no financial or other conflicts of interest related to the contents of the paper. Lastly, indicate that you are the corresponding author, and provide your full contact information.

Journal Responses

You will likely receive an electronic acknowledgment of your submission shortly after the process has been completed. Your manuscript will then undergo an initial screening by an editor or editorial assistant to verify that it falls within the area of interest for the journal and perhaps also to ensure that it conforms to the formatting requirements. If it passes muster, it will be sent out for peer review by **external reviewers**. Many journals notify the corresponding author when the article has successfully passed the initial review and has been sent out for peer review. If the article does not pass the initial screening, a rejection letter will soon make its way into your inbox.

If your article passes the initial screening, reviewers will be asked to critique your manuscript and make recommendations about publication to the editor. The editor will then make a decision. Journals vary as to how long these steps may take. Once your article has been peer-reviewed, you will receive one of the following types of responses from the editor.

- *Rejection.* It is common for a manuscript to be rejected by a journal. Your best response to a rejection letter is to focus on resubmitting your manuscript to another journal without undue delay. Do, however, pay attention to the reviewers' comments to see if they can help you to improve the paper prior to resubmitting it elsewhere.
- *Revise and resubmit.* This is a common "nonrejection" response. Here, the editor and reviewers are recommending that major and/or minor revisions be made to the article before they will consider publishing it. You will be given a period of time in which to respond to comments and make any required and optional revisions to the manuscript. The article will then be reviewed again, and the editor will make a final determination.
- *Acceptance pending revision.* If your article is accepted with revisions, rejoice! This is great news. You will "simply" need to respond to the reviewers' comments (see the next section).
- *Acceptance without revision.* This response is rare and obviously requires little further action on your part.

Responding to Reviewers' Comments

In the majority of cases, successfully getting your article published is dependent upon your ability to respond thoughtfully and effectively to the reviewers' comments. All journals require a cover letter for resubmission that details how you responded to the comments. Before you begin addressing the comments, find out whether a point-by-point response is required or whether the editor is looking for a more general response describing your revisions. (This information is typically provided in the editor's email with the response to your initial submission.) Keep a record of how you have addressed each comment as you go; it will save time later if you can avoid reconstructing your revisions for the sake of the cover letter.

Some comments are straightforward to address. For example, a reviewer might request:

- Additional background information on a topic
- A more detailed explanation of the methods used for analysis
- Additional illustrative quotes
- Revision of phrasing or word choice to improve clarity
- Deletion of redundant text
- Additional information, for example, about a participant who was quoted in the paper or about what the participant meant by a given comment

However, other comments are trickier. Sometimes, it may appear that the reviewers were quantitative researchers with little experience in qualitative research. Clues may be in requests such as:

- Justify the small sample size
- Specify the power or minimum sample size calculation
- Describe how "validity" was determined
- Specify how many focus group participants expressed a particular idea or preference
- Provide profile information on focus group participants who are quoted in the article
- Justify why a study whose findings have limited generalizability is of interest to readers
- Provide a hypothesis (e.g., when the study was actually exploratory or formative and not hypothesis driven)
- Reduce the word count from 5,000 to 3,000 while retaining all of the substantive content

Responses to some of these comments, such as reviewers' application of quantitative terminology and concepts to qualitative research, may be a matter of clarifying norms for qualitative research. For example, to justify the small sample size for in-depth interviews, you could cite research, such as Guest, Bunce, and Johnson (2006), that shows that data saturation is reached at 12 in-depth interviews. For requests for more information about focus group participants, you could explain that focus group data are not normally tallied, or that it may not be possible to link a comment to an individual profile. For critiques of generalizability, you could explain that qualitative research by definition seeks an in-depth perspective on context-specific phenomena, including culturally specific, ethnic group-specific, gender-specific, country-specific, and regionally specific issues. You could also add to your Discussion section an explanation of how your study could be replicated in other populations and how the findings may be applicable to other, similar populations or in other geographical regions.

Other challenging reviews may include preferences for how data are presented. For example, combining data from different categories of participants under a given theme might be confusing for reviewers who want separate sections for each type of participant, even if it means repeating the themes.

It is not uncommon to receive conflicting recommendations from reviewers. For example, in one mixed-methods study, one reviewer took issue with the authors' having combined their presentation of the qualitative and quantitative results and objected to alternating between the two types of data. The other reviewer commended the authors for their effective presentation of the combined data. In another example, one reviewer appreciated that a detailed description of the study population provided context for understanding the results that followed, whereas a second reviewer said it was unnecessary detail and should be incorporated more briefly into the Discussion.

To address conflicting and other challenging comments, you will need to make a decision about how to proceed and then justify to the editor and reviewers in your cover letter why you chose that particular solution, presentation format, and so forth.

When to Stop Writing

Qualitative studies tend to generate vast amounts of textual data. How do you decide what to report on in initial and subsequent articles?

The answer lies in your research objectives. Your first priority should be to report on the answers to your research objectives. Depending on how many objectives you have and how they fit together, you will potentially be able to write more than one article from your primary analysis. Later, you might also conduct and write up secondary analyses of data that may also be of interest. However, part of responsible conduct of research is not slicing up your data into small segments to be reported separately simply to publish more articles.

External Review: Assessing the Product

As a qualitative researcher, your obligation is "to gather the most highly credible information possible within the constraints of your situation and to present your conclusions in a form that makes them... understandable and useful" (Morris, Fitz-Gibbon, & Freeman, 1987, p. 8). Whether or not you communicate effectively with specific audiences will influence whether those groups will consider your study credible. Policymakers, fellow researchers, and community members will determine their confidence in your study by examining both what you say and the manner in which you say it.

You can use three basic strategies to enhance the credibility and communicability of your study article or report:

1. Make sure the study question and results matter to your intended readers (relevance).
2. Understand the needs of your audience (length, level of complexity, conventions regarding credibility).
3. Attend to the basics of good writing (clarity, accuracy, logical development of ideas).

Individuals and agencies that use qualitative results to achieve their objectives are likely to have developed their own frameworks to help them evaluate what they receive from investigators. Similarly, publishers, professional societies, thesis committees, conference committees, evaluators, and government monitors all have their criteria for establishing the quality of proposals or written accounts of research. Donors and journal editors provide their reviewers with checklists and guidelines that reflect their priorities. The essential points for ensuring quality range from stating the problem through design decisions and analysis, and finally putting the whole process and outcome in writing. The checklists in Tong, Sainsbury, and Craig (2007; see Recommended Readings) provide useful reviews of these steps.

No matter whom you communicate with, your readers will consider your text in light of their own needs and interests, both personal and professional. For example, if you report on in-depth interviews with civil society advocates, the Ministry of Health, and policymakers on implementation of universal health care, your intended readers will interpret and act on the text by relating what you present to their own views on the subject. These may concern positions on human rights, government transparency, or even the value they assign to qualitative as opposed to quantitative approaches to studying health systems strengthening. In order to convince readers that your findings hold merit, you will need to achieve a balance between challenging their assumptions and reiterating the familiar—in terms of the format, style, and content of your report.

Take care that what you say and the evidence you marshal to support your insights will seem realistic to your intended audiences, as well as to those you interviewed or observed in your study. Does your writing convey to readers "a sense of familiarity and relevance as well as a sense of distinction and innovation" (Golden-Biddle & Locke, 1999, p. 374)? Most readers will judge your written presentation as a direct reflection of the quality of your research. To convince the reader that you have accurately recorded and understood the meaning of what study participants said, present detailed descriptions and key quotations, and back up your argument with evidence (Rubin & Rubin, 1995). Then check your work by reviewing the content checklist in Box 8.2. If you follow these steps, you will go a long way toward convincing your readers of your report's credibility.

An important related issue is effective communication—writing that engages your readers intellectually and emotionally. The goal of qualitative writing is "to represent the world of your interviewees accurately, vividly and convincingly" (Rubin & Rubin, 1995, p. 261). Your results will be important "if your report is read and its vividness influences decision-makers" (p. 53). Writing has the potential to motivate readers to change practices, to explore new avenues of research, to inform health advocacy efforts, or to spur communities into action. Your responsibility is to make your study report as accessible, credible, and engaging as possible. Vivid stories can provide convincing descriptions of health conditions or issues, touching your readers more profoundly than abstract discussions alone. Hearing health experiences in people's own words is gripping and powerful. Individual stories convey excitement, fear, drama, and realism. Do not be afraid to share emotion in bringing the interviewees' insights to life for your readers (Rubin & Rubin, 1995).

The ultimate interpreter of the quality and usefulness of your work is the reader, who interacts with what you have communicated and decides whether to integrate it into his or her work and worldview or to dismiss it. Your study's credibility and communicability will determine to a large extent whether readers will use your findings and whether the findings will have an impact on health policies, practices, and behaviors.

Summary

Many researchers think of writing as an extension of the data analysis because it requires careful attention to relationships that have emerged and their clear expression in the conclusions. Writing up the results of your findings allows you to look back on the whole research process. As a writer, you are now, in effect, speaking to your audience, explaining what you have found in words that will excite their interest and stimulate new thinking.

Scientific writing conventions developed for quantitative research can provide an organizational roadmap for researchers writing up qualitative or mixed-method results. Social scientists and health practitioners using qualitative methods also need to share information introducing their study, explaining the methods used, summarizing key results, and providing an interpretation of meaning. But it is critical to report accurately those components of the research that distinguish the qualitative study from the quantitative and that influence how the data are interpreted. In reporting their results, qualitative writers must be attuned to these differences, including how they have selected and incorporated quotes from transcripts, how they organized and presented results where the iterative nature of the research must be conveyed, the importance of addressing reflexivity, and issues related to generalizability. This chapter addresses these considerations. It also provides concrete advice on aspects of the writing process, including selecting a writing format, identifying an appropriate journal, authorship issues, internal review of manuscript drafts, and responding to comments from peer reviewers.

Whether you find the writing process itself to be arduous or a pleasure, publishing your article or disseminating your report is part of the responsible conduct of research, giving stakeholders the opportunity to apply your findings in ways that may improve the health of the public. By sharing your findings with the public health community and other stakeholders, you will also have made a substantive contribution to the knowledge base in your field of study.

Key Terms

1. **Peer-reviewed journal:** A journal that publishes articles based on the recommendations of external reviewers.
2. **Internal reviewer**: Someone from within the organization(s) of the author(s) who reviews a manuscript/article prior to the author(s) submitting it to a journal or to its intended audience (e.g., policymakers, funders, etc.)
3. **External reviewer**: Someone requested by a peer-review journal to review a submitted manuscript/article, provide comments, and advise on whether the journal should publish the manuscript.

Review Questions

1. What are the four criteria that qualify someone to be listed as author on a scientific article? Based on these four criteria, develop an authorship agreement. What issues may come up as you debate author order?
2. What does IMRAD stand for, and what belongs in each section of this format? Which section do you think you would find the most challenging and why?
3. To what extent is it appropriate to provide interpretation of results in the Results section versus the Discussion section, and how does this relate to study design?

Recommended Readings

Belcher, W. L. (2009). *Writing your journal article in 12 weeks: A guide to academic publishing success.* Thousand Oaks, CA: Sage.

Day, R. A., & Gastel, B. (2011). *How to write and publish a scientific paper* (7th ed.). Santa Barbara, CA: Greenwood.

Tong, A., Sainsbury, P., & Craig, J. (2007). Consolidated criteria for reporting qualitative research (COREQ): A 32-item checklist for interviews and focus groups. *International Journal for Quality in Health Care, 19*(6), 349–357. doi:10.1093/intqhc/mzm042

References

Amin, R., De Oliveira, T. J., Da Cunha, M., Brown, T. W., Favin, M., & Cappelier, K. (2013). Factors limiting immunization coverage in urban Dili, Timor-Leste. *Global Health: Science and Practice, 1*(3), 417–427. doi:10.9745/GHSP-D-13-00115

Barnett, B., & Stein, J. (1998). *Women's voices, women's lives: The impact of family planning*. Research Triangle Park, NC: Family Health International.

Blanchet, K., & James, P. (2013). The role of social networks in the governance of health systems: The case of eye care systems in Ghana. *Health Policy and Planning, 28*(2), 143–156. doi:10.1093/heapol/czs031

Cáceres, C. F. (1999). *La (re)configuracion del universo sexual*. Lima, Peru: REDESS Jóvenes.

Cope, M., & Elwood, S. (2009). Conclusion: For qualitative GIS. In M. Cope & S. Elwood (Eds.), *Qualitative GIS: A Mixed Methods Approach* (pp. 171–177). London, England: Sage. doi:10.4135/9780857024541.d16

Denzin, N. K., & Lincoln, Y. S. (Eds.). (2000). *Handbook of qualitative research* (2nd ed.). Thousand Oaks, CA: Sage.

Flick, U. (1998). *An introduction to qualitative research*. Thousand Oaks, CA: Sage.

Global Network of People Living With HIV. (2013). *Understanding the perspectives and/or experiences of women living with HIV regarding Option B+ in Uganda and Malawi*. Rebekah Webb Consulting. Available at http://www.gnpplus.net/assets/2013-Option-B+-Report-GNP-and-ICW.pdf

Golden-Biddle, K., & Locke, L. (1999). Appealing work: An investigation of how ethnographic texts convince. In A. Bryman & R. G. Burgess (Eds.), *Qualitative research: Vol. 3. Analysis and interpretation of qualitative data* (pp. 369–396). London, England: Sage.

Greenhalgh, T., Helman, C., & Chowdhury, A. M. (1998). Health beliefs and folk models of diabetes in British Bangladeshis: A qualitative study. *British Medical Journal, 316*(7136), 978–983. doi:10.1136/bmj.316.7136.978

Guest, G., Bunce, A., & Johnson, L. (2006). How many interviews are enough? An experiment with data saturation and variability. *Field Methods, 18*(1), 59–82. doi:10.1177/1525822X05279903

Hardee, K., Irani, L., & Rodriguez, M. (forthcoming). Linking family planning/reproductive health policies to health programs and outcomes: The importance of the policy implementation space. *International Journal of Gynecology and Obstetrics.*

Janesick, V. J. (2000). The choreography of QR design: Minuets, improvisations, and crystallization. In N. K. Denzin & Y. S. Lincoln (Eds.), *Handbook of qualitative research* (pp. 379–399). Thousand Oaks, CA: Sage.

Lincoln, Y. S., & Guba, E. G. (1985). Establishing trustworthiness. In Y. S. Lincoln & E. G. Guba (Eds.), *Naturalistic inquiry* (pp. 289–331). Beverly Hills, CA: Sage.

Lofland, J. (1974). Styles of reporting qualitative field research. *American Sociologist, 9*(3), 101–111.

Miller, W. L., & Crabtree, B. F. (2000). Clinical research. In N. K. Denzin & Y. S. Lincoln (Eds.), *Handbook of qualitative research* (pp. 605–648). Thousand Oaks, CA: Sage: 607–631.

Morris, L. L., Fitz-Gibbon, C. T., & Freeman, M. E. (1987). *How to communicate evaluation findings.* Newbury Park, CA: Sage.

Mounier-Jack, S., Burchett, H. E., Griffiths, U. K., Konate, M., & Diarra, K. S. (2014). Meningococcal vaccine introduction in Mali through mass campaigns and its impact on the health system. *Global Health: Science and Practice, 2*(1), 117–129. doi:10.9745/GHSP-D-13-00130

Northern Illinois University. (2004). *Responsible conduct in data management.* Washington, DC: Office of Research Integrity, Department of Health and Human Services. Available at http://ori.hhs.gov/education/products/n_illinois_u/datamanagement/dprtopic.html

Richardson L. (1990). *Writing strategies: Reaching diverse audiences.* Newbury Park, CA: Sage.

Ronai, C. R. (1995). Multiple reflections of child sex abuse: An argument for a layered account. *Journal of Contemporary Ethnography, 23*(4), 395–426. doi:10.1177/089124195023004001

Rotter, J. B. (1966). Generalized expectancies for internal versus external control of reinforcement. *Psychological Monographs, 80*(1). doi:10.1037/h0092976

Rubin, H. J., & Rubin, I. S. (1995). *Qualitative interviewing: The art of hearing data.* Thousand Oaks, CA: Sage.

Sylla, A. H., Robinson, E. T., Raney, L., & Seck, K. (2012). Qualitative study of health information needs, flow, and use in Senegal. *Journal of Health Communication, 17* (Suppl 2), 46–63. doi:10.1080/10810730.2012.666624

Ulin, P. R., Cayemittes, M., & Metellus, E. (1995). *Haitian women's role in sexual decision-making: The gap between AIDS knowledge and behavior change.* Research Triangle Park, NC: Family Health International. Available at http://citeseerx.ist.psu.edu/viewdoc/download?doi=10.1.1.466.1974&rep=rep1&type=pdf

van Kessel, G., Gibbs, L., & MacDougall, C. (2014). Strategies to enhance resilience post-natural disaster: A qualitative study of experiences with Australian floods and fires. *Journal of Public Health, 37*(2), 328–336. doi:10.1093/pubmed/fdu051

Wolcott, H. F. (1990). *Writing up qualitative research: Qualitative research methods* (Vol. 20). Newbury Park, CA: Sage.

APPENDIX 1

CASE STUDIES

CASE STUDY 1
PREVENT: HUMAN–ANIMAL EXPOSURE STUDY

Country: Uganda

Topic: Zoonoses (naturally occurring diseases that can be transmitted between vertebrate animals and humans)

BACKGROUND

A majority of the infectious agents implicated in newly emerging diseases have a zoonotic origin (Taylor, Latham, & Woolhouse, 2001). Animals that are natural reservoirs for pathogens that can be transmitted to humans include domestic and wild animals, ungulates, carnivores, rodents, bats, and birds (Woolhouse, 2006). Overall, an estimated 70% of zoonotic pathogens that cause disease in humans come from wild animals (Cutler, Fooks, & Van der Poel, 2010). Bats, nonhuman primates, and rodents have been most frequently implicated in the transmission of high-impact infectious diseases.

AIMS

As part of USAID's Emerging Pandemic Threats (EPT) program, this two-stage, mixed-methods study sought to understand and address the risks of transmitting EPT viruses from animals to humans, with the ultimate aim of developing feasible and acceptable interventions to reduce these risks. The overall goals of

(Continued)

the study were to: (1) indicate which specific human activities are associated with particularly high rates of exposure, and (2) describe how exposure to animals is modified by different social factors and by the environmental context.

Before the study could systematically measure human's exposure to animals, formative research was needed to determine how to quantify risk by better understanding how, where, and when people interact with animals. The specific aims of the formative research were to:

- Understand the overall context of the human–animal interface including how culture, societal roles, physical space, time, and resources affect the way people interact with specific animals.
- Collect information to be used to adapt the standard human–animal exposure survey questionnaire to local conditions.
- Identify any circumstances that might result in over- or underreporting of certain exposures.
- Explore different factors that may have implications for the implementation of the survey or for sample design.

THEORY OR APPROACH USED

A premise of the human–animal exposure study is that disease transmission is not a purely biological process. Opportunities for transmission depend on human activity: how, where, and when people interact with animals (Woldehanna & Zimicki, 2015). Human activity, which occurs in and is modulated by the physical environment, is influenced by social factors including culture, gender, age, socioeconomic status, and occupation. For example, culture determines which, if any, animals are considered acceptable to eat. Gender, age, and socioeconomic status affect division of labor, and thus the amount of time people engage in specific activities; occupations related to animals (hunting, butchering, caring for animals) obviously place their actors at special risk compared to the general population. Finally, the variety and number of animals that can be contacted is affected by both the seasonality of human activities and the location where contact occurs (urban/rural, agricultural/forest, disturbance zones).

METHODS

The study was conducted in two areas of southwestern Uganda, in and near the sites where a second project (the PREDICT project) was sampling animals. These

(Continued)

areas were chosen because they present interesting factors (proximity of a protected forest to a densely populated and cultivated area, possible cross-border issues) that may illuminate some of the complex dynamics involved in increased risk of zoonotic disease emergence.

Two phases of research were conducted:

Phase 1

Formative qualitative data were collected to gain an in-depth understanding of the human–animal interface. Data collection methods were:

- Key informant interviews with nine district officials, village elders, local animal health workers, and people who hunt frequently. The key informant interviews aimed to obtain initial information about local animal names, community perceptions about local animal taxonomies, groups most exposed to animals, and any local sensitivities around animals.
- Individual interviews with approximately 60 adult men and women from the two study areas using two structured tools. The interviews aimed to assess animal recognition and further assess how community members categorize animals. Focus group discussions using participatory appraisal techniques were conducted with separate groups of men, women, girls, and boys.

More than 400 individuals participated in the formative phase of the study.

Phase 2

- The validity and reliability of a subsequent quantitative survey was first assessed through cognitive interviews with about 30 individuals selected from each ethnic group.
- A representative survey was conducted with a total of 1,294 individuals to quantify and compare different subgroups' exposure to animals.

CONTRIBUTIONS OF THE METHODOLOGICAL APPROACH

The formative research resulted in materials used to adapt the survey and included:

- A dictionary of local animals in the local language, with the phonetic spelling of the local name in English and comments with respect to the use of the animal name

(Continued)

- A dictionary of key terms critical for accurate understanding of the survey (e.g., butchering, kill, hunt, spaces, seasons), with the term in the local language, phonetic spelling of the local name in English, and comments on context of use

Other products of the analysis included seasonal calendars and community maps with notes relevant for the adaptation and implementation of the survey.

Key staff: Susan Zimicki, Sara Woldehanna, Marga Eichley (FHI 360)

References

Cutler, S. J., Fooks, A. R., & Van der Poel, W. H. (2010). Public health threat of new, reemerging, and neglected zoonoses in the industrialized world. *Emerging Infectious Diseases*, *16*(1), 1–7.

Taylor, L. H., Latham, S. M., & Woolhouse, M. E. (2001). Risk factors for human disease emergence. *Philosophical Transactions of the Royal Society B: Biological Sciences*, *356*, 983–989.

Woldehanna, S., & Zimicki, S. (2015). An expanded one health model: Integrating social science and one health to inform a study of the human-animal interface. *Social Science and Medicine*, *129*, 87–95.

Woolhouse, M. E. J. (2006). Where do emerging pathogens come from? *Microbe*, *1*(11), 515.

CASE STUDY 2
ENGAGING MALE PARTNERS IN WOMEN'S MICROBICIDE USE

Countries: South Africa, Kenya, Tanzania

Topic: Microbicides, male engagement

BACKGROUND

Microbicides, which are substances that can be inserted into the vagina or rectum to reduce women's risk of HIV, are still being tested in clinical trials to see if they are effective. Microbicides were developed as a woman-controlled method of HIV prevention. While women appreciate a method they can use without their partner's knowledge, many women—particularly those in steady relationships—prefer to discuss microbicides with their male partners. Moreover, male partners' awareness and acceptance of product use influenced women's product acceptance and self-reported adherence in clinical trials. In some cases, women also reported that involving their partners in microbicide use benefitted their relationships by improving communication and promoting shared responsibility for HIV protection. Studies and experience from women-centered health programs, such as family planning and prevention of mother-to-child transmission (PMTCT), suggest that efforts to secure the involvement and support of male partners are critical to the success of these programs. Future microbicide studies and eventual product introduction must carefully consider how to constructively engage men while protecting women's rights to decide on their own whether to use the product.

AIMS

The aims of the study were to determine: (1) whether/how women and men want men to be involved in microbicide use, (2) whether/how trial participants communicated with their partners about microbicide use and women's and men's preferred communication and decision-making processes, (3) existing gender norms that could facilitate or hinder constructive male engagement in microbicide use, and (4) potentially effective ways to engage men in women's microbicide use.

THEORY OR APPROACH USED

Transformative approach

(Continued)

METHODS

Qualitative

The study design was unique in that it involved synthesizing findings from six qualitative studies that investigated men's role in their partners' microbicide use during clinical trials in sub-Saharan Africa. FHI 360, the lead research organization, collected new qualitative data in Kenya with former microbicide trial participants, their partners, and community members. FHI 360 also partnered with investigators from five completed qualitative studies conducted in conjunction with microbicide trials. Investigators from each study analyzed their data to answer a common set of research questions on partner communication about microbicides, men's role in women's microbicide use, and potential strategies for engaging men in future microbicide introduction. Collectively, the analyses included data from 535 interviews and 107 focus groups with trial participants, male partners, and community members in South Africa, Kenya, and Tanzania. After analyzing the data, the researchers participated in a two-day meeting to present and discuss results from each study, identify central themes and key findings, and discuss programmatic implications of the data.

KEY FINDINGS

The majority of women in steady partnerships wanted agreement from their partners to use microbicides. Women used various strategies to obtain their agreement, including using the product for a while before telling their partners, giving men information gradually, and continuing to bring up microbicides until resistant partners acquiesced. Among men who were aware their partners were participating in a trial and using microbicides, involvement ranged from opposition, to agreement/noninterference, to active support. Both men and women expressed a desire for men to have access to information about microbicides and to be able to talk with a health care provider about microbicides.

CONTRIBUTIONS OF THE METHODOLOGICAL APPROACH

This study was designed to inform recommendations on engaging male partners in future microbicide trials and eventual product introduction. Synthesizing data from multiple studies was useful for identifying common themes emerging from the studies, with the recommendations potentially having more validity and generalizability than if they were developed based on findings from just one study. Clinical trials are a unique environment, so men's roles may differ in the context of real-world use of microbicides; nevertheless, the data provide a starting point for

(Continued)

identifying potentially effective ways to engage male partners in future research and eventual microbicide introduction.

Additionally, using existing data was a good use of resources. Data for five of the studies had already been collected, and this study provided an opportunity to analyze and use these data that may not have been used otherwise.

Key staff: Michele Lanham, Rose Wilcher, Robyn Dayton, Sidney Schuler, Rachel Lenzi (FHI 360); Elizabeth Bukusi, Betty Njoroge (Kenya Medical Research Institute); Elizabeth Montgomery (RTI International); Robert Pool (University of Amsterdam); Barbara Friedland (Population Council)

Supplemental Case Study Materials

Lanham, M., Wilcher, R., Montgomery, E. T., Pool, R., Schuler, S., Lenzi, R., & Friedland, B. (2014). Engaging male partners in women's microbicide use: Evidence from clinical trials and implications for future research and microbicide introduction. *Journal of the International AIDS Society, 17*(3, Suppl 2), 19159. doi:10.7448/IAS.17.3.19159

CASE STUDY 3
LINCS 2 DURHAM: LINKING COMMUNITIES AND SCIENTISTS TO DURHAM HIV PREVENTION

Countries: United States

Topic: HIV prevention

BACKGROUND

The HIV epidemic in the United States disproportionately affects Black Americans, who represented 12% of the U.S. population but 44% of new HIV infections in 2010 (Centers for Disease Control and Prevention, 2015a). There are also geographic disparities, with states in the South and the Northeast reporting the highest rates of new infections (Centers for Disease Control and Prevention, 2015b). In North Carolina in 2011, 68% of persons newly diagnosed with HIV disease were Black. Durham County, NC had the fourth highest three-year average HIV disease rate among the state's 100 counties (29.9 per 100,000 population) in 2011 (N.C. Department of Health and Human Services, 2012).

LinCS 2 Durham HIV Prevention was a 5-year community-based participatory research project (funded by National Institute of Nursing Research/NIH Grant RO1 NR011232) that brought together members of Durham's Black community and HIV prevention scientists in the region to develop community support and program capacity in support of new HIV prevention technologies. Scientists globally and locally are developing and testing new methods of HIV prevention including vaccines, microbicides, and pre-exposure prophylaxis (PrEP). In order to successfully evaluate and eventually implement these new methods, communities affected by HIV and scientists need to collaborate.

AIMS

LinCS 2 Durham sought to foster collaboration and dialogue about HIV, and to generate interest in and evaluate the suitability of biomedical HIV prevention strategies and research in the local community. The specific aims of the study were to:

1. Implement and conduct a process evaluation of a systematic community-based participatory research model to build support for new HIV prevention technologies in the African American community;

(Continued)

2. Describe the communities and group affiliations that exist among young (ages 18-30) at-risk African Americans, and measure the relationship among experiences of discrimination, levels of trust, and support for new HIV prevention technologies in this population; and

3. Identify priorities for evaluating and implementing new HIV prevention technologies in the African American community.

THEORY OR APPROACH USED

The research design was informed by a conceptual framework with four dimensions:

1. An overarching framework, the prevention science research continuum, that integrates research with policy, community, behavior, and programs (MacQueen & Cates, 2005);

2. Principles of community-based participatory research (Israel et al., 1998);

3. Ethnography to generate empirical evidence on community processes, structures, and functioning in the research community, to inform the design of research and to provide a bridge between local residents, the research team, and other stakeholder groups; and

4. Principles of group theory based in empirical evidence from psychology, sociology, and anthropology to support the community-based participatory research (CBPR) approach; refine the structure of stakeholder involvement; avoid problems such as group-think, complacency, and co-optation; and foster inclusiveness, creativity, and active problem-solving.

METHODS

The LinCS 2 Durham Collaborative Council (CC), a partnership among Durham stakeholders and the research team, was the heart of the project and guided the development and implementation of study activities. CC members included representatives from community grassroots organizations, public health and health research organizations, academia, and other fields in addition to representatives from the Durham community at large including Black young adults ages 18-30 recruited through a series of community events. The CC met monthly to discuss the status of study activities and plan next steps.

(Continued)

The project included a wide range of activities including participant observations; focus groups; a community survey on HIV attitudes, beliefs, and behaviors; development and piloting of an HIV prevention research literacy curriculum; and an ongoing process evaluation of the CC. As with all elements of the project, the community survey was based on a participatory approach inclusive of the development of the data collection methods, materials, recruitment efforts, interpretation of study data, and dissemination within the local community.

Qualitative

- Participant observations were conducted at 33 venues where Black young people socialized, including nightclubs, sports bars, and shopping centers.
- Focus group discussions ($n = 4$) were conducted with Black men and women ages 18 to 30 to understand patterns of sexual behavior and partnerships and the best ways to conduct community outreach. Community survey questions and participant recruitment were informed by the focus group data.

Quantitative

- The Community survey was conducted with 508 sexually active Black men and women ages 18 to 30 to better understand their HIV beliefs, attitudes, and behaviors. The survey had quantitative and qualitative components and was completed using Audio Computer-Assisted Self-Interview software (ACASI) and face-to-face interviewing.
- Two pilot sessions ($n = 26$) of the research literacy curriculum were conducted to determine curriculum effectiveness in changing knowledge, attitudes, and self-confidence related to HIV; research; ethics and human subjects; clinical research; community roles in research; and HIV prevention.

CONTRIBUTIONS OF THE METHODOLOGICAL APPROACH

LinCS 2 Durham drew on established principles for CBPR such as recognizing the importance of community identity, building on community strengths and resources, promoting co-learning and capacity building, and involving partners equitably throughout the research. The participatory approach utilized within the development and implementation of the study activities helped to ensure that the process and results were relevant to both researchers and the local community.

(Continued)

The research team used participant observations as an opportunity to raise awareness of the study, pass out condoms, and invite community members to join the Collaborative Council. Findings from the focus groups informed the development of the community survey. The survey findings were disseminated through an innovative, multi-dimensional plan intended to reach community members as well as academic and professional audiences. One unique dissemination method used to reach community members was a month-long art exhibit at a popular Black-owned coffee shop; the exhibit opening included poetry and musical performances. The Collaborative Council worked with local artists, who used different art mediums to portray key survey findings in creative, visually compelling, and memorable ways. Survey findings were also disseminated through established electronic newsletters, social media, public service announcements, flyers, and professional presentations.

One of the important accomplishments of the Collaborative Council was development of an HIV prevention intervention concept to address the challenges being faced in Durham and elsewhere with regard to linking those at greatest risk for HIV and newly diagnosed to services and care to keep them healthy and support them in achieving positive life goals.

Key staff: Kathleen MacQueen, Natalie T. Eley, Monique P. Mueller, Mario Chen (FHI 360); David Jolly, LaHoma Smith Romocki, Michelle Laws, Brett Chambers, Eunice Okumu (North Carolina Central University); Ronald Strauss, Kia Caldwell, Malika Roman Isler, Vanessa White, Allison Mathews (University of North Carolina at Chapel Hill); Randy Rogers, Mary DeCoster, Tekola Fisseha, Annette Carrington Johnson (Durham County Department of Public Health); David Napp (Independent Evaluator)

Supplemental Case Study Materials

MacQueen, K. M., Chen, M., Jolly, D., Mueller, M. P., Okumu, E., Eley, N. T., . . . , & Rogers, R. C. (2015). HIV testing experience and risk behavior among sexually active Black young adults: A CBPR-based study using respondent-driven sampling in Durham, North Carolina. *American Journal of Community Psychology, 55*(3), 433–443. doi:10.1007/s10464-015-9725-z

Isler, M. R., Brown, A. L., Eley, N., Mathews, A., Batten, K., Rogers, R., . . . , & MacQueen, K. M. (2014). Curriculum development to increase minority research literacy for HIV prevention research: A CBPR approach. *Prog Community Health Partnership, 8*(4), 511–521. doi:10.1353/cpr.2014.0059

(Continued)

References

Centers for Disease Control and Prevention. (2015a). *HIV among African Americans*. Available at http://www.cdc.gov/hiv/risk/racialethnic/aa/facts/index.html

Centers for Disease Control and Prevention. (2015b). *HIV and AIDS in the United States by geographic distribution*. Available at http://www.cdc.gov/hiv/statistics/basics/geographicdistribution.html

Israel, B. A., Schulz, A. J., Parker, E. A., & Becker, A. B. (1998). Review of community-based research: Assessing partnership approaches to improve public health. *Annu Rev Public Health, 19*,173–202. doi: 10.1146/annurev.publhealth.19.1.173

MacQueen, K. M., & Cates, W., Jr. (2005). The multiple layers of prevention-science research. *American Journal of Preventive Medicine, 28*(5), 491–495. doi:10.1016/j.amepre.2005.02.020

North Carolina Department of Health and Human Services. (2012). *Epidemiologic profile for HIV/STD prevention & care planning*. Raleigh.

CASE STUDY 4
SUSTAINED ACCEPTABILITY OF VAGINAL MICROBICIDES

Country: India

Topic: Acceptability of and adherence to new ARV-based prevention methods

BACKGROUND

In the early years of studies on microbicides, social scientists were focused on acceptability of the attributes of the products, while clinical researchers were focused on proving efficacy rather than on effectiveness outside of the clinic setting, where dynamics of variable use would be at play. In addition, there was the strong belief that microbicides would be female controlled and able to be used clandestinely; thus, there was little attention to the role of male partners or the dynamics of decision making about sexual practices. To address these gaps that would affect women's ability to sustain use of a product over months or years, this study integrated qualitative and quantitative data collection methods in a longitudinal study of microbicide acceptability among married men and women in Pune, India.

AIMS

The overall objectives of the study were to:

1. Identify and describe factors that enable individuals and couples to use microbicides consistently and long term.
2. Account for the effects of clinical trial and acceptability research participation on microbicide use, including motivations for joining the trial and the importance of counseling and support provided by study staff in maintaining product use.

THEORY OR APPROACH USED

The researchers developed a conceptual model that was informed by the AIDS Risk Reduction Model and constructs drawn from other theories, including sexual power and couple harmony.

(Continued)

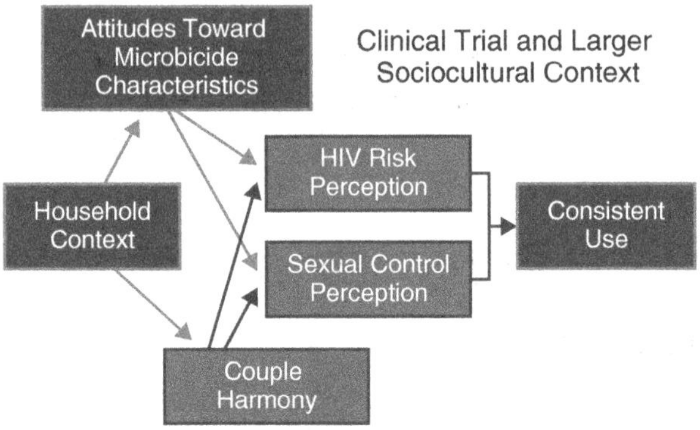

METHODS

Formative Stage: Qualitative

During the first phase of data collection, two to three in-depth interviews were conducted with 30 women (15 women at high risk of HIV because a husband was HIV positive or they or their partner had a history of sexually transmitted infections, and 15 women at low or unknown risk) and 15 husbands. Interviews focused on key concepts believed to influence risk-reduction behaviors, including HIV risk perception, self-efficacy, couple harmony, and sexual communication. In-depth interview data were used to identify individual, couple related, or environmental domains likely to influence microbicide use. Qualitative analysis highlighted how women's perceptions of HIV risk were often contingent on having physical evidence of a partner's infidelity. Textual data provided the basis for construction of approximately 130 draft items for a later structured survey representing HIV risk perception, couple harmony, and sexual power and control.

During a second formative phase, the face and content validity of the domains and items were assessed through cognitive interviews with 16 women and 8 men, followed by a review by a panel of 12 U.S. and South Asian experts in sexual and reproductive health issues.

Formative Stage: Quantitative

Finally, the revised domains and items were then included in a structured survey instrument and administered to 305 women and 151 husbands. The items were

(Continued)

factor analyzed using exploratory factor analysis procedures. Resulting factors were further assessed for construct validity by examining associations with other theoretical variables, identified *a priori* and included in the scale survey. The formative research produced scales measuring couple harmony, perceived partner infidelity, and protection efficacy.

Assessment Stage: Mixed Method

Once the acceptability scales were developed, they were used in a longitudinal study of microbicide acceptability. The acceptability study enrolled 100 women who were concurrently participating in a clinical trial to assess the safety of a microbicide gel; 100 nonparticipating women and 103 male partners (evenly distributed between the clinical trial and nonclinical trial cohorts) were also enrolled. Participants were asked to respond to structured questions at baseline and during follow-up visits scheduled at 8, 16, and 24 weeks, or until discontinuation. A small cohort of couples also participated in qualitative interviews conducted at 12 and 20 weeks after joining the study. The study identified important differences between women and their partners who joined and did not join the clinical trial. It also found that condom use, but not gel use, was predicted by couple harmony.

CONTRIBUTIONS OF THE METHODOLOGICAL APPROACH

The mixed-method approach to this study provided valuable insight into factors associated with microbicide acceptability and use. The scales produced through the project have been used in other contexts and further validate the utility of this approach to better measure difficult or nuanced cultural concepts.

Key study staff: Elizabeth Tolley, Sharon Tsui (FHI 360); Sanjay Mehendale, Rewa Malhotra-Kohli (National AIDS Research Institute)

Supplementary Case Study Materials

Marlow, H. M., Tolley, E. E., Kohli, R., & Mehendale, S. (2010). Sexual communication among married couples in the context of a microbicide clinical trial and acceptability study in Pune, India. *Cult Health Sex 12*(8): 899–912. doi:10.1080/13691058.2010.508843

(Continued)

Tolley, E. E., Eng, E., Kohli, R., Bentley, M. E., Mehendale, S., Bunce, A., Severy, L. J. (2006). Examining the context of microbicide acceptability among married women and men in India. *Culture, Health & Sexuality*, *8*(4), 351–369. doi:10.1080/13691050600793071

Tolley, E. E., Tsui, S., Mehendale, S., Weaver, M. A., & Kohli, R. (2012). Predicting product adherence in a topical microbicide safety trial in Pune, India. *AIDS and Behavior*, *16*(7), 1808–1815. doi:10.1007/s10461-011-0036-6

CASE STUDY 5
ADOLESCENT WOMEN AND MICROBICIDE TRIALS: ASSESSING CHALLENGES AND OPPORTUNITIES TO THEIR PARTICIPATION

Countries: Tanzania, India

Formative Phase: Dar es Salaam, Tanzania, and Pune, India

Mock Clinical Trial: Dar es Salaam, Tanzania

Topic: Microbicides, young women, sexual and reproductive health, HIV risk characteristics, proxy product acceptability

BACKGROUND

Women need new HIV prevention methods that they control, including oral and topical microbicides, to reduce their vulnerability to HIV. However, adolescent girls are often excluded from studies of these methods, and regulatory bodies are unlikely to allow these methods to be marketed to adolescents without research on the effectiveness and acceptability of microbicides among this age group. To address the challenges in recruiting and retaining young women in HIV prevention trials, FHI 360 and its collaborators conducted a multiphase study that included formative research in both India and Tanzania and a mock clinical trial in Tanzania.

AIMS

This study conducted formative community-level research in India and Tanzania and a pilot prospective clinic-based study in Tanzania to investigate the challenges and opportunities related to including young women aged 15 to 21 in future HIV prevention trials, more specifically, topical and oral microbicide trials. The specific aims of this study were as follows:

1. Determine whether and how HIV risk characteristics of young women differ by younger (15–17) versus older age groups (18–21) and by country context.
2. Evaluate the legal, sociocultural, and service delivery factors that hinder young women's participation in topical or oral microbicide trials—and by extension, other HIV prevention clinical trials—and make specific recommendations to enhance their participation.
3. Examine and compare, by age and country, young women's (aged 15–17 and 18–21) understanding of and ability to adhere to the requirements of trial participation in the context of a prospective clinic-based study.

(Continued)

4. Determine young women's acceptability and use of a proxy gel or a proxy pill, including circumstances in which participants apply the gel and take the pill; reasons for nonuse of gel or pill; for the gel, negotiations about use with partners; and for the gel, the influences of use on sexual satisfaction for themselves and their partners.

THEORY OR APPROACH USED

Bandura's social cognitive theory (SCT) is the principal health behavior theory informing the domains of inquiry for this study. SCT theorizes a dynamic and continuous interaction between three components in determining health outcomes: the person, his or her behaviors, and the environment. SCT acknowledges the important influence of *situation* on behavior. Situation may even be applied to encompass the laws or policies regulating adolescent access to health services; the timing and physical location of a study clinic; and the social interactions of

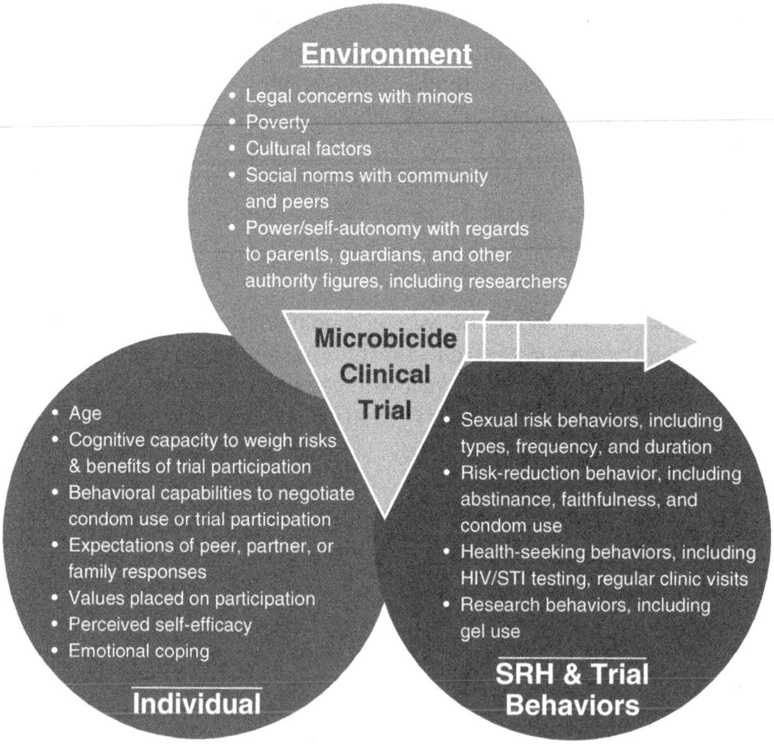
Environment
• Legal concerns with minors
• Poverty
• Cultural factors
• Social norms with community and peers
• Power/self-autonomy with regards to parents, guardians, and other authority figures, including researchers
Microbicide Clinical Trial
• Age
• Cognitive capacity to weigh risks & benefits of trial participation
• Behavioral capabilities to negotiate condom use or trial participation
• Expectations of peer, partner, or family responses
• Values placed on participation
• Perceived self-efficacy
• Emotional coping
Individual
• Sexual risk behaviors, including types, frequency, and duration
• Risk-reduction behavior, including abstinance, faithfulness, and condom use
• Health-seeking behaviors, including HIV/STI testing, regular clinic visits
• Research behaviors, including gel use
SRH & Trial Behaviors

(Continued)

peers, sexual partners, or family members relating to trial participation. The concept also acknowledges perceived self-efficacy, yet recognizes at the same time that excessive fear, or *affective states,* may derail an individual's ability to undertake a protective behavior. SCT also incorporates *reciprocal determinism,* which is the notion that characteristics of the person, behavior, and environment are constantly interacting and that a change in one component will have an impact on others.

METHODS

A formative community research phase was conducted to determine how risk characteristics vary by age group and context/venue (aim 1) and to assess the sociocultural, legal, and service delivery challenges and opportunities to their recruitment in microbicide trials (aim 2). A series of workshops was conducted to elaborate a set of youth-friendly procedures for a pilot clinic-based study and to make any necessary adjustments to its design. Next, a pilot clinical study (PCS) was conducted with 6 months of follow-up to prospectively examine adolescent women's changes in sexual risk and risk reduction behaviors (aim 1) and their understanding of and willingness and ability to adhere to the PCS procedures (aim 3). Prospective study participants could elect to participate in a 2-month randomized trial of a topical microbicide or oral pill proxy product to provide additional information on their acceptability and use of a vaginal gel or oral pill (aim 4). We engaged the collaboration of a youth advisory group and other community stakeholders throughout the study.

CONTRIBUTIONS OF THE METHODOLOGICAL APPROACH

In-depth interviews with adolescents and key informants and focus group discussions with partners (mother, fathers, and representative male sexual partners) were effective for revealing adolescent risk characteristics and the broader challenges of including and opportunities to include adolescents in microbicide trials.

The workshops held with adolescents, parents, and key community members, including those in the health sector, were beneficial based on feedback provided on informed consents and procedures to include within the PCS. The PCS provided a mock trial environment in which recruitment, retention, and acceptability could be assessed.

Key study staff: Elizabeth E. Tolley, Joy Noel Baumgartner, Jennifer Headley (FHI 360); Sylvia Kaaya (Muhimbili University); Gowri Sastry (Maharashtra Association of Anthropological Sciences)

(Continued)

Supplementary Case Study Materials

Baumgartner, J. N., Kaaya, S., Karungula, H., Kaale, A., Headley, J., & Tolley, E. E. (2015). Domestic violence among adolescents in HIV prevention research in Tanzania: Participant experiences and measurement issues. *Maternal and Child Health Journal, 19*(1), 33–39. doi:10.1007/s10995-014-1492-1

Tolley, E. E, Kaaya, S., Kaale, A., Minja, A., Bangapi, D., Kalungura, H., Headley, J., & Baumgartner, J. N. (2014). Comparing patterns of sexual risk among adolescent and young women in a mixed-method study in Tanzania: Implications for adolescent participation in HIV prevention trials. *Journal of the International AIDS Society, 17*(Suppl 2), 19149. doi:10.7448/ias.17.3.19149

CASE STUDY 6
A FIELD ASSESSMENT OF ADOPTION OF IMPROVED COOK STOVE PRACTICES: FOCUS ON STRUCTURAL DRIVERS

Country: Indonesia

Topic: Reduction of indoor air pollution to improve health

BACKGROUND

Over 3 billion people on the planet use biomass to fuel their cook stoves, and over 4 million deaths each year are attributable to the effects of indoor air pollution (IAP) caused by the smoke from inefficient cook stoves (World Health Organization, 2014). In Indonesia, the number of estimated deaths is 45,000 (World Health Organization, 2009). Much effort has been expended to develop improved cook stoves and teach people cleaner cooking practices (CCP) for the purpose of improving health, but there has been great variability in the willingness of people to engage in cleaner practices. In particular, an Indonesian development organization in Yogyakarta, Dian Desa, has been working to introduce CCP to many villages in their catchment area, with great variation by village in adoption and correct use. To Dian Desa, these villages were very similar and they were not sure how to change their intervention to increase uptake.

Two villages from the Koulon Progo District of Yogyakarta—where Dian Desa had worked to introduce cleaner wood burning stoves and other cleaner practices—were included in this assessment. The Koulon Progo District was a rural area where the primary means of income was in the harvesting and processing of palm sugar, and thus, cook stoves were used for household *and* industrial purposes. Though Dian Desa found strong uptake of the improved cook stoves in most villages in KP, there was one village in particular where there was resistance: Hargowillis.

AIMS

To increase understanding of the reasons for variability in adoption of cleaner cooking practices among similar villages in Jogyakarta, Indonesia, for the purpose of developing/adapting interventions to increase cleaner cooking practices.

(Continued)

THEORY OR APPROACH USED

A general framework was developed to guide the formative research based on the assumption that the increased adoption of cleaner cooking practices will lead to reduced exposure to indoor air pollution, and this will lead to improved health outcomes. We sought to increase our understanding of the influences or drivers of adoption, shifting our intervention target from the individual to the potential modification of social conditions that drive cooking behaviors. Based on a literature review and discussions with Dian Desa staff, we identified eight potential drivers that would form the basis of our IDI and FGD guides. (See diagram in Box 3.1 in Chapter 3.)

METHODS

To determine what was different about the village of Hargowillis compared to other villages in the district where cook stoves were used for similar purposes, the qualitative assessment included IDIs and FGDs with a variety of stakeholders at various administrative levels, including the central government (Ministry of Education, Ministry of Health) and district, village, and sub-village officers. Of special interest were village residents, including both women and men; gender plays a strong role in CCP because women do most of the cooking, but men are responsible for many household decisions.

CONTRIBUTIONS OF THE QUALITATIVE APPROACH

Open-ended formative research methods were used to collect information from a wide variety of stakeholders because there was very little known about why uptake of cleaner cook stoves was higher in some villages than in other similar villages. In Yogyakarta, CCP usually are introduced at the village or sub-village level, and often through women's or trade associations. In Hargowillis, the researchers found that conflict between groups caused resistance to the acquisition of new stoves. In contrast, in the villages where introduction efforts met with nearly universal uptake and use, more cohesive organizations with influential community leaders—especially in the women's associations—were present. Potential barriers, such as cost of the new stoves, were met with community solutions and pooling of resources for loans or labor.

Researchers also found that though people in these villages acknowledged that improved cook stoves (ICSs) created less smoke and soot, they had little concern about the health effects of smoke on respiratory illnesses. Although both clinic records and self-reports of villagers confirmed that respiratory illnesses were the most frequent reasons for seeking health care, neither doctors nor villagers

(Continued)

attributed respiratory illnesses to household smoke. Households that had reduced IAP through CCP, however, reported that they felt better when there was less smoke in the house. Though this lack of consciousness about the health effects of IAP did not differentiate between villages who used CCP and those that did not, this was considered to be a modifiable structural driver that could improve uptake in all villages.

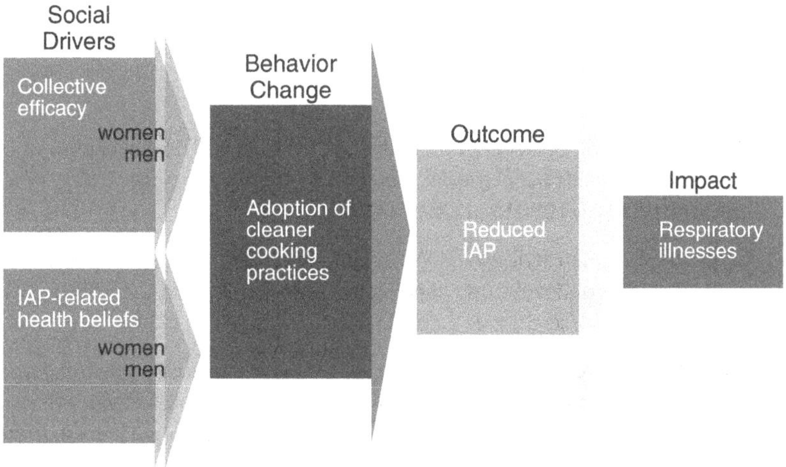

Based on findings from this assessment, we believe the relevant social drivers requiring intervention are collective efficacy (CE) and IAP-related health beliefs. Gender was not included as a modifiable driver in the new intervention framework but as a factor that should be taken into consideration when developing messages and activities to influence the two drivers in the model. CE is the belief that individuals can work as a group to achieve a collective goal, similar to the concept of self-efficacy but at a collective level. Social cohesion and social control are two dimensions measured by CE scales (Sampson, Raudenbush, & Earls, 1997). CE has relevance for adoption of CCP because it fosters social learning among community members when new ideas are communicated in a group forum, similar to what we observed in communities where there had been the greatest uptake of CCP. Activities to improve CE would encourage greater community cohesion around relevant common goals and mentor potential leaders.

The second key intervention strategy would be changing people's IAP-related health beliefs. Awareness raising campaigns could be facilitated by local clinic doctors identified as trusted sources of information during routine health education presentations held monthly at the subvillage health posts. Local health

(Continued)

data disaggregated by sex and age would inform local residents of health disparities in respiratory illnesses. The Health Belief Model (Rosenstock, Stretcher, & Becker, 1988) provides a framework for developing messages salient to women's and men's perceived susceptibility to and severity of illnesses caused by IAP and addressing barriers to and perceived benefits of adoption of CCP.

Key study staff: Cynthia Geary and Ciptasari Prabawanti (FHI 360)

References

Rosenstock, I. M., Strecher, V. J., & Becker, M. H. (1988). Social learning theory and the health belief model. *Health Education & Behavior, 15*(2), 175–183. doi:10.1177/109019818801500203

Sampson, R. J., Raudenbush, S. W., & Earls, F. (1997). Neighborhoods and violent crime: A multilevel study of collective efficacy. *Science, 277*(5328), 918–924. doi:10.1126/science.277.5328.918

World Health Organization. (2009). *Country profiles of environmental burden of disease: Indonesia*. Public Health and the Environment. Geneva, Switzerland. Available at http://www.who.int/quantifying&uscore;ehimpacts/national/countryprofile/indonesia.pdf

World Health Organization. (2014). *Household air pollution and health*. Fact sheet no. *292*. Available at http://www.who.int/mediacentre/factsheets/fs292/en/

CASE STUDY 7
EXPLORING GENDER-BASED VIOLENCE AMONG MEN WHO HAVE SEX WITH MEN, MALE SEX WORKERS, AND TRANSGENDER COMMUNITIES

Countries: Bangladesh and Papua New Guinea

Topic: Gender-based violence

BACKGROUND

In the Asia Pacific region, violence and harassment among men who have sex with men, male sex workers, and transgender populations are monitored primarily through national HIV surveillance systems. Though limited, existing data indicate that the prevalence of gender-based violence in these populations is high. In Bangladesh, for example, the 2006–2007 behavioral surveillance survey reported that 36% of men who have sex with men, 28% of transgender individuals, and 45% of male sex workers were raped or beaten in the previous year (Ministry of Health and Family Welfare of Bangladesh, 2009).

Despite this evidence, gender-based violence and its consequences for these populations are rarely addressed. Most gender-based violence efforts to date have focused on women and girls, resulting in limited expertise and a lack of clear and targeted recommendations for conducting gender-based violence interventions with other populations. Gaining a better understanding of the nature of gender-based violence among men who have sex with men, transgender individuals, and male sex workers is essential to inform the development of interventions for these populations.

AIMS

The aims of the study were to (1) explore gender-based violence among men who have sex with men, male sex workers, and transgender individuals; (2) identify current programs, policies, and donor funding and gaps in programs, policies, and funding; and (3) explore potential intervention recommendations for interventions design to prevent gender-based violence and to provide services for victims of violence.

THEORY OR APPROACH USED

Modified version of the Gender Based Violence/HIV Program Implementer's Wheel, which uses an ecological model to illustrate the multilevel causes of gender-based

(Continued)

violence and takes into consideration the multisectoral collaborations (e.g., health, justice, and social services) that are needed to develop interventions. This model is also informed by theories on gender constructs that perpetuate gender-based violence and the social cognitive theory to illustrate the importance of individual and collective efficacy in transforming gender norms (Gardsbane, 2010).

METHODS

Qualitative

- Focus group discussions with men who have sex with men, male sex workers, and transgender individuals ($n = 18$ focus groups with 115 individuals)
- In-depth interviews with key informants ($n = 28$), including:
  - Stakeholders and informal leaders from men who have sex with men, male sex workers, and transgender communities
  - Representatives from community-based organizations who work with these populations
  - Law enforcement officers
  - Health service providers
  - Legal service providers
  - Managers and owners of establishments (e.g., bars, discos)
  - Key local policymakers
  - Donors

RATIONALE FOR THE METHODOLOGY

Focus group discussions were conducted with men who have sex with men, male sex workers, and transgender individuals to gather data on how they are treated by the community, experiences of gender-based violence, and suggestions for future intervention strategies. In-depth interviews would usually be more appropriate for a sensitive topic like gender-based violence, but participants were recruited from established support groups, so groups had already established rapport and could support each other in discussing a difficult topic.

In-depth interviews were conducted with key informants, many of whom were service providers and informal leaders in the community, to also understand their perspective on these populations and their needs; assess what services are available for gender-based violence prevention and support; and learn about the challenges service providers face in implementing these services. In-depth interviews were conducted with key informants instead of focus group discussions because participants had varying job functions and roles in the community.

(Continued)

KEY FINDINGS

Study participants reported that men who have sex with men, transgender individuals, and male sex workers in Bangladesh and Papua New Guinea face numerous types of gender-based violence, ranging from being teased by people on the street to being raped and murdered. The violence reported by study participants was grouped into four types: physical violence, sexual violence, verbal violence, and other types of violence. Examples of other types of violence include stigma, discrimination, exclusion, harassment, blackmail, clients refusing to pay after having sex, rejection or nonacceptance by family or community members, disrespect, police ignoring gender-based violence complaints, health care staff refusing to provide care, and humiliation. "Other types of violence" were the most commonly discussed, indicating that while direct, easily identifiable (physical, sexual, and verbal) violence directed at individuals in these populations is common in these settings, of equal importance are other, less obvious and less easily categorized forms of violence. Moreover, many individuals experienced multiple forms of gender-based violence.

Gender-based violence was perpetuated against sexual minorities from a wide variety of sources, including one's own family members and sexual partners, transactional sex clients, and community members. Two key sources of violence were police officers and health care providers, thus creating barriers to accessing legal and health care services.

The primary reason identified by study participants for gender-based violence toward sexual minorities was that these individuals have identities or exhibit behaviors that violate existing societal norms, for example, displaying feminine behaviors. Additionally, engaging in sex work was noted as a major cause of gender-based violence.

Participants named a variety of programs and service providers in their communities working either to prevent violence or to assist survivors, including health care and counseling services, human rights advocacy, legal support, and skills training. However, they also listed numerous obstacles to effective implementation of gender-based violence interventions and services, including religious beliefs and ongoing political and legal barriers, such as the criminalization of men having sex with men.

OTHER CONSIDERATIONS

Recruiting sexual minorities can be challenging because self-identifying as a member of one of these populations can present legal and social risks. In both

(Continued)

countries, the research team worked with local nongovernmental organizations, community-based organizations, and networks for men who have sex with men, transgender individuals, and male sex workers. Organization staff and network members invited clients and contacts to participate in the study. Using this approach, the research team was able to successfully recruit participants into the study.

TAKE-HOME POINTS

Formative research can be used to inform programming for hard-to-reach populations. Working with local organizations and networks that are already connected to these individuals can help identify individuals who meet the recruitment criteria. Because potential participants already trust these organizations and networks, they may be more likely to participate in the study than if approached by the research team directly.

Key staff: Christina Wong and Shanti Noriega (FHI 360)

Supplemental Case Study Materials

Wong, C. M., & Noriega, S. (2013). Exploring gender based violence among men who have sex with men (MSM), male sex worker (MSW) and transgender (TG) communities in Bangladesh and Papua New Guinea: Results and Recommendations. Available at http://www.fhi360.org/explore/content?f%5B0%5D=type%3Aresource&f%5B1%5D=field_practice_areas%3A278

References

Gardsbane, D. (2010). *Gender-based violence and HIV* (p. 2). Arlington, VA: USAID AIDSTAR-ONE PROJECT.

Ministry of Health and Family Welfare of Bangladesh. (2009). *Behavioral surveillance survey 2006–2007: Technical report*. Dhaka, Bangladesh: National AIDS/STD Program.

CASE STUDY 8
SOCIOBEHAVIORAL RESEARCH AND COMMUNITY PLANNING TO DEVELOP SITE-SPECIFIC PLANS FOR PREP ROLLOUT

Country: Kenya

Topic: Implementation of pre-exposure prophylaxis (PrEP) for HIV prevention

BACKGROUND

Extensive planning is required before new health interventions can be implemented in developing and developed countries alike. Research and planning activities were carried out in Bondo, Kenya, during the FEM-PrEP clinical trial testing emtricitabine/tenofovir disoproxil fumarate as PrEP for HIV prevention. The purpose was to help facilitate preparations for the rollout of PrEP in Kenya if the drug was found to be effective at reducing the chance of HIV infection.

AIMS

1. To conduct qualitative research to inform planning for a pilot social marketing intervention for PrEP that could be implemented if PrEP was demonstrated to reduce the chance of HIV infection. This research included identification of:
   a. Country priorities for PrEP use
   b. Appropriate target populations
   c. Factors relevant for integrating PrEP into the local HIV prevention context
   d. Barriers and facilitators to successful intervention implementation and uptake
2. To facilitate community planning of pilot social marketing interventions for PrEP

THEORY OR APPROACH USED

A social marketing methodological approach was used.

(Continued)

METHODS

- Semistructured interviews were conducted with local civil society leaders, public health stakeholders at multiple administrative levels, members of local potential target populations for PrEP, and FEM-PrEP trial participants to learn their views on the use of PrEP in Kenya.
- Stakeholder consultations were conducted with district, provincial, and national public health stakeholders to disseminate preliminary findings and to problem-solve with regard to local PrEP implementation. Researchers used structured guides with open-ended questions to generate discussion among the attendees.

CONTRIBUTIONS OF THE METHODOLOGICAL APPROACH

Triangulation of interviews and consultations with public health stakeholders of different administrative levels was effective for eliciting a range of concerns with respect to the future implementation of PrEP in Kenya. Consultations, in particular, proved to be an effective way to engage public health officials because the consultations acknowledged them as experts rather than treating them as research "subjects." It also provided more time than a focus group would have allowed for educating stakeholders about PrEP, informing them of interim study results, and having discussions. Thus, the consultations were a combination of research dissemination and data collection.

In addition, individual interviews with members of potential target populations for PrEP provided data on sensitive topics, including women's perceptions of their risk of HIV infection and their descriptions of any behavioral risk-reduction methods they had tried or would potentially try in the next year. These behavioral methods included condoms, with consistent use described as difficult; partner reduction, but this was described as difficult to sustain due to poverty and the need for financial support from partners; and abstinence, which was also described as impossible as a long-term solution.

Key study staff: Natasha Mack, Christina Wong (FHI 360); Kawango Agot, Jacob Odhiambo (Impact Research and Development Organization)

(Continued)

Supplemental Case Study Materials

Mack, N., Odhiambo, J., Wong, C. M., & Agot, K. (2014). Barriers and facilitators to pre-exposure prophylaxis (PrEP) eligibility screening and ongoing HIV testing among target populations in Bondo and Rarieda, Kenya: Results of a consultation with community stakeholders. *BMC Health Services Research, 14,* 231. doi:10.1186/1472-6963-14-231

Mack, N., Wong, C., McKenna, K., Lemons, A., Odhiambo, J., & Agot, K. (2015). Human resource challenges to integrating HIV pre-exposure prophylaxis (PrEP) into the public health system in Kenya: A qualitative study. *African Journal of Reproductive Health, 19*(1), 54–62.

CASE STUDY 9
EVALUATION OF MALAWI MALE MOTIVATOR INTERVENTION

Country: Malawi

Topic: Engaging men in family planning decision making

BACKGROUND

The 1994 International Conference on Population and Development in Cairo, Egypt, reemphasized that family planning interventions should engage men and acknowledge their role in reproductive health services as a means to improve the reproductive health of women and men. However, family planning interventions for men have not been rigorously evaluated. Malawi has a high fertility rate at 6.34 children per woman of reproductive age and low contraceptive prevalence at 26%. The Malawi Male Motivator intervention was implemented by Save the Children to increase use of family planning among young Malawian couples. Building upon research showing that men tend to get reproductive health information from peers, the intervention relied on a male outreach worker, referred to as a *male motivator,* to target husbands.

AIMS

To examine the effect of the Malawi Male Motivators' intervention on couples' contraceptive uptake

THEORY OR APPROACH USED

Information-motivation-behavioral skills model

METHODS

Quantitative

- Intervention participants completed pre- and post-intervention surveys ($n = 289$)

Qualitative

- Ten percent of participants in the intervention arm were randomly selected for post-intervention semi-structured interviews ($n = 14$)

(Continued)

- Female partners of intervention participants were randomly selected for semi-structured interviews 1 year after the intervention ($n = 30$)

CONTRIBUTIONS OF THE QUALITATIVE APPROACH

This explanatory study was designed to determine whether the intervention had an effect on contraceptive uptake. However, the research team also used mixed-methods data collection to assess *how* and *why* the intervention affected contraceptive uptake. Pre- and post-intervention surveys used scales based on the information-motivation-behavioral skills model to assess changes in family planning knowledge, family planning attitudes, gender norms, family planning self-efficacy, and couples' communication about family planning.

Semi-structured interviews with intervention participants assessed participants' perception of the study, whether they and their wives or girlfriends were using contraception and the rationale for their use or nonuse, thoughts on the information shared during intervention visits, and their comfort discussing family planning with their wives or girlfriends and friends.

Building off the key finding that couples' communication played an important role in the intervention's effectiveness, the research team decided to conduct follow-up semi-structured interviews with the female partners of male participants 1 year after the intervention to further explore how couples' communication played into the intervention's success.

KEY FINDINGS

The intervention resulted in a significant increase in self-reported contraceptive use in both the intervention and control arms ($P < .01$) and a significantly greater increase in contraceptive use in the intervention arm compared with the control arm ($P < .01$). The quantitative survey data indicated that increased ease and frequency of communication within couples were significant predictors of contraceptive uptake ($P < .01$). Qualitative interviews with men supported and provided additional explanations of these findings. Many men who were interviewed said their interactions with the male motivator made them more comfortable discussing family planning with their wives, and more than half of the men said the intervention had provided an opportunity to talk with their wives or girlfriends about family planning. Interestingly, the semi-structured interviews with men indicated that men found financial reasons for family planning the most persuasive: nearly all of the men interviewed discussed the relationship between use of family planning and economic benefits.

(Continued)

Women reported improvements in couples' communication, increased frequency of communication, and increased shared decision making as a result of the study, which they said contributed to their family planning use. They said reduced male opposition to family planning also helped promote their family planning use. Finally, there was a shift away from traditional communication and decision-making roles, typically dominated by men, toward more joint decision making and equitable communication. The findings suggest that men often lack information and experience discussing family planning with their partners, and interventions that help to develop these skills are necessary to facilitate open and equitable discussion.

TAKE-HOME POINT

By using a mixed-methods study design, the research team was able to show not only that the intervention was effective but also explain how and why it was effective, which will inform replication, adaptation, and scale-up of the intervention in Malawi and other countries.

Key study staff: Dominick Shattuck, Greg Guest, Miriam Hartmann (FHI 360)

Supplementary Case Study Materials

Hartmann, M., Gilles, K., Shattuck, D., Kerner, B., & Guest, G. (2012). Changes in couples' communication as a result of a male-involvement family planning intervention. *Journal of Health Communication, 17*(7), 802–819. doi:10.1080/10810730.2011.650825

Shattuck, D., Kerner, B., Gilles, K., Hartmann, M., Ng'ombe, T., & Guest, G. (2011). Encouraging contraceptive uptake by motivating men to communicate about family planning: The Malawi Male Motivator project. *American Journal of Public Health, 101*(6), 1089–1095. doi:10.2105/AJPH.2010.300091

CASE STUDY 10
REASONS FOR CONTRACEPTIVE NONUSE IN RWANDA

Country: Rwanda

Topic: Acceptability of and adherence to contraceptive products

BACKGROUND

Like many other developing countries, Rwanda has been committed to achieving the Millenium Development Goals (MDGs) by 2015. With a population density of 365 people per square kilometer and an estimated fertility rate of 5.5 children per woman in 2008, the country faces severe demographic pressure (INSR & ORC Macro 2008; Thaxton, 2015). Government efforts to decentralize the health care system and integrate family planning into all health services have met with some success, with contraceptive prevalence increasing from 4% in 2000 to 45% in 2010 (USAID/Africa Bureau, USAID/Population and Reproductive Health, Ethiopia Federal Ministry of Health, Malawi Ministry of Health, & Health RMo, 2012). However, to reach the country's target of 70% by 2015, major increases remain necessary. This study sought to identify why women in Rwanda may not be using contraception.

AIMS

The objectives of the study were to:

- Identify reasons for current nonuse of modern contraceptive methods.
- Examine barriers to use.
- Explore psychosocial factors influencing use of contraception.

The study focused on understanding user demand for and use of contraception rather than supply side issues, as some women and couples may never have made contact with service providers or availed themselves of contraceptive services.

THEORY OR APPROACH USED

The stages of change theory provided a point of reference for data collection. This theory suggests that people move through stages—from precontemplation,

(Continued)

preparation, and action—before being able to achieve long-term adherence to more complex behaviors. In this study, participants were asked about their current, past, and/or ever use of contraception in in-depth interviews, and these data were captured on a brief form that could be used to stratify participants by their "stage of change" vis-à-vis contraceptive use. Qualitative data helped to better understand the psychological and social factors that influenced never-use (similar to precontemplation), interest in future use (preparation), and various durations of contraceptive method use.

METHODS

The community-based, cross-sectional, mixed-method study was conducted in 5 of 30 districts. It included a survey with 637 women and in-depth interviews with 54 women and 27 male partners. Participants were selected through a multistage random sampling process. One woman was randomly selected per household at the last stage.

- Women participating in the quantitative survey provided information on social and demographic characteristics, fertility intentions, sources of contraceptive information, contraceptive use history, psychosocial and cultural factors, partner support, and service delivery environment.
- In every eighth household, the randomly selected woman was invited to participate in an in-depth interview. The male partner of every other female participant was also invited to participate in a separate qualitative interview after permission was received from the woman.
- In-depth interviews explored in greater depth women's and their partners' fertility desires, their attitudes toward and experiences with different contraceptive methods, and the nature of discussions with each other, with other community members, and with health care providers.

CONTRIBUTIONS OF THE METHODOLOGICAL APPROACH

In-depth interviews with women were effective for revealing misperceptions about fertility that led to gaps in contraceptive coverage, particularly postpartum. The interviews also highlighted how provider practices, including screening for pregnancy through direct observation of menses, may hamper contraceptive use. Interviews with male partners revealed some conflict in men's attitudes toward contraceptive use; men were clear about the benefit of using contraception given the economic and educational challenges of raising children. However, they may

(Continued)

be reluctant to encourage their partners to continue using contraception if they experienced side effects affecting sexual relations.

Key staff: Aurélie Brunie, Elizabeth E. Tolley, Emmanuel Munyambanza (FHI 360)

Supplementary Case Study Materials

Brunie, A., Tolley, E. E., Ngabo, F., Wesson, J., & Chen, M. (2013). Getting to 70%: Barriers to modern contraceptive use for women in Rwanda. *International Journal of Gynecology & Obstetrics, 123*(Suppl 1), e11–e15. doi:10.1016/j.ijgo.2013.07.005

References

Institut National de la Statistique du Rwanda (INSR) & ORC Macro. (2008). *Rwanda interim Demographic and Health Survey 2007–2008: Preliminary report*. Calverton, MD.

Thaxton, M. (2015). *Integrating population, health, and environment in Rwanda.* Population Reference Bureau. Available at http://www.prb.org/pdf09/phe-rwanda.pdf

USAID/Africa Bureau, USAID/Population and Reproductive Health, Ethiopia Federal Ministry of Health, Malawi Ministry of Health, & Health RMo. (2012). Three successful sub-Saharan Africa family planning programs: Lessons for meeting the MDGs. Washington, DC: USAID Africa Bureau.

CASE STUDY 11
PERSONAL INVOLVEMENT OF YOUNG PEOPLE IN HIV PREVENTION CAMPAIGN MESSAGES: THE ROLE OF MESSAGE FORMAT, CULTURE, AND GENDER

Countries: Brazil, Kenya, Nepal, and Senegal

Topic: Health communications

BACKGROUND

In 2002, MTV International, the world's largest youth-brand media network, in partnership with FHI (now FHI 360), the Kaiser Foundation, and the Gates Foundation to produce, broadcast, and distribute a campaign that included an hour-long Staying Alive documentary in conjunction with a panel discussion, seven public service announcements (PSAs), a website linked to MTV.com, and live concerts held on World AIDS Day in Seattle, Washington, and Johannesburg, South Africa. The PSAs and the documentary focused on different aspects of AIDS prevention. The PSAs focused exclusively on reducing condom stigma, whereas the documentary focused on issues related to people living with HIV or at risk of HIV infection. As part of an evaluation of the campaign, FGDs were conducted in four countries where the campaign was aired to find out more about young people's perspectives on the documentary and PSAs. Because it was a global campaign reaching 789 million households in 166 countries, there was concern about whether young people in diverse cultural contexts would find the materials for the campaign to be personally relevant. FGD data allowed researchers to examine reactions to and interpretations of content across four culturally diverse countries. The FGD transcripts were analyzed to examine participants' involvement with the message content as it related to message format—PSA (short) or documentary (long)—culture and gender. Personal involvement was of interest because it has been shown to mediate the effects of persuasive messages.

AIMS

The specific objectives of the analysis described here were: (1) to determine the broad themes that surfaced in discussions of the various materials and how self-referential statements were expressed within these themes; (2) to determine whether there were differences in the amount and type of self-referential

(Continued)

statements with respect to program format (PSA or documentary); (3) determine the degree to which themes identified and types of self-referential statements varied by cultural context (country site) and participant gender; and (4) to consider the implications of these findings for future programming of global HIV prevention campaigns for youth.

THEORY OR APPROACH USED

The Elaboration Likelihood Model (ELM) (Petty & Cacioppo, 1981) served as the theoretical basis of the analysis. According to the ELM, there are two paths to persuasion. The central route produces message-relevant thinking and the peripheral path relies more on cues that will persuade the viewer in absence of message elaboration: source attractiveness, source credibility, humor, visual or audio aesthetics, or associations with pleasure. Persuasion resulting from the central route is more stable and is more likely to foster behavior change. A key factor in one's motivation to think about the message is personal involvement or relevance, which leads to great self-referential thinking during a persuasive appeal (Petty, Cacioppo, & Goldman, 1984). Researchers believed that a focus on self-referential thinking would indicate a mechanism for persuasion that might vary by message format, culture, and recipient gender. The data were exploratory, but researchers found this to be a useful framework for examining the potential persuasive impact of the campaign materials.

METHODS

All data were collected through FGDs in four sites several months after the campaign had aired. The four sites were São Paulo, Brazil; Kathmandu, Nepal; Dakar, Senegal; and Nairobi, Kenya. In each site, FGDs of six to ten 16- to 25-year-olds (MTV's target audience) were convened to provide audience perspectives on two types of campaign materials: PSAs (short form) and the documentary (long form). About one third of the groups were composed of females only, one third were composed of males only, and one third were mixed-gender groups. Specifically, 167 male and 168 female participants took part in this study. Gender was the only consistent segmentation across sites. The number of FGDs in each site represented two FGDs per gender, class, and/or other variable classifications, which we felt would give us saturation of new ideas. The viewing environment created by the FGDs facilitated more attention to the campaign materials than there might have been if viewing them at home with more possible distractions. This might have reduced the ecological validity, but studying audience reactions in multiple countries increased our confidence in similar findings across sites.

(Continued)

Study participants were recruited through local youth-serving organizations by local researchers and were thus samples of convenience. Participants were asked questions about their knowledge and beliefs about HIV/AIDS. They were then shown videotaped PSAs; each was shown twice. A set of standardized questions guided the post-viewing discussions, though moderators were free to follow up and probe as necessary. After the PSA discussions, they were shown a videotape of the documentary, followed by questions about the documentary. Campaign materials were shown in the language they would have been shown on their local station. The PSAs were mostly nonverbal except for a tagline at the end. All FGDs were audiotaped and then transcribed by the local research team in each site. All transcripts were translated into English by professional translators in the United States, Dakar, Nairobi, and Kathmandu.

Data were analyzed in several layers of iteration. First, all transcripts were read in English by three U.S.-based qualitative researchers trained in qualitative analysis and media effects. General codes were assigned for gender composition of the FGD and study site. A coding tree was developed to identify general themes that surfaced from the first reading. Second, two analysts completed the initial coding using the coding tree; the coding tree was revised during this process based on discussions between the analysts. One coder went through all the transcripts to incorporate any changes needed based on coding tree revisions. Reports were generated by site and FGD, generally focusing on discussions of specific PSAs or documentary "characters." A second layer of codes was created by a third analyst for several specific types of self-referential statements: personal connections, lessons learned, and emotional response. These codes were examined by message format, site, and respondent gender.

CONTRIBUTIONS OF THE QUALITATIVE APPROACH

Researchers found several consistent responses to the campaign materials across cultures and genders. The PSAs, which focused on condoms, were found to be entertaining and relevant, and viewers said they could connect to them on a personal level. The documentary elicited many common responses of sympathy to the characters who were living with AIDS. They felt sympathy for the young mother in Cambodia who was shunned by her neighbors and had a difficult time accessing drugs to treat her illness. Respondents felt anger at her husband who infected her. They felt admiration for the young man from Latvia who was struggling against his drug addiction. The larger themes identified were tolerance for people living with

(Continued)

HIV, the struggle of people living with HIV, fidelity and trust, the need for access to medicine, and everyone's personal responsibility for the fight against AIDS.

Additional findings demonstrated relationships between self-referential statements (indicating message involvement) and message format, culture, and gender. Researchers found differences in the proportion of personal connections related to type of programming; in general, respondents made more connections between their own lives and the longer format programming. Respondents were more likely to express changes in attitudes and intentions to change behavior in response to the long form compared to the short form materials. Emotional reactions tended to be more intense for the documentary stories than for the PSA stories. Some PSAs elicited more personal connections from young men than young women because they related more directly to the experience of young men than of young women. Female respondents often rallied around strong female characters and railed against men who were mistreating women. The PSAs elicited more negative reactions due to cultural inappropriateness than did the documentary. There was more resistance to condom messages in culturally conservative sites and more resistance from young women than young men.

Thus, researchers found greater central processing of the documentary stories. These long form stories strongly resonated with audiences across genders and cultures and seemed to be appropriate for a diverse global audience. The resistance found to the PSAs was primarily context specific; short messages, which are less expensive and can be shown frequently over a short period of time for greater impact, might be best left to local production.

Key study staff: Cynthia Geary, Holly Burke, Laura Johnson, Jennifer Liku (FHI 360); Laure Castlenau (IBOPE, Sao Paulo, Brazil); Shailes Neupane (Valley Research Group, Kathmandu, Nepal); Cheik Niang (Institute for Environmental Sciences, Dakar, Senegal)

Supplemental Case Study Materials

Geary, C. W., Burke, H. M., Johnson, L., Liku, J., Castlenau, L., Neupane, S., & Niang, C. (2006). Personal involvement of young people in HIV prevention campaign messages: The role of message format, culture and gender. *Health Education & Behavior*, *35*(2), 190–206. doi:10.1177/1090198106288252

(Continued)

References

Petty, R., & Cacioppo, J. T. (1981). *Attitudes and persuasion: Classic and contemporary approaches*. Dubuque, IA: W.C. Brown.

Petty, R., Cacioppo, J. T., & Goldman, R. (1984). Personal involvement as a determinant of argument-based persuasion. *Journal of Personality and Social Psychology*, *41*(5), 847–855. doi:10.1037/0022-3514.41.5.847

CASE STUDY 12
VOLUNTARY MEDICAL MALE CIRCUMCISION IN KENYA

Country: Kenya

Topic: Voluntary medical male circumcision (VMMC) for HIV prevention

BACKGROUND

Three randomized controlled trials conducted in Uganda, Kenya, and South Africa between 2002 and 2006 demonstrated that VMMC partially protects men against HIV infection acquired through vaginal sex (Auvert et al., 2005; Bailey et al., 2007; Gray et al., 2007; Irin News, 2012). VMMC services are now being scaled-up in sub-Saharan Africa, including Kenya (Mwandi et al., 2011). However, the uptake of VMMC among adult men has been lower than desired in Nyanza Province, Kenya, where the prevalence of HIV is the highest at 13.9% and the prevalence of male circumcision (44.8%) is lowest (Kenya National Bureau of Statistics [KNBS] & ICF Macro, 2010). The largest increase in HIV prevalence among men occurs between ages 20 and 29 with prevalence peaking at 10.4% among men aged 35 to 39, indicating the importance of targeting adult men with HIV prevention efforts like VMMC (KNBS and ICF Macro, 2010). From 2010 to 2012, Kenya's Rapid Results Initiatives—the periodic, intensive programmatic efforts to provide VMMC services—increased the number of VMMCs among men over age 15; however, the number of men over 24 who have been circumcised remains lower than desired with only approximately 10% of men 25 and older circumcised in Nyanza (Hankins, Forsythe, & Njeuhmeli, 2011; Herman-Roloff, Llewellyn, and others 2011; KNBS & ICF Macro, 2010; Mwandi et al., 2011). Given this age group's high risk of acquiring HIV, increasing VMMC uptake in this age group is likely to have an immediate impact on population-level HIV incidence in Nyanza. In order to increase uptake, the identification of barriers to seeking VMMC and evidence-informed interventions to address those barriers were needed (Gray, Wawer, & Kigozi, 2013; Hankins et al., 2010; KNBS & ICF Macro, 2010). Previous research identified several barriers to uptake, but qualitative exploration of barriers has been limited and interventions informed by evidence have not been fully developed.

AIMS

The purpose of this study was to:

- Increase understanding of the factors that serve as primary barriers to uptake of VMMC.

(Continued)

- Develop interventions to increase uptake of VMMC among high-risk men between the ages of 18 and 35 in Nyanza Province, Kenya, based on the identified barriers.

METHODS

- Semi-structured interviews and focus group discussions were conducted with circumcised and uncircumcised men to learn their barriers to uptake of VMMC.
- Pile sorts in which men were asked to rank a list of 18 reasons why men might not want to get circumcised were used in the focus groups to learn about group norms surrounding barriers to circumcision. Reasons for the rankings were then discussed.
- Semi-structured interviews were conducted with female partners, peers, community and religious leaders, health care providers, and employers to examine the role others may play in inhibiting and motivating men to seek VMMC.
- Once preliminary results from the interviews were available, a workshop was held with representatives of the Ministries of Health, VMMC service providers, demand creation partners, and agencies funding VMMC efforts. During the workshop, these stakeholders identified and prioritized the most feasible and acceptable interventions for addressing the main barriers to VMMC uptake.

CONTRIBUTIONS OF THE METHODOLOGICAL APPROACH

The pile sort exercise during the focus groups enabled men to give responses drawing on both their personal experiences and those of friends or community members, going beyond individual experiences to capture stories or broader memes. During the discussion of the pile sort results, researchers learned how men ranked their barriers to VMMC and how much agreement there was on the rankings. Researchers identified men's financial concerns about lost wages as a primary barrier to uptake of VMMC during the semi-structured interviews. In the subsequent workshop, stakeholders prioritized VMMC interventions addressing these financial concerns.

Previous research on barriers to VMMC was limited to mostly quantitative, closed-ended questions. This study used qualitative methods to broaden the understanding of men's barriers and identify strategies to address those barriers. Additionally, interviews with female partners, employers, community and faith leaders, and health care providers enabled researchers to investigate the role that influential others play in men's decisions to seek, or not seek, VMMC. Data on the social, cultural, physical, and economic factors that influenced men's decision

(Continued)

making informed the development of successful interventions to address barriers to VMMC and capitalize on facilitating factors.

Key study staff: Emily Evens, Michele Lanham, Catherine Hart, Mores Loolpapit, Isaac Oguma (FHI 360); Walter Obiero (Nyanza Reproductive Health Society)

Supplemental Case Study Materials

Evens, E., Lanham, M., Hart, C., Loolpapit, M., Oguma, I., & Obiero, W. (2014). Identifying and addressing barriers to uptake of voluntary medical male circumcision in Nyanza, Kenya among men 18–35: A qualitative study. *PloS ONE*, *9*(6), e98221. doi:10.1371/journal.pone.0098221

References

Auvert, B., Taljaard, D., Lagarde, E., Sobngwi-Tambekou, J., Sitta, R., & Puren, A. (2005). Randomized, controlled intervention trial of male circumcision for reduction of HIV infection risk: The ANRS 1265 trial. *PLoS Med*, *2*(11), e298. doi:10.1371/journal.pmed.0020298

Bailey, R. C., Moses, S., Parker, C. B., Agot, K., Maclean, I., Krieger, J. N., . . . , & Ndinya-Achola, J. O. (2007). Male circumcision for HIV prevention in young men in Kisumu, Kenya: A randomized controlled trial. *The Lancet*, *369*(9562), 643–656. doi:10.1016/S0140-6736(07)60312-2

Gray, R., Kigozi, G., Serwadda, D., Makumbi, F., Watya, S., Nalugoda, F., . . . , & Wawer, M. J. (2007). Male circumcision for HIV prevention in men in Rakai, Uganda: A randomized trial. *The Lancet*, *369*(9562), 657–666. doi:10.1016/S0140-6736(07)60313-4

Gray, R., Wawer, M. J., & Kigozi, G. (2013). Programme science research on medical male circumcision scale-up in sub-Saharan Africa. *Sexually Transmitted Infections*, *89*(5), 345–349. doi:10.1136/sextrans-2012-050595

Hankins, C., Forsythe, S., & Njeuhmeli, E. (2011). Voluntary medical male circumcision: An introduction to the cost, impact, and challenges of accelerated scaling up. *PLoS Med*, *8*(11), e1001127. doi:10.1371/journal.pmed.1001127

(Continued)

Herman-Roloff, A., Llewellyn, E., Obiero, W., Agot, K., Ndinya-Achola, J., Muraguri, N., & Bailey, R. C. (2011). Implementing voluntary medical male circumcision for HIV prevention in Nyanza Province, Kenya: Lessons learned during the first year. *PLOS ONE*, *6*(4), e18299. doi:10.1371/journal.pone.0018299

Irin News. 2012. *KENYA: Push to meet 2013 male circumcision targets. IRIN humanitarian news and analysis*. Available at http://www.irinnews.org/report/96717/kenya-push-to-meet-2013-male-circumcision-targets

Kenya National Bureau of Statistics & ICF Macro. (2010). *Kenya Demographic and Health Survey 2008–2009*. Calverton, MD: KNBS and ICF Macro.

Mwandi, Z., Murphy, A., Reed, J., Chesang, K., Njeuhmeli, E., Agot, K., . . . , & Bock, N. (2011). Voluntary medical male circumcision: Translating research into the rapid expansion of services in Kenya, 2008–2011. *PLOS Med*, *8*(11), 001130. doi:10.1371/journal.pmed.1001130

CASE STUDY 13
ALIVE & THRIVE

Country: Vietnam

Topic: Infant and young child feeding (IYCF)

BACKGROUND

The time between birth and 24 months provides a unique window of opportunity to positively affect the long-term health and development of children through nutrition. The World Health Organization (WHO) and UNICEF issued a Global Strategy for Infant and Young Child Feeding in 2003 as a guide for action to develop comprehensive programs (World Health Organization/UNICEF, 2003). At that time, few field-tested, documented examples of the design of large, multicomponent IYCF programs existed. However, global IYCF indicators, monitoring tools, counseling materials, training manuals, and programmatic lessons were available (World Health Organization/UNICEF, 2006, 2007). In this study, formative research was conducted on IYCF practices as part of a larger effort to improve rates of exclusive breastfeeding and improving complementary feeding practices.

AIMS

The formative research sought to:

- Identify existing breastfeeding and complementary feeding practices and their facilitators and barriers.
- Understand the roles of mothers, family members, health providers, policymakers, and institutions in these feeding practices.

THEORY OR APPROACH USED

The formative research examined the behaviors, opportunities, and constraints to improved IYCF at multiple levels (following the social-ecological model), including direct observations and interviews with mothers, fathers, grandmothers, and health providers who most immediately influence such behaviors. Opinion leaders were also interviewed to assess policy and advocacy needs and efforts.

Design of the subsequent behavior change program drew upon several behavioral models, including the individual stages of behavior change, the theory of reasoned action, and a socioecological model.

(Continued)

METHODS

- Semi-structured interviews with pregnant women and mothers of infants to elicit their perceptions and practices on IYCF
- Opportunistic observations of mothers breastfeeding, preparing food, and feeding and interacting with their children
- Food attribute exercises with mothers to elicit beliefs about the quality and adequacy of each food item for young children
- Semi-structured interviews with fathers to explore male involvement in IYCF
- Focus group discussions with grandmothers
- Semi-structured interviews with health providers
- Trials of improved practices (TIPS) and 24-hour dietary recalls

FINDINGS

The research identified several key barriers to optimal infant feeding practices. One important barrier was the misperception that mothers have insufficient milk, both in terms of quantity and quality. Health care providers and mothers alike were often unaware of the role that early initiation of breastfeeding, exclusive breastfeeding, and the practice of emptying one breast of milk before switching to the other breast had on milk production. A second barrier related to the common practice of giving infants water just after nursing to clean a child's mouth or quench thirst, especially during summer. Other barriers included concerns about how to initiate breastfeeding after a delivery by cesarean section, how to continue giving breastmilk when a mother needed to return to the workplace, and the belief that a combination of breastmilk and formula milk was the best nutrition for a young infant.

Based on TIPS, during which pregnant and new mothers were invited to try out "small doable actions" that could improve their infants' nutrition, the study found that (1) pregnant women were more likely to initiate breastfeeding within 1 hour of birth if they were counseled about it before delivery, and (2) mothers were more committed to exclusively breastfeeding their infants (below the age of 6 months) once they understood that breastmilk was 88% water and that giving additional water could displace breastmilk. Finally, the TIPS interviews noted ongoing difficulties with accommodating breastfeeding practices upon return to work. While some women attempted to express milk and store it for their infants, having sufficient privacy to express milk and refrigeration for milk storage were difficult challenges to overcome.

(Continued)

CONTRIBUTIONS OF THE QUALITATIVE APPROACH

The results of the formative research were used to inform the development of Alive & Thrive program strategies and activities, including an innovative social franchise model to provide good quality infant and young child feeding counseling services, a media campaign, and a workplace lactation support program that were successful in improving exclusive breastfeeding practices. Significant policy changes were achieved with paid maternity leave being extended from 4 to 6 months and a strengthened national code for the marketing of breastmilk substitutes.

Key study staff: Nemat Hajeebhoy, Giang Huong Nguyen, Chau Hai Vu, Ann Jimerson (FHI 360)

Supplementary Case Study Materials

Alive & Thrive. (2012a). *Formative research on infant & young child feeding in Viet Nam: Phase 1 summary report*. Ha Noi, Viet Nam.

Alive & Thrive. (2012b). *Formative research on infant & young child feeding in Viet Nam. Phase 2 summary report: Trials of improved practices*. Ha Noi, Viet Nam.

Baker, J., Sanghvi, T., Hajeebhoy, N., Martin, L., & Lapping, K. (2013). Using an evidence-based approach to design large-scale programs to improve infant and young child feeding. *Food & Nutrition Bulletin, 34*(Suppl 2), 146S–155S.

References

World Health Organization/UNICEF. (2003). *Global strategy for infant and young child feeding*. Geneva: World Health Organization.

World Health Organization/UNICEF. (2006). *Infant and young child feeding: An integrated course. Trainer's guide*. Geneva, Switzerland: World Health Organization. Available at http://whqlibdoc.who.int/publications/2006/9789241594769_eng.pdf

World Health Organization/UNICEF. (2007). *Planning guide for national implementation of the global strategy for infant and young child feeding*. Geneva, Switzerland: World Health Organization.

CASE STUDY 14
COMMUNICATING ABOUT MICROBICIDES WITH WOMEN IN MIND

Date: 2012–2014
Country: Kenya
Topic: Vaginal microbicides, new ARV-based HIV prevention for women

BACKGROUND

Globally, women continue to be disproportionally affected by HIV, despite widespread HIV knowledge and availability of condoms. To curb the epidemic, HIV prevention products that work for women are needed. In 2010, the clinical trial CAPRISA 004 provided proof of concept that pericoital, vaginal use of tenofovir 1% microbicide gel can reduce HIV acquisition among women. Efforts to develop and assess other female initiated products, including vaginal rings, are ongoing. Given the potential challenges to positioning new ARV prevention products so that women can use them, now is the time to think strategically about demand generation.

Along with product efficacy, price, and availability, women's social and sexual contexts will shape their interest in and ability to use microbicides. Communication campaigns will also play a key role in generating demand and educating women about correct use. For example, by framing microbicide-related messages exclusively on HIV prevention, or on other benefits such as sexual pleasure and empowerment, communication strategies could either facilitate or impede a woman's interest in their use. Moreover, because the current pericoital gel use regimen is complicated, and because microbicides are not likely to be as effective as condoms, in-depth education will be necessary to ensure proper use and understanding of efficacy.

AIMS

This project aimed to develop a minimum package of microbicide-related communication materials and then test their efficacy in generating awareness of and demand for microbicides among women, male partners, and providers.

THEORY OR APPROACH USED

Two theories were consulted. Based on the social cognitive model, messages were developed to target the individual and environmental barriers and facilitators of

(Continued)

microbicide-related behaviors for different audiences. Additionally, the elaboration likelihood model informed pretesting and materials assessment. This theory suggests that communication materials influence audiences through two routes to persuasion: (1) peripheral cues (based on positive/negative "cues" such as attractiveness) and (2) central processing (based on relevance of topic to individual). The project developed and tested two sets of awareness-raising materials.

METHODS

Phase 1: Kenyan stakeholders and representative audiences were consulted to identify priority audiences, determine what types of materials to develop, and inform message content. Activities included a national policy consultation with Kenyan policymakers, program implementers, and researchers to determine which audiences should be prioritized for microbicide-related communication; 12 workshops in four regions with target audiences to provide input on draft messages and visual images; and a national message development workshop to draft audience profiles and key audience-specific messages.

Phase 2: A local design firm was identified to develop materials, which included materials for awareness-raising (posters, TV storyboards, and radio spots) and in-depth education (flip charts, an informational brochure, and counseling algorithm). Two versions of awareness-raising materials were developed: one with microbicides framed as HIV prevention, and one with microbicides framed primarily as a product with other benefits in addition to HIV prevention. Two rounds of pretesting were conducted with target audiences in four regions to refine messages and materials prior to formal research assessment.

Phase 3: A mixed-method design was used to assess materials. The ability of awareness-raising materials to general interest in and demand for microbicides was assessed via a quantitative intercept survey with 200 men and 800 women, randomized to (1) microbicide information only, (2) HIV-framed materials, or (3) non-HIV-framed materials. At the conclusion of the survey, participants were asked an open-ended question regarding their final thoughts about microbicides and the materials they viewed. NGOs tested in-depth educational materials to determine how well flipcharts addressed women's informational needs and generated microbicide interest. In addition, in-depth interviews were conducted with health care providers to assess providers' acceptability of vaginal microbicides, ability to appropriately use materials to counsel women on microbicides, and their thoughts on the content and usefulness of materials.

(Continued)

CONTRIBUTIONS OF THE QUALITATIVE APPROACH

Qualitative analysis of the mock discussion groups revealed that participants were engaged in the discussion about microbicides. Moreover, research assistants were able to document questions that participants had, either about microbicides or about the flip charts. They were also able to identify areas where additional training might be required for facilitators.

Analysis of the in-depth interviews with health care providers revealed that materials were well-received and effective in educating providers about microbicides and at helping providers deliver appropriate counseling for hypothetical scenarios involving women in different sexual contexts.

Key study staff: Elizabeth Tolley, Elizabeth Ryan, Allison Pack, Emily Bockh, Samuel Field (FHI 360 USA); Caroline Mackenzie, Alice Olawo (FHI 360 Kenya); George Githuka (National AIDS and STI Control Programme)

Supplementary Case Study Materials

Ryan, E., Bockh, E., Tolley, E. E., Pack, A. P., Mackenzie, C., Olawo, A., & Githuka, G. (2015). Positioning microbicides for HIV prevention in Kenya: A case study. *Social Marketing Quarterly*, *22*(2), 100–114. doi:10.1177/1524500415583058

Sidibe, S., Pack, A. P., Tolley, E. E., Ryan, E., Mackenzie, C., Bockh, E., & Githuka, G. (2014). Communicating about microbicides with women in mind: Tailoring messages for specific audiences. *Journal of the International AIDS Society*, *17*(Suppl 2), 19151. doi:10.7448/IAS.17.3.19151

APPENDIX 2

EXAMPLES OF ORAL CONSENT FORMS

Example 1: Acceptability of Six-Month Injectable Contraception

Informed Consent for Policymaker and Program Manager Consultations

Hello. My name is ________________. I am working with FHI 360, an NGO that works on health and development projects. FHI 360 has an office in [Nairobi, Kenya, or Kigali, Kenya].

Introduction

FHI 360 has been awarded a grant from the Bill & Melinda Gates Foundation (BMGF) to develop a longer-acting injectable contraceptive method. An injectable contraceptive that lasts for at least 6 months would provide women with greater choice and simplify use of injectable contraception, thus improving continuation and increasing typical use effectiveness. The main goal of the overall project is to identify and obtain proof of Concept (POC) for several potential innovative injectable approaches that could be developed to provide at least 6 months of contraceptive protection (LA6+).

Reason for This Research

We are seeking interest in and guidance from family planning and reproductive health officials in two priority countries to assess acceptability, potential demand, and policy issues related to development of an injectable contraceptive method lasting six months or longer. In addition, we plan to talk to about

20 health providers, program managers, and administrators and to interview approximately 80 to 100 women who used contraception, including women who have used injectable contraception.

Your Part in This Research

If you agree to take part in the research, I will ask you about your attitudes toward the development of a longer-acting injectable contraceptive method. Specifically, we would like input on the potential positioning of a 6-month injectable within your current method mix, as well recommendations on individual or institutional policymakers, program implementers, or potential user groups who should be included in data collection activities. I will also ask your opinion about possible characteristics of a new, longer-acting injectable method. The discussion will take approximately one hour.

Possible Benefits and Risks

Although there are no direct benefits for your participation in this consultation, we will share any ideas that you have about a new method with product developers. By understanding your concerns or product preferences, we hope to identify and develop a new method that is acceptable and easy to use.

Confidentiality

Before we begin, I would like to ask you whether we have permission to identify you directly in our internal reports. If you would prefer, we can keep your identity anonymous. Whether you are willing to be cited or prefer to remain anonymous, we will share a transcript of this interview with you so that you can review it and provide any clarifications or revisions before we use it in our analysis. You will be invited to suggest changes or identify content that you would prefer be removed from the transcript. We will let you know when we need these edits when we send you the transcript.

Digital Recording

I would like to digitally record the interview so that I can remember all the information you provide. Afterward, I will listen to the recording and write down the discussion. The information from this and other interviews and group discussions may be presented at professional meetings or in written articles. We will not mention your or anyone's name in any presentations or written papers. We will erase digital recordings once the study has been completed.

If You Have a Problem or Have Other Questions

If you have any questions about this interview, or about the study more generally, you can contact me, [name, provide business card] or [local site investigator], principal investigator of the study, at [local investigator telephone number and email address].

Ethical Review

This research has been reviewed and approved by the institutional review board (IRB) of FHI 360 and the [Kenya/Rwanda IRB].

• • •

Are you willing to proceed with the interview?

____

Signature of person obtaining consent   Date

____

Printed name of person obtaining consent

Example 2: Communicating About Microbicides With Women in Mind

Informed Consent for Young Women Participating in FGDs to Test Materials

Interviewer: Please read the following.

Hello. My name is _______________. I'm working with FHI 360 on a research study to test materials that teach people about a new HIV prevention product that is being developed. We would like to know what you think about these materials. The product they describe is not yet available for use, but it may be available in the future. We want to plan for that possibility.

If you do not want to talk to me, you do not have to. We will ask about 1,000 men and women in Kenya to take part in the study. We would like to include you in our focus group discussion.

We will not record your name or any other information that can be used to identify you. If you agree to participate:

- We will first give you a short survey. The survey will ask you about yourself and what you think about HIV. You can either complete this by yourself, or, if you need help filling out the survey, we can help you. When you are finished, we will put it in a manila envelope. We will not share your answers with the group.

- Next, we will tell you and the group a little about the product being developed. We will also show you some of the materials that have been developed. A researcher will take notes.
- Finally, we will give you one more short survey. This time, we will ask you what you think about the materials you saw and the product they described. Again, we can help you if you need assistance. We will also put this survey in a manila envelope. We will not share your answers with the group.

This process should take about an hour and a half. We will give you a light snack. We will also give you a transport reimbursement of up to 1,000 Kenyan shillings.

There are no major risks participating in this study. However, some questions might make you feel uncomfortable. If that happens, you may refuse to answer any question, or you may stop participating at any time.

There are also no direct benefits from participating in this study. But, the results of this study will teach us about the kind of information that women and couples need to decide if the product is useful for them.

This study has been reviewed and approved by the Kenya Medical Research Institute (KEMRI). It has also been approved the Protection of Human Subjects Committee (PHSC) at FHI 360. These committees review research studies in order to help protect participants. If you have any questions about this project, you may contact [name of Principal Investigator and email] or [Local investigator name, email and telephone number]. You may also keep a copy of this form if you'd like.

Do you have any questions for me?

Can you please describe in your own words what you will be doing if you participate in this study?

Confirmation of Oral Consent

I certify that the nature and purpose, the potential benefits, and the possible risks associated with participating in this project have been explained to this individual. The individual has also voluntarily agreed to participate.

____

Signature of person who obtained consent   Date

____

Printed name of person obtaining consent

APPENDIX 3

PARTICIPANT OBSERVATION NOTES

Notes from field observations conducted by site data collectors provided by Kathleen M. MacQueen, FHI 360.

Example 1

Observer ID No.: ITE06

Site Code: ASH03

Date: 16 and 19 September 2016

Day: TUESDAY & FRIDAY

Time: 11:00 am–1:00 pm/9:00 am–10:30 pm

XXX BAR

A report on Participant Observation carried out at XXX Guest Inn (pub), at XXX on 16 and 19 September 2003.

The observation was carried out on Tuesday 16 and Friday 19 September 2003 based on the activities of commercial sex workers during day and night.

XXX Guest Inn is located about 400 meters behind the XXX Divisional Police Quarters. The area is known as XXX. The road leading to the place from the main road is rough and not motorable. The environment is littered with rubbish all over and there was stagnant water in between the houses. Most of the structures found at this site were either wooden or made from aluminum sheets. However, the XXX Guest Inn was built with cement and painted in pink and blue.

During the day, the place was somehow quiet with few people around. Most of the people found around were children and women. The children were of school-going age, however they were just loitering about and were also in dirty clothing.

Inside the XXX Guest Inn itself there were about 10 people, all men between the ages of 25 and 45 years busily smoking and drinking hard liquor. Most of the people around were either speaking XXX or XXX. One of the customers around told me that we can find people around only in the night because the area is noted for its nocturnal activities such as prostitution, drug peddling, and other crime-related activities.

When we visited there again on Friday 19th September between 9:30 p.m. and 11 p.m., the situation was completely different. The place was very dark; only [establishment] XXX and a few houses around had electricity. When we got to the place, even before the car stopped, my colleagues and I were given a very strong warning by a group of young men who were smoking something believed to be Indian hemp to put our headlights off. During the night, the place was very busy with a lot of people, both women and men. Most of the men were smoking and were dirty with a very bad body odor. The ladies were shabbily dressed. About 50 to 75 ladies were counted just around the XXX Guest Inn area. Some were sitting on benches, some squatting, and others were just walking around waiting for clients. The XXX Guest Inn was closed to customers who were there to buy liquor or cigarettes. However, one is allowed to enter if he or she is going to book a room. I was approached by a lady who asked me whether I am looking for a lady for the night. I asked how much does she charge for her services and she said 15,000 [local currency] for a short time and 100,000 for a full night. She also said a room at the XXX Guest Inn cost 10,000 for short time and 25,000 for a full night.

Example 2

Archival No. : AA001

Address: XXX

Observer ID: RB1

Date: 3 October 2016

Time: 11:15 p.m.–8:00 a.m.

I. Profile of settings hosting interactions that may expose people to HIV infection

1.1. Physical profile of the sector (description of characterizing and bordering physical references like streets, landscape, urban settings, and so on).

XXX Street is a sector that is framed by XXX Avenue westward, XXX Street southward, XXX Boulevard eastward, and XXX Street northward. Some reference sites are XXX Motel and Hotel XXX on

XXX Street, XXX Motel, and Motel XXX on XXX Street. There are some big buildings and the road network is quite orderly, segmenting the sector into six blocks. The landscape is homogeneously flat plain some blocks eastward from the XXX River.

1.2. Entertainment and socializing profile of the sector/area

1.2.1. Entertainment and socializing profile of the sector/area
Different leisure and socializing sites are found at XXX Street including motorcycles-taxi stops, bars; dancing clubs, hotels; games and gambling sites; grocery stores; inns; small traders (manufactured products and cooked food including beef kebab, roasted fish, and fritters). The sites host alcohol consumption, chatting, food consumption, commercial sex, playing games, etc.

1.2.2. Hosting capacity of entertainment and socializing sites (number of seats/tables)
Leisure and socializing sites at XXX Street have an estimated average capacity of about 75 seats. At the bar selected for observation, there were 80 seats.

1.2.3. Density of potential high transmission sites within the sector by 10 minutes of ordinary walk
During a 10-minute walk, we encountered 34 entertainment/socializing sites along the main road. They included 17 bars/dancing clubs, 6 restaurants, 3 hotels, and 8 inns.

II. Interaction between research staff and key informants of targeted sites

2.1. Identifying gatekeepers and potential key informants of the target sites
One male gatekeeper and potential key informant was identified. We talked with him in front of the bar where we were conducting the observation. He is a resident of the sector.

2.2. Establishing relationship with gatekeepers and potential key-informants of the target sites
Rapport was established with the above gatekeeper/key informant, who agreed to help with any future components of the study. He promised to take part in in-depth interviews should we solicit him and to help with the recruitment of sex workers.

III. Sociodemographic profile of actors and site

3.1. Presence of at-risk socioprofessional groups
It appeared that about five local socioprofessional groups are at risk of HIV infection. Among these are sex workers, staff of the

leisure sites, residents, motorbike-taxi drivers, small merchants (manufactured and cooked food products). The presence of sex workers was observed in or around different leisure/socializing sites and on the streets. The profiles of some of the above categories of persons include:

- Managers of snack bars who are young females and males between 20 and 35 years old
- Small merchants, female holders of roasted fish stands aged 25 to 40 years; sellers of boxes containing new manufactured products aged 20 to 35 years
- Servants of hotels or snack bars, females and males between 18 and 30 years of age
- Hotel and inn receptionists, both females and males between 25 and 40 years of age
- Motorcycle-taxi drivers, all males aged 20 to 30 years.

3.2. Profiles of subjects in the respective socioprofessional groups

3.2.1. Who are clients of sex workers?
It was reported that clients at the observation site are people of different ages and professions. Among said clients are workers (office staff), rickshaw movers, and expatriates. An informant reported that it only takes affording the money in order to get sex services from a sex worker. The client's socioeconomic background does not matter. He further said that seeking the services of sex workers is not specific to any given category of persons.

3.2.2. Age of sex worker, their clients, and others in sector
Sex workers are females aged 16 to 45 years. The age range of clients is 20 to 65 years.

3.2.3. Sex of sex workers
The majority of sex workers are female. A few men are found looking for clients at the same observation site.

3.2.4. Look of sex workers in the sector
Sex workers were seen wearing clothing that is rather "sexy" (extravagant and ostentatious) including disclosure of body shapes and nakedness of some parts of the body like the back, the breast, the belly, the thighs, and legs. Hairstyles are

ostentatious, made of grafts of synthetic hair of striking colors (including red, blond, and purple).

3.2.5. Years of activity (sex worker only)

It was reported that experience in the business varies from 0 to 15 years depending on the age of the sex worker.

3.2.6. Socioeconomic status of sex worker

The socioeconomic background of sex workers is poor, whereas their clients appear rather well off.

3.2.7. Professional status of sex worker (whether amateur or professional)

The sex workers that we observed were all professionals. Some were reported to have been renting rooms at a nearby motel for as many as three years, living exclusively on commercial sex income.

3.2.8. Residence: stability and migration (sex worker and clients)

Sex workers are made up of both residents and migrants. Among residents there women who live in the area and others who are inn dwellers. Among migrants there are immigrants from other areas of the country and [country]. Some transitory sex workers like to move to different sectors where they wish to benefit from the privileges of newness. Similar information was tough to collect about the clients because the environment appeared hostile.

3.3. Demographic density and social conditions in the neighborhood

3.3.1. Proximity between houses

The sector is somewhat crowded. Fencing is not common. A number of houses are tight against each other. From the streets, very narrow paths are the most prevalent ways leading to residences and for people walking within the settlements. This demonstrated the close proximity of houses.

3.3.2. Intimacy of family life

Some of the residential neighborhoods behind the commercial and leisure sites of the roadsides lack necessary conditions for the preservation of the intimacy of family life. Where fences are absent and houses stand close one to the other, households' daily life scenes, including the most intimate, are exposed (by sight, hearing, etc.) to the neighbors or passers-by, whether happening inside or outdoors. Furthermore, up to three houses are sometimes using the same bathing room and WC.

3.3.3. Social distance among neighbors

Under such conditions as above described, neighbors of the observation site cannot maintain sensible social distance. They are rather embarked in a remarkable level of togetherness and solidarity.

3.3.4. Socioeconomic status of the site (administrative, commercial, academic, industrial, etc.)

The area is a commercial sector, although it is also residential because of the houses found behind the commercial and leisure sites that stand on streets sides and in buildings.

3.3.5. Profile and role of allies of sex worker

Allies of sex workers are men whose roles consist of protecting sex workers against insolvent clients. Generally called XXX, allies intervene and would sometimes take away all of the client's belongings.

IV. Social dynamic within the site

4.1. Social behaviors

Neighbors maintain mutual civilities and solidarity in the face of hardship or bad fate (e.g., the death of a household member or family member). In such circumstances there is a high turnout of neighbors.

4.2. Sexual behaviors

A couple walking out of a hotel room (after sexual intercourse said the informant. A man talking with a woman and framing her legs with his). Sex workers do hail clients and chat them up.

4.3. Use of psychotropic substances

Our informant said that he could provide us with some cannabis if we were ready to pay for it. He said that men and women consume it in the search for more courage in the face of challenges. Dealing is secret, as our informant refused to disclose any sales point or contact to us. When approaching him for the informal discussion, his body seemed to diffuse an odor of hashish.

4.4. Verbal behavior

Neighbors were seen holding talks in compounds/yards. Sex workers were either discussing gently here or shouting at each other there.

A dispute between two sex workers about the reimbursement of a debt was overheard.

4.5. Organization within groups of sex workers

4.5.1. Are sex workers linked by organizational rules? Describe
There is no structured hierarchical organization linking sex workers together. Competition is allowed in client approaching strategy.

4.5.2. Are sex workers teaming or working individually?
At the observation site, sex workers carry on their business individually. Collaboration is casual and will happen in special circumstances like a client asking for an orgy. Sometimes sex workers do have sex between themselves.

4.6. Social perception of sex work
Commercial sex was reported not to have a negative social image in the sector. It is practiced and benefits from indulgence by local inhabitants and in the local community at large. Our informant (local inhabitant) underlined that he is sometimes involved as a mediator between clients and sex workers.

V. Intensity of at-risk activities within the site

5.1. Number of person spending time on the site per 20 minutes
Over a period of 20 minutes, we recorded the presence of 40 persons, including 20 females and 20 potential clients.

5.2. Estimate frequentation of site by hours, days, and months per annum
It was reported that frequentation of the job sites/sector fluctuates according to the residence area of the sex worker. Residents (of houses or inns) of the sector and of immediate neighborhoods are available for the business at any time, including the daytime. The arrival of immigrants would commence at 7 p.m. and reach its peak at 11 p.m. during on-duty days (Mondays–Thursdays). Over the weekends (Fridays–Sundays), arrival times are around 8 p.m. and they peak at 12 a.m. Departure is at 6 a.m. at the latest.

5.3. Cost/charges for sexual services
It was reported that at the observation site, copulation with condom concluded by an ejaculation is priced at 1.500. 5,000–10,000 are charged per service/hour without condom. Sex is performed in rented sites (e.g., inns, hotels). The client covers such costs in addition.

VI. Future prospects for further components of the study

6.1. Potential subjects for further components of the research

Staff of inns and restaurants, residents/residents, small merchants, bar or dancing clubs owners/managers/attendants, motorbike-taxi drivers, sex workers and clients are advisable informants to be considered for samples of relevant further components of the formative study.

APPENDIX 4

TOPIC GUIDES WITH PICTURES

Topic Guide for Consultations With Program Implementers and Service Providers

Study to Assess Acceptability and Potential Demand for a 6-Month Injectable Contraceptive Method

I. Current injectable landscape

1. Which injectable contraceptive products are available (in your program/clinic)?
   a. If more than one brand, which product is most preferred? Why?
2. What, if any, issues are there in ensuring that stocks of injectables are available?
   a. Any problems with stock-outs? If so, why do you think this happens?
3. What kinds of providers are authorized to provide injectable contraception in your program/at this clinic (e.g., in Marie Stopes Clinics; through public sector clinics supported by the MoH)?
   a. What kind of training or certification is required? Can you describe how you were trained to provide injectables?
4. How would you describe women who obtain injectable contraception through your program/clinic?
   a. How do they differ from users of other modern methods?
   b. How do they differ from users of traditional methods? Or from women who are not using contraceptives?

5. What are some of the common beliefs about injectable contraception?
   a. What concerns do clients raise related to injectable side effects?
      i. (If bleeding side effects mentioned) How important is it to most women to have regular menstrual periods? How do you counsel women about bleeding side effects?
   b. What concerns do you or other service providers have about injectable contraception?
   c. How common is the belief that injectables may lead to sterility? Who has these kinds of concerns? How do you counsel women that may have this concern?
   d. Once injected, pregnancy protection cannot be reversed until the effect of the drug has worn off. How does this affect attitudes toward injectables?
   e. What aspects of injectable contraception do you believe are the most beneficial?
   f. How much traction have recent reports about HC–HIV interaction received in Kenya?
6. What do you consider to be the most important information/counseling messages to provide before a woman decides to use an injectable?
7. How easy or difficult is it for women to remember to get another injection on time?
   a. What, if anything, does your program/clinic do to assist women in obtaining their next injection?
   b. When would a woman be considered "late" to obtain her next injection?
   c. What happens if a woman returns late for her next injection?

Interviewer Reads: As described during the consent process, the goal of this project is to develop a longer-acting injectable contraceptive method. Our clinical and product development colleagues are conducting a landscape analysis to identify promising candidates. There are several ways that a longer-acting injectable might be developed. I'd like to get your feedback on some of the possible approaches.

II. Potential product approaches

8. One possibility would be to use a higher dose of a known drug.
   a. How acceptable would this be to current users of DMPA?

b. What concerns might they have about receiving a higher dose of the drug?

c. What side effects would they anticipate from this higher dose injectable?

d. How are those concerns balanced by a perceived benefit of longer duration of effectiveness?

9. A second approach would be to identify new chemical entities that might have longer duration of effect.
   a. What questions or concerns would you have about contraceptive options that were steroidal?

   b. What questions or concerns would you have about a longer-acting injectable that was nonhormonal?

10. A longer-acting injectable might be achieved by changing the injection site or type of injection.
    a. What preferences would providers or clients have for injections that were either intramuscular (deep into the muscle tissue) or subcutaneous (injected just under the skin)?

    b. To what degree would the site of injection influence provider and/or client preferences, for example, if the injection was administered in the arm versus abdomen or thigh/hip for a subcutaneous injection? Or if it were administered in the arm versus thigh/hip for intramuscular injection?

III. Refer to Target Product Profile (TPP)[1] activity for this section

Interviewer Reads: I'd like to get some feedback from you about potential characteristics of a new longer-acting injectable. For each characteristic, I will show you a card. After discussing all the different characteristics, I will ask you to think about which characteristics you believe to be most important—and least important—to target for a new, longer-acting injectable contraceptive method.

IV. Interest in a longer-acting injectable

11. Who are current users of longer acting methods (IUDs, implants, sterilization)?

[1]The TPP guides the product development process. It includes a list of product characteristics (e.g., efficacy level, demographic profile of intended users, likely side effects) and the ideal and minimally acceptable range for each characteristic.

12. What kinds of women do you believe would be interested in a longer-acting injectable method?
13. If this new contraceptive method were to be introduced through your program/in your clinic, what key steps would need to be taken?
    a. What kinds of training would need to take place?
    b. What, if any, changes would you need to make to monitoring/ tracking systems?
14. How would provision of this new method affect the current work load?
    a. If an injectable user only needed to return every 6 months, instead of every 3 months, how would this change affect your (program/daily work load)?

Thank you very much for you time and for the thoughtful information you have shared with me today!

Topic Guide for FGDs With End Users

Study to Assess Acceptability and Potential Demand for a Six-Month Injectable Contraceptive Method

I. Warm-up

1. In general, how easy or difficult is it for a woman [in Kenya/Rwanda] to obtain and use a contraceptive method if she wants to delay or avoid a next pregnancy?
    a. What are some of the barriers to contraceptive use that women generally face?
    b. Which method(s) do you feel women in [Kenya/Rwanda[most prefer to use? Why do you say that?
    c. Which method(s) are least preferred? Can you explain why?

II. Injectable contraception attitudes

2. I'd like to talk specifically about injectable contraception. Several contraceptive methods currently exist that are delivered through a syringe or injection. One method (DMPA) requires a new injection every 3 months. Several others require a new injection every 2 months or are given on a monthly basis. Which injectable methods are available in [Kenya/Rwanda]?
    a. What different kinds of clinics make this method available? (Explore public/private sources.)

3. What do you think about this/these method(s)?

4. What aspects of injectable contraception do you believe are the most beneficial?
   a. Why do you think some women choose to use injectables instead of other methods?

5. What concerns do you have about injectable contraception?
   a. What kinds of side effects do people associate with injectable contraception?
      i. (If bleeding side effects mentioned) How important is it to most women to have regular menstrual periods?

   b. How common is the belief that injectables may lead to sterility? Who has these kinds of concerns? Why do these beliefs exist?

   c. Once injected, pregnancy protection cannot be reversed until the effect of the drug has worn off. How do you feel about this?

   d. What, if anything, have you heard about women's ability to get pregnant after using injectables? How important is it for women to be able to get pregnant immediately or within a predictable period of time after stopping a contraceptive method?

   e. How appropriate is injectable use if a woman is concerned about both pregnancy and HIV? What method or methods should she use in this case?

6. For nonuser FGD: Which contraceptive method(s) have you used? Why did you choose this/these methods?
   a. Have you ever considered using the injectable yourself? Why or why not?

7. For current/past Injectable user FGD: Why did you first decide to use an injectable? (Ask several women to describe their decision-making process.)

III. Injectable contraception experiences (for current and past injectable user FGDs only)

8. Overall, how much have you liked using the injectable? Why?

9. Was the injection given in the arm, the hip, or another part of the body? Do you like it? If not, where would you prefer to get the injection?

10. What experiences have you had with side effects?
    a. How much, if at all, did these experiences affect your desire to continue using the method?

11. How easy or difficult has it been to remember to get another injection on time?
    a. When would you be considered "late" to obtain your next injection?
    b. Have any of you ever returned to the clinic past your appointment date for your next injection? What happened?
    c. In what ways did the clinic staff help you to remember your next injection?
12. Have you ever gone to the clinic for an injection and been told that they were out of stock? If so, what did you do?
13. In your experience, what do you consider the most important information/counseling messages that a woman needs to know before using an injectable?
14. (For discontinuers) What was the main reason that you stopped using the injectable?
15. (For current users) Have you ever thought about stopping injectable use or switching to a different method? Why do you say this?

Interviewer Reads: As described during the consent process, the goal of this project is to develop a longer-acting injectable contraceptive method. Our clinical and product development colleagues are conducting a landscape analysis to identify promising candidates. There are several ways that a longer-acting injectable might be developed. I'd like to get your feedback on some of the possible approaches.

IV. Potential product approaches

16. One possibility would be to use a higher dose of a known drug.
    a. What concerns would you have, if any, about using an injectable with a higher dose of a drug if it increased the duration of protection?
    b. What side effects would you worry about, if any?
    c. Would you accept two injections instead of one if they increased the duration of protection?
17. A second approach would be to identify new drugs/chemicals that might have a longer duration of effect.
    a. Which would you prefer: new options that were based on hormones (like the pill or current injectables) or new options that didn't contain hormones? Why do you say this?

b. What if the new chemical made a longer-acting injectable a bit more painful than the current injectable method?

18. A longer-acting injectable might be achieved by changing the site of injection. For example, the injection might be delivered in the hip or the abdomen. How would you feel about these options? What would be preferred site of injection? Why?
    a. What if it were given just under the skin with a shorter needle instead of deeper in the arm muscle?

19. How interested would you be in using a longer-acting method that you could inject yourself instead of needing a clinic provider to give you the injection?

20. What information would you need before deciding to use a new product, if it were available?

V. Refer to Target Product Profile activity for this section

Interviewer Reads: I'd like to get some feedback from you about potential characteristics of a new longer-acting injectable. For each characteristic, I will show you a card. After discussing all the different characteristics, I will ask you to think about which characteristics you believe to be most important—and least important—to target for a new, longer-acting injectable contraceptive method.

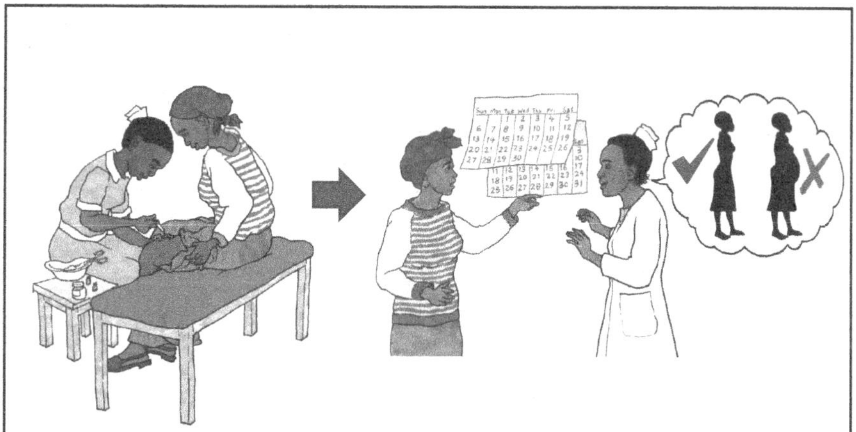

99% EFFECTIVE

UZUIAJI WA MIMBA WA KIWANGO CHA 99%

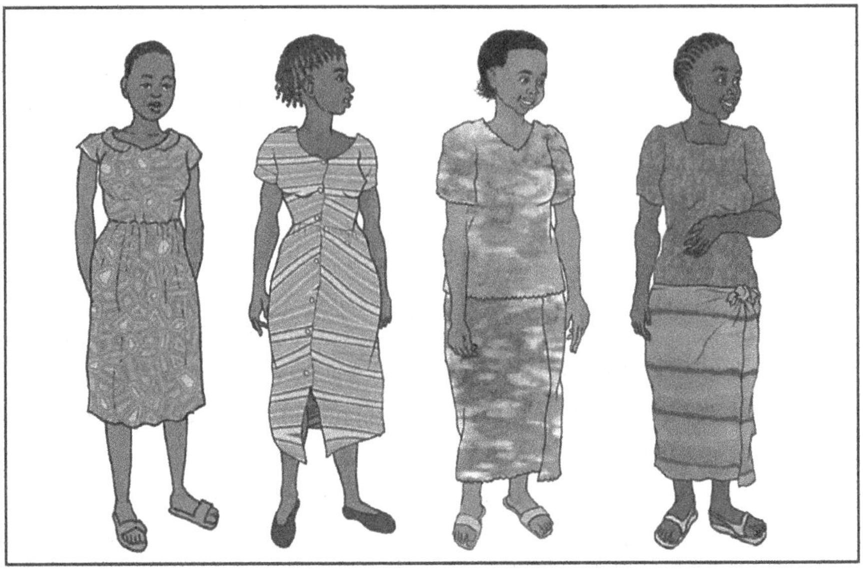

WOMEN OF ALL REPRODUCTIVE AGES

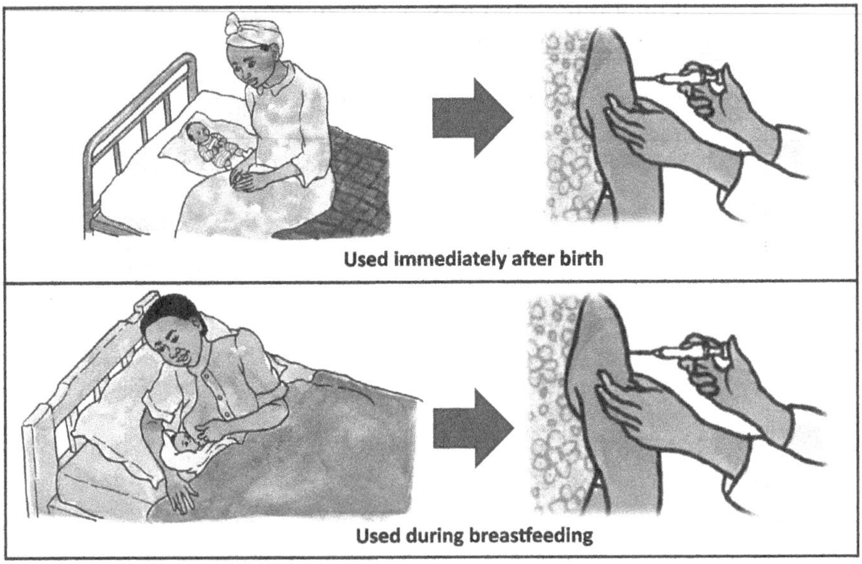

SAFE FOR NEW MOTHERS

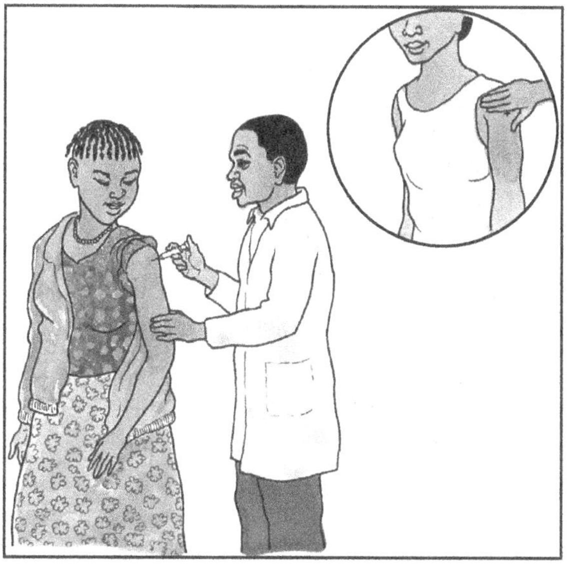

INJECTION IN ARM

INADUNGWE KWA MKONO

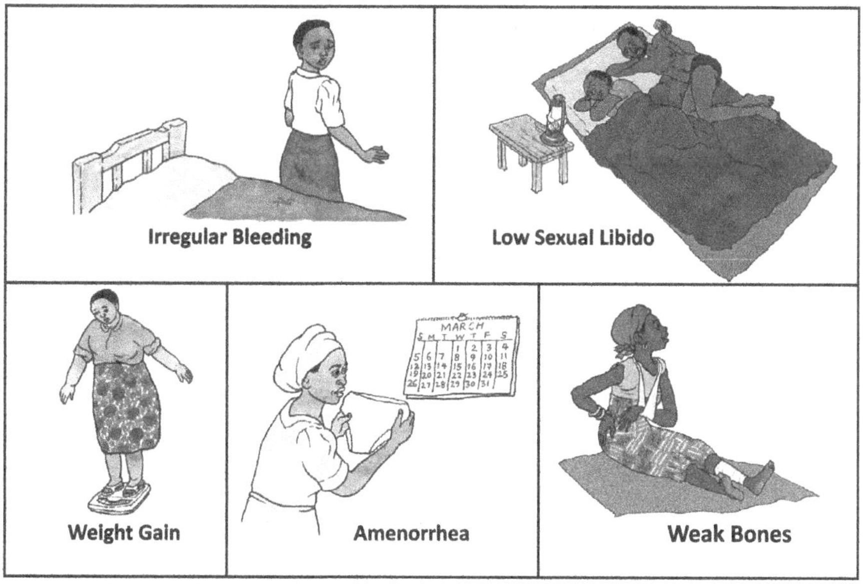

SIDE EFFECTS NO WORSE THAN CURRENT INJECTABLES

VI. Interest in a longer-acting injectable

21. How interested would you be in using a longer-acting injectable method?
    a. What benefits would there be in using a longer-acting method like this?
    b. What disadvantages could there be?
22. If an injectable user only needed to return every 6 months instead of every 3 months, how easy or difficult would it be to remember to come for your next injection?
23. How much would you be willing to pay for an injectable method that protected you from pregnancy for 6 months? What if it prevented pregnancy for 1 year?
    a. How much do you pay for your current method?
    b. How much would a longer-acting injectable save you, in terms of travel or child care costs? In terms of the time needed to get to and from the clinic?
24. What other questions or comments do you have before we end our discussion today?

Thank you very much for you time and for the thoughtful information you have shared with me today!

APPENDIX 5

SAMPLE INTERVIEWER TRAINING PROGRAM AGENDAS AND TRAINING SCHEDULES

Techniques for Conducting In-Depth Interviews and FGDs

27–29 January 2014

Facilitator: Christina Wong, FHI 360

Training Objectives

Upon completion of the training, participants will be able to:

- Develop a semi-structured in-depth interview/focus group discussion question guide.
- Conduct in-depth interviews (IDIs) and focus group discussions (FGDs).
- Document and manage data collected.

Training Outline

Designing semistructured interview/focus group guides

- Framing qualitative questions
- Stages of IDIs/FGDs useful to note for the design of IDI/FGD guides

Techniques for conducting in-depth interviews

- What is an in-depth interview (IDI)?
- Responsibilities of an in-depth interviewer
- Effective techniques of in-depth interviewing
- How to handle different situations in an in-depth interview
- Steps in conducting in-depth interviews

Techniques for conducting focus group discussions

- What is a focus group discussion (FGD)?
- Differences between a FGD and an in-depth interview
- Roles in FGD
- Stages of the FGD
- Listening roadblocks and active listening
- How to deal with different personalities
- Steps in conducting FGD

Data documentation

- Reasons for note-taking
- Types of note-taking
- How to document data from IDIs and FGDs
- How to take notes
- Guidelines for writing up transcripts and expanded notes

Data management and storage

- Converting raw data to computer files
- Organizing data storage

Day 1

Time	Session	Materials
8:30–9:00	Introductions and training overview	
9:00–10:00	Overview of qualitative data collection methods used in public health	PowerPoint
10:00–10:15	Break	
10:15–10:45	Values exploration exercise	Handout
10:45–12:00	Designing semi-structured interview/focus group guides	
	Practice: Develop an interview guide in small groups	PowerPoint
12:00–1:00	Lunch	
1:00–2:30	Practice: Develop an interview guide in small groups (continued) and present back to the big group	PowerPoint
2:30–3:00	Techniques for conducting in-depth interviews	PowerPoint and handouts
3:00–3:15	Break	
3:15–4:30	Techniques for conducting in-depth interviews (continued)	PowerPoint and handouts

Day 2

Time	Session	Materials
8:30–10:00	Techniques for conducting in-depth interviews (continued)	PowerPoint and handouts
10:00–10:15	Break	
10:15–11:30	Techniques for conducting in-depth interviews (continued)	PowerPoint and handouts
12:00–1:00	Lunch	
1:00–2:30	Data documentation, data management and storage	PowerPoint and handouts
2:30–3:00	Practice: Conducting in-depth interviews and transcribing	
3:00–3:15	Break	
3:15–4:30	Practice: Conducting in-depth interviews and transcribing (continued)	

Day 3

Time	Session	Materials
8:30–9:30	Review transcripts and debrief	
9:30–10:00	Techniques for conducting focus group discussions	PowerPoint and handouts
10:00–10:15	Break	
10:15–12:00	Techniques for conducting focus group discussions	PowerPoint and handouts
12:00– 1:00	Lunch	
1:00–3:00	Practice: Conducting focus group discussions and transcribing	
3:00–3:15	Break	
3:15–4:00	Practice: Conducting focus group discussions and transcribing (continued)	
4:00–4:30	Training debrief Training evaluation and certificates	Training evaluation Certificates

Required Reading

Mack, N., Woodsong, C., MacQueen, K. M., Guest, G., & Namey, E. (2006). *Qualitative research methods: A data collector's field guide*. Durham, NC: Family Health International. Available for free download at http://www.fhi360.org/sites/default/files/media/documents/Qualitative%20Research%20Methods%20-%20A%20Data%20Collector's%20Field%20Guide.pdf

SAMPLE BUDGET CATEGORIES FOR PLANNING QUALITATIVE DATA COLLECTION

Evaluation of Integration of Nutrition Curricula in Secondary Schools*

Sites: 5 Districts in Nepal
Estimated Total Duration: 2 Years
Last Revised: 10/15/2015

* *This template and the figures are illustrative only and serve as a guide to the budgeting process.*

Instructions: Please use this template to help guide the complete budgeting process. We have provided some broad categories to help you and your team think through all of the potential costs associated with implementing a study in the field. This list is not exhaustive. For smaller studies and smaller teams, some categories here may be extraneous. Each category should be broken down into smaller sub-categories in order to obtain an accurate estimate of the cost of each individual item. The individual quantities (column C) should be multiplied by the individual annual costs (column D) and then multiplied by the number of years (Column E) to obtain the total cost (column F). Values in the total cost columns can be summed to reach an overall estimate of the budget for the study. The Notes column (G) should be used to indicate any additional information for the items in the budget. Note that local currency conversions will have to be factored in.

A	B	C	D	E	F	G
Budget Item / Sub Item	**Unit**	**Quantity**	**Cost Per Year**	**Years**	**Total Cost**	**Notes**
Staffing						
PI						
Study Manager					$ -	
Subcontractors					$ -	
Consultants					$ -	
Data Manager					$ -	
Data Analysts					$ -	
Data Collector					$ -	
Moderators					$ -	
Note takers					$ -	
Transcriptionist					$ -	
Translator					$ -	
Driver					$ -	

(continued)

A Budget Item / Sub Item	B Unit	C Quantity	D Cost Per Year	E Years	F Total Cost	G Notes
Activities						
IRB Approvals					$ -	
Study Sponsor IRB					$ -	
Local Collaborator IRB						
Travel (to/from site)					$ -	
Per Diems					$ -	
Travel (local)					$ -	
Per Diems					$ -	
Vehicles					$ -	
Training					$ -	
Materials					$ -	
Facility					$ -	
Per Diems					$ -	
Food and Beverage					$ -	
Community Introduction					$ -	
Materials					$ -	
Facility					$ -	
Food & Beverage					$ -	
Data Collection					$ -	
Participant Observation					$ -	
IDIs					$ -	
FGDs					$ -	
Materials					$ -	
Digital Recorders					$ -	
Participant Incentives					$ -	
Transport Reimbursements					$ -	
Facility					$ -	
Food and Beverage					$ -	

(continued)

A	B	C	D	E	F	G
Budget Item / Sub Item	**Unit**	**Quantity**	**Cost Per Year**	**Years**	**Total Cost**	**Notes**
Activities						
Community Dissemination					$ -	
Materials					$ -	
Facility					$ -	
Food and Beverage					$ -	
Other Dissemination					$ -	
Conference Fees					$ -	
Publication Fees					$ -	
Other						
Study Office Space						
Security					$ -	
Laptops					$ -	
File Storage					$ -	
Transcription Machines					$ -	
Data Entry / Analysis Software Licenses					$ -	
Office Supplies					$ -	
TOTAL COST						

APPENDIX 7

CODING SUMMARY REPORT

Project: Adolescents and MCTs, Tanzania

Generated: 11/17/2010 9:34 p.m.

Free Nodes/Risk Perception

Internals\FGD\FGD#1 with Mothers in Tanzania

Reference 1

M: IS THERE ANYONE ELSE WHO WORRIES? TO WHAT DEGREE ARE YOU WORRIED? SISTER, CAN YOU TELL US TO WHETHER YOU WORRY ABOUT HIV/AIDS FOR YOUR DAUGHTER?

P4: I thank you, I thank you so much. All parents have worries - as all others (in the FGD) have just said. The world is declining. Because as a parent, you can talk to your children at home, but when they go out, they use public transport; they meet with men or older boys. Who knows how they (men) will talk to them (daughters) in convincing ways. We ask ourselves, 'I don't know. Will our children get it (HIV)?' Eeh!!! We really do not have much peace. Because you see, as others said before, people are using these ARV drugs. They (people infected with HIV) become attractive - they get well, so that person keeps spreading it (HIV). So all of us stay worried and we pray to God, because we are not sure if our children will really get to where we have gotten (in life).

Reference 2

M: THANK YOU, SO I WILL CONTINUE BY ASKING ABOUT GIRLS AGED 15 AND 17 YEARS. WHAT ARE YOUR WORRIES IN GENERAL? CAN ANOTHER PERSON SHARE WITH US WHAT THEIR WORRIES ARE?

P6: The disease is like that, you cannot rely on the hope that your child will survive or not.

Reference 3

P6:	XXX is like YYY [names], she had friends who were not girls. She had many boyfriends also, but the other YYY [name] she is not settled.
M:	DO YOU HAVE FEARS ABOUT DAUGHTERS HAVING BOYFRIENDS?
P6:	I worry about her.
PARTICIPANTS:	LAUGHTER
M:	HOW DID YOU HANDLE YOUR WORRIES?
P6:	She might go out to visit men. I trust the older one to be sensible, but not the younger one.
M:	YOU DON'T TRUST HER? HOW OLD IS SHE, THE YOUNGER ONE?
P6:	She is 13 years old.

Internals\FGD\ FGD#1 With Sexual Partners in Tanzania

Reference 1

I: TO WHAT DEGREE ARE YOU WORRIED ABOUT HIV/AIDS FOR YOURSELF?

RI: On my side, my worry about HIV is very high because of (the way) transmission happens. For example, during sexual intercourse there are several ways a person can get HIV. Also, in a road accident you can get injured and come into contact with an infected person, so you can get it. Another worry is when you share sharp tools like razor blades and needles. So in the community, there is a lot of fear that people can get HIV.

R2: On my side, my worry is I have never checked my health status. Also there some tools like those my friend mentioned that we normally share. In short, because I have never tested HIV, I worry that I may have it.

Reference 2

I: HOW MUCH ARE YOU WORRIED ABOUT HIV/AIDS FOR YOUR PARTNERS?

R8: My worry with my partners, first they are not satisfied with their partner because you can go to work and return with some money – if you give her some, she says it's not enough. When you are at work, she can go to another man, so if you have sex with her, she feels that you don't satisfy her. I mean, (you may) not satisfy her when you have sex with her, because she went to another man who satisfied her(more). So when you are at work, you worry that your partner may go to another man.

R3: My worry is that you cannot trust your partner – that she is with you alone, because even me, I have other women. If I have another women, I believe that even her, she may have another man, so what's needed here is (always) to use condoms.

Reference 3

I: WHAT ARE YOUR CONCERNS IN GENERAL FOR GIRLS AGED 15 TO 17?

R3: Mhh, due to lack of education about HIV transmission for girls of this age. Second, we have to look at ourselves. We men, we should not trust them (girls), that they are safe and they don't have HIV. A girl of 15 can be positive, maybe she was born with HIV. A large percent of us, we trust that she is negative so we have sex with her without using condoms. Also, we have to stop (our) bad behaviors. Taking a young girl 15 years old and having sex with her without protection is immoral, because if you have unsafe sex you can infect her with HIV. So, we have to look at ourselves.

Reference 4

I: OK I AM STILL ASKING, HOW IMPORTANT IS IT FOR MEN TO BE SEXUALLY EXPERIENCED BEFORE MARRIAGE?

R2: There is no importance for men to have sexual experience before marriage. Personally, I have done research on this matter and have come to the conclusion that most men who have a tendency of having sex frequently before marriage, even when they marry, they cannot be faithful to their partners. You can see a married man in a secluded area (of a bar or club) with a lady and after some time he goes back to his wife. I used to ask people about this issue and come to the conclusion that a man who is used to having sex with different women, cannot get settled even if he is married. He is used to having different tastes in sex making, so his wife will give him one taste.

Internals\KI\Tanzania Key Informant #6, From Education

Reference 1

INTERVIEWER: WHAT PUTS GIRLS AT GREATER RISK FOR THESE NEGATIVE SEXUAL AND REPRODUCTIVE HEALTH OUTCOMES?

Interviewee: I see that they are in greater risk... poverty which causes that. We also talk about this issue – I talk with girls when I go to the high schools and you are also a witness. Being a girl today is very expensive compared to our parents' times. During our parents' times, they (girls) just took coconut oil mixed with jasmine and applied it to their bodies. They just plaited their hair in three lines and it was enough. Right now there are special cosmetics for the face; there is something to make the hair grow fast etc. There are different lotions... you might find your monthly budget in cosmetics alone reached 70,000 (Tanzania shillings) and that is a minimum. But if you want to use designer cosmetics, they are expensive. So that is the danger. And girls see those things not only from international celebrities, but also local celebrities. They look at how they (celebrities) dress, the salon they visit etc. and someone would like to be that way but her income is low or she has no income at all. That is where problems begin. For me, what puts adolescents at greater risk is this.

Internals\MTN\1st of Several Interviews With a Tanzania Married Teen #11

Reference 1

HOW CONCERNED ARE YOU ABOUT PREGNANCY, SEXUALLY TRANSMITTED DISEASES, HIV IN YOUR LIFE?

In short, I am not afraid of pregnancy, because I gave birth What worries me is disease. At least other diseases can be treated, but it (treatment) is not easy for AIDS. Yes, you can get treatment, but you can pass away any day.

Internals\MTN\2nd Interview With the Same Married Teen #11

Reference 1

I: OK, TALKING ABOUT FIDELITY, HOW IMPORTANT IS FIDELITY TO YOU?

R: Fidelity is very important because it keeps me from getting diseases – because I trust him with everything and he trusts me too. But if we don't trust each other, I will do what he does and the result is disease.

I: YOU SAID FIDELITY PREVENTS YOU FROM DISEASES. WHAT KIND OF DISEASES?

R: Suppose I found my lover just sitting with a girl, maybe they are just talking like the way we were friends before we became lovers [her and her partner], then I start suspecting them as lovers and I say they can't be just talking. I also must do something. That is when you bring diseases to each other.

I: WHAT DISEASES ARE YOU TALKING ABOUT?

R: There are a lot of diseases – like HIV, I don't know, Syphilis. You might not have it, but your partner might do it (have sex with someone) and get it; you won't know if he already has it.

I: DO YOU WORRY ABOUT YOUR PARTNER'S FIDELITY?

R: No I don't have any worries, because he does not have any "women stories."

I: WHAT DO YOU MEAN WHEN YOU SAY HE DOES NOT HAVE WOMEN STORIES?

R: I mean he is not thinking of being with other women. In short, people don't even know that he has a woman. They don't even know if I am his woman. Everyone is asking him about his woman; in short, he keeps it secret so you won't know.

I: I AM SORRY FOR THIS QUESTION, BUT IF HE CAN HIDE ABOUT YOU, THAT HE IS WITH YOU BUT OTHERS DON'T KNOW THAT HE IS WITH YOU, DON'T YOU THINK HE MIGHT HAVE SOMEONE ELSE AND HIDE IT? EVEN YOU WON'T KNOW IT?

R: No, at their home they all know that I am with him, but other people are asking him 'Who is your girlfriend? Why don't we see you with a woman?'

Reference 2

I: DO YOU USE CONDOMS WITH YOUR CURRENT PARTNER?

R: No.

I: WHY DON'T YOU USE CONDOMS?

R: We trust each other.

I: OKAY, WHOSE IDEA IS IT NOT TO USE CONDOMS?

R: It is ours, because he was sick and he got tested, and I got tested when I was pregnant. And, at the last point, when the baby was sick, we tested me and the child. They thought maybe they tested us wrong, so we had to test again. When we tested, they found us to be negative. That is when the child was sick until the time when she died. So we are all tested, that is why we trust each other.

APPENDIX 8

EXAMPLE OF DATA ANALYSIS MEMO

MEMO: Adolescent risk context

DATA USED: Repeated in-depth interviews with 23 adolescents in Tanzania

ANALYST: BT

DATE: 3/24/2013

• • •

Based on our data from Tanzania, the family and partner relationship dynamics of young women in our different risk groups appeared to vary in several ways.

Family backgrounds: It was surprising that many of the adolescents and young women in this study described fragmented or broken households. Among young women engaged in sex work or married, almost none had lived with a biological parent for many years.

- Engaged in sex work ($n = 5$): Three of five women were single or double orphans. The other two had parents who divorced when they were very young; these girls appeared to be left to their own devices. All but one currently live on their own or with a girlfriend. One 16-year-old lives with her mother.
- Married ($n = 8$): Five of eight young married women were single or double orphans. One, whose parents were separated and described her father as a "drunkard," lived with an aunt to go to school. Two lived with

parents (in one case, the stepfather) but appeared to have good enough home lives. They both got pregnant in seventh standard (equivalent to last year of U.S. primary school) and decided to get married. All but one married women currently live most of the time with their husbands. One adolescent had a quarrel with her husband at the time of the first interview and was living with her mother.

- Out-of-school youth ($n = 5$): Two of five women were single orphans; in both cases the father had died. In two additional cases, the parents were divorced. One of these women described her father as being harsh. Currently, four of the five live with relatives (grandmother, uncle, etc.) and one lives with both parents.
- In-school youth ($n = 5$): None of these young women had lost a parent, however for two of five, the parents had divorced. Two young women live with both parents and the third lives with her mother only. (Her parents met in college and had her but didn't stay together.) All live with one (two with mother) or both (three) parents.

Education: Married girls have the lowest level of education (less than seventh standard, on average) compared to other groups. In-school youth have the highest education (10 years equivalent to about form three or the advanced cycle of U.S. secondary school) and the other two groups have similar levels—a bit over 8 years.

Circumstances around sexual debut: Age of sexual debut is similar across groups (15.5–15.6) except for in-school youth, who started sex on average a half year later than the other groups (16).

Sexual partnerships: Young women's sexual behaviors and their attitudes toward their sexual partners also vary by risk context. While young women engaged in sex work have much more frequent acts of sex, their relationships with their main sexual partner (a lover or boyfriend) appear much more loving and harmonious compared to young married women.

- On average, most participants describe having three or more partners. Married women are the only exception, with an average of just over two partners.
- Sexual frequency: Female sex workers (FSWs) may have several clients a day, but not all describe sex every day. Married women describe sex two to four times per week. In-school youth describe having sex less frequently, from once weekly for one young woman with a lover who is local, to once every month to three months for a young woman whose boyfriend is studying elsewhere. For out-of-school youth, it varies from one to two times per month to two to three times per week. Most often several times a month.

Attitudes toward main sexual partner: Those engaged in sex work and in-school youth describe better relationships.

- FSWs: Describe the highest levels of couple harmony, followed by in-school youth. In three of five cases, the boyfriend/lover is described as "not a hooligan," "generous, calm," or the woman says she "loves his walk."
- Married: Described the lowest levels couple harmony and concern about partner fidelity. All describe circumstances when the husband has been abusive; in six of eight cases, the husband has beaten her. In two others, they deny being beaten but express fear that he might. Five of eight women are worried or very worried about their husband's behavior because they can't monitor him.
- Out of school: In two cases, the partner is seen as a womanizer, so they feel little trust. Three other participants have found a new partner who is described as attractive and as someone who satisfies their monetary/ sexual needs. In two of five cases, the partner has been abusive.
- In school: No reports of abuse. Relationships are generally described in positive terms, though some are long distance. All seem to recognize the possibility that a partner could be cheating, but two of five have seen no evidence and two of five are somewhat worried because monitoring may be difficult. One young woman acknowledges he could have 50 partners, but that is okay because they are not engaged. (He is White, provides her with lots of comforts, and is kind.)

Condom use and experience with reproductive tract or sexually transmitted infections:

- FSWs: All currently use condoms with at least some of their sexual partners. Only one woman in this group reported symptoms of an RTI/STI.
- Married: This group was the least likely to use condoms; only two of eight currently used them, and both described their use as preventing pregnancy and disease. (Both describe not trusting their husbands.) The lack of condom use by the other married women was due to trust issues or because the husband refuses condom use within marriage. Three women in this group had experienced some symptoms of an RTI/STI, and one woman was very concerned that she might get HIV.
- Out of school: Two of five report condom use; both describe using condoms for pregnancy and HIV protection. Only one woman described symptoms of an RTI/STI.
- In school: Two of five use condoms, both to prevent pregnancy. In one case, the partner suggested they use condoms for that reason. Three of these young women described RTI/STI-like symptoms. The most frequent descriptions included the word "fungus."

Fertility and contraceptive use: Only 4 of 23 participants currently want to get pregnant; 3 in the married group (and 1 of them already is pregnant). Others do not want to get pregnant soon. Nevertheless, few participants have used contraceptives other than condoms, or they try to "count safe days." Two FSWs, two out-of-school youth, and two married participants are using or have used a hormonal method, although several are no longer using hormonals, having switched because of concerns about side effects. Two in-school youth relied on abortion and two others on the calendar method.

APPENDIX 9

MAKING STUDY FINDINGS ACCESSIBLE TO OTHER RESEARCHERS

You can make your study findings more accessible to other researchers nationally, regionally, and internationally in four important ways:

1. Add standardized cataloging information to the title page or inside cover of your report.
2. Submit your report or article to bibliographic indexing databases and information clearinghouses.
3. Make your study report or dataset available to other researchers through physical and electronic libraries.
4. Ask a health organization or research partner organization to post your report on its website.

Following are some general guidelines based on advice from qualitative researchers and librarians. Where you submit your materials may depend on your study topic and region.

Cataloging Information

International Standard Book Number (ISBN). If your institution is registered as a publisher with the ISBN system, assign an ISBN number and print the number with other title page or cover information in your document.

U.S. Library of Congress (LOC). People throughout the world searching for information on publications use the LOC database. There are two options for getting your book into the LOC database. Both require providing information to the LOC before publication:

1. Register the book electronically by completing the LOC preassigned control number program form before publication. You will receive an LOC control number (LCCN) that should be printed in the book, usually on the back of the title page. You are required to send a copy of the book to the LOC when it is published. When the LOC receives the book, it will catalog the book and add it to its database. The LCCN and the database make it much easier for libraries and dealers to find your book and the catalog information. For more information and electronic registration forms, go to http://www.loc.gov/publish/pcn

2. Register with the LOC Cataloging-in-Publication (CIP) program. Before printing, generally at the final draft stage, you send the complete text of the book in electronic form to the LOC for cataloging. The LOC will send you the complete bibliographic record of your book, including classification numbers and subject headings. This information should be printed in the book when it is published. Having the catalog record in the book makes it much easier for libraries to process the book and for anyone to select, locate, and order it. You must send a copy of the book to the LOC once it is published. For more information on the CIP, contact

   Cataloging-in-Publication Division (CIP)

   Library of Congress

   101 Independence Avenue, S.E.

   Washington, DC 20540-4320

   For online submission, fill in the blank fields at http://www.loc.gov/publish/cip/contact

   For general information or to view the forms and register, go to http://www.loc.gov/publish/cip/

Bibliographic Indexing Databases and Information Clearinghouses

Most databases such as PubMed, the Social Sciences Index, and others automatically get citations from journal publishers, so if you publish in a journal, your article should be included in those databases. However, consider submitting your report or article to bibliographic indexing databases and information clearinghouses, such as the following:

Population Information Online (POPLINE). POPLINE (http://www.popline.org) is the world's largest bibliographic database on population, family planning, and related health issues. POPLINE provides citations with abstracts for over 370,000 records representing published and unpublished literature in the field.

POPLINE provides authoritative, accurate, and up-to-date reproductive health information in electronic formats for developing-country health professionals and policymakers. Full-text copies of most of the documents cited in POPLINE are available free of charge to individuals or institutions in low- and middle-income countries who have little or no Internet access, upon request. POPLINE also provides full-text documents on the Internet.

To submit your article or report for inclusion in the POPLINE database, contact

POPLINE Acquisitions

Center for Communication Programs

Johns Hopkins Bloomberg School of Public Health

111 Market Place, Suite 310

Baltimore, MD 21202

Tel: 410-659-6300

Fax: 410-659-6266

Email: popline@jhuccp.org

Zunia. Zunia (http://zunia.org) is a website and knowledge exchange platform that accepts citations and abstracts related to international development issues, including health. To submit a new ítem, visit https://zunia.org/?q=member-log-in&destination=%2Fnew-post. Zunia is managed by Development Gateway.

Development Gateway, Inc.

1110 Vermont Avenue, Suite 500

Washington, DC 20005

Tel: 202-572-9200

Email: info@developmentgateway.org

Development Experience Clearinghouse (DEC). If your research is done with support from the U.S. Agency for International Development

(USAID), you may submit your study reports or documents for inclusion in the DEC Development Experience System (DEXS). This database was developed to ensure that valuable USAID experience is preserved and gains wider exposure. Once processed into the DEXS system, your documents will be searchable and accessible online, and the public can order paper copies at any time. For general information, visit https://dec.usaid.gov/dec/home/Default.aspx. For instructions on how to submit your material, see https://dec.usaid.gov/SSO/Login.aspx?returnURL=fi9jb250ZW50L3N1Ym1pdC5hc3B4, or contact

Document Acquisitions

USAID Development Experience Clearinghouse

Knowledge Services Center (KSC)

1300 Pennsylvania Avenue, NW

RRB M.01-010

Washington, DC 20523

Tel: 202-712-0579

Email: ksc@usaid.gov

U.S. Library of Congress (LOC). The size and variety of its collections make the LOC the largest library in the world. Collections include research materials in more than 450 languages. By sending a copy of your research report to the LOC, you contribute to the preservation of knowledge and public access to your materials, whether available in hard copy or in a full-text electronic version. To submit your report, send a copy to

Beacher Wiggins, Director

Acquisitions and Bibliographic Access Directorate

Library of Congress

101 Independence Avenue, S.E.

Washington, DC 20540-4170

Tel: 202-707-5325

Email: bwig@loc.gov

For more information, see http://www.loc.gov/rr/coll-general.html

U.S. National Library of Medicine (NLM). The NLM (http://www.nlm.nih.gov/hinfo.html) provides online access to MEDLINE, PubMed, and other specialized databases on HIV/AIDS, bioethics, public health, and health services research. To request that your publication or document be cataloged and made accessible through the NLM, contact

The National Library of Medicine

Cataloging Section

8600 Rockville Pike

Bethesda, MD 20894

Tel: 301-594-5983

Fax: 301-402-1384

Email: custserv@nlm.nih.gov

Depositing Datasets

To make your research permanently available to the international community, seek opportunities to deposit your dataset at a national or regional university library or faculty of social sciences.

Inter-University Consortium for Political and Social Research (ICPSR). ICPSR, established in 1962, is the main repository for social science research in the United States. ICPSR is an international consortium of more than 700 academic institutions and research organizations, and it provides leadership and training in data access, curation, and methods of analysis for the social science research community. ICPSR preserves data to ensure that data resources are available to future generations of scholars, maintaining a data archive of more than 500,000 files of research in the social sciences, and migrating the data to new storage media as changes in technology warrant. In addition, ICPSR provides user support to assist researchers in identifying relevant data for analysis and in conducting their research projects.

ICPSR, a unit within the Institute for Social Research at the University of Michigan, encourages researchers to deposit their own computer-readable data in the archive for long-term preservation and for use in secondary analysis by other social science researchers.

For instructions on how to prepare a dataset for deposit, visit the ICPSR website at http://www.icpsr.umich.edu/icpsrweb/deposit/index.jsp;jsessionid=1659949BF45AB3C62DE8717CC4F9451E. For more information, visit https://www.icpsr.umich.edu/icpsrweb/landing.jsp, or contact

The Inter-University Consortium for Political and Social Research

University of Michigan

Institute for Social Research

P.O. Box 1248

Ann Arbor, MI 48106-1248

Tel: 734-615-8400

Email: mshukait@icpsr.umich.edu

The Australian Data Archive. The Social Science Data Archive (SSDA) was established in 1981 to collect and preserve computer-readable data and make the data available for further analysis. SSDA actively sought deposit of datasets from research by academic, government, and private organizations in order to preserve them for future use. Now the datasets are in the Australian Data Archive (ADA) central facility, which is hosted at the Australian National University within the Australian Centre for Applied Social Research Methods (AusCen) in the College of Arts and Social Sciences. For information on how to deposit data, visit http://www.ada.edu.au/ada/data-deposit, or contact

Australian Data Archive

18 Balmain Lane

Australian National University

ACTON ACT 0200

Tel: 61 2 6125 2200

Fax: 61 2 6125 0627

Email: ada@anu.edu.au

Dublin Core Metadata Initiative. The Dublin Core is a directory of directories (http://dublincore.org). One way to help other researchers find your report or locate your datasets, if these materials are available on the Internet, is to make sure the final HTML webpages are annotated with Dublin

Core metatags or indexing information. Dublin Core metadata supplement existing methods for searching and indexing Web-based metadata, regardless of whether the corresponding resource is an electronic or physical document. Adding Dublin Core metatags promotes greater access to your information by anyone searching the World Wide Web. Even if your study report will not immediately be posted on the Internet, you can add bibliographic descriptors to your dataset or report using the Dublin Core metadata element set. Some people also use Dublin Core elements for cataloging.

To download the Dublin Core metadata, see http://dublincore.org/documents/2000/07/16/usageguide. For a copy of this guide in other languages, see http://dublincore.org/resources/translations.

Websites

Ibiblio If your organization—or a research partner's organization—has posted your material on a website, explore the group's interest in permitting a major Web hub such as ibiblio.org to replicate the material in the social or applied sciences sections of its collections. Ibiblio, a collaboration of the Center for the Public Domain and the University of North Carolina at Chapel Hill, is home to one of the largest collections of freely available full-text online information used for teaching, research, and public service. For more information, visit http://www.ibiblio.org/share.

AMEDEO If you own the copyright to your research report, do not plan to submit your data to a peer-review journal, and would like to see your findings made freely available to the public, consider submitting your text electronically to AMEDEO.com, the Medical Literature Guide, at http://www.amedeo.com. The editors will post your report on the following website, which archives scientific research and ideas: http://www.FreeMedicalJournals.com. They will also send a citation of your article to subscribers to its weekly e-bulletin.

APPENDIX 10

DISSEMINATION MATERIALS FOR COMMUNITY STAKEHOLDERS

Research Briefs

Many researchers communicate findings through 1–2 page briefs or factsheets that explain the context, purpose, methods, and results of their studies. These are sometimes presented as chronological narratives, and other times in a standard scientific IMRAD format (with Introduction, Methods, Results, and Conclusions/Recommendation sections). Examples of these two approaches to writing research briefs follow.

Example 1. Narrative Format

Economic Vulnerability and Women's Risk of HIV

By Emily E. Namey, MA

FHI 360

In many countries around the world, HIV infection is concentrated among small segments of the population. These "key populations"—sex workers, people who inject drugs, and men who have sex with men, for example—participate in risk behaviors that increase their chances of acquiring HIV. Much of the HIV prevention work with key populations, understandably, focuses on changing knowledge or attitudes to reduce specific HIV risk behaviors. However, the men and women who comprise "key populations" often face a range of other economic and social issues in addition to the health risk of HIV infection. In the case of female sex workers, the larger socio-economic context of women's lives is often a driving motivation for participation in sex work. In an environment of limited economic opportunities for women, where women often rely on men for financial support, a divorce, death of a parent or spouse, or social unrest can substantially reduce a woman's ability to financially support herself and her dependents, compelling her to consider sex work as an income generating activity. Viewed in this broader context, HIV prevention activities that address only the sexual risk behaviors of female sex workers ignore the root cause of these women's HIV risk: economic vulnerability.

In an attempt to address the underlying drivers of HIV risk behaviors of female sex workers (FSWs), program development staff in a West African capital decided to attempt an intervention with FSWs that focused on economic strengthening activities, rather than purely HIV education and behavior change. But the range of economic strengthening approaches is wide: Should the intervention involve some kind of cash transfer to female sex workers, giving women money for a period of time to help them to pay off debt and get on their feet without sex work? Or would small loans for alternative income-generating activities work? Or perhaps community-based savings groups might be effective? Though there was not a substantial literature base of evidence to help inform the decision about which approach might work, there was a substantial pool of experts available to weigh in on the issue: the community of FSWs in the city.

The program staff retained an experienced team of qualitative researchers to help them better understand what the financial lives of FSWs looked like. Did they have substantial debt? Were they working for pimps or madams? How much were they earning and what were they spending money on? All of this information was essential for both selecting an approach and tailoring it to the population.

The researchers embarked on a relatively rapid assessment of the situation, using participant observation and interviewing methods, along with more structured financial diaries, to gain both a comprehensive and detailed view of the ways FSWs managed their money. The results were surprising—to both the researchers and the FSWs themselves. The average weekly income of FSWs in this city was relatively substantial, and while a majority of it went to "routine" expenses of daily life such as food, water, and shelter, FSWs identified money management as a large problem. Whatever money came in almost immediately went out, without regard or thought to "need." And nearly a quarter of earnings were "re-invested" in sex work-related products: new clothes, make-up, hair, nails, etc. Most of the FSWs had plans for other activities they'd rather do—small time vending, opening a restaurant—but little ability to plan or save for these dreams. Banks were viewed as places for wealthy people to keep their riches, and the documentation requirements for opening an account were seen as similarly exclusionary.

Based on this information, the program staff developed a pilot economic strengthening curriculum with three pillars: financial management (income allocation and budgeting), life skills (goal setting, confidence building), and entrepreneurship (business planning). Cash hand-outs and small business loans were seen as both unnecessary and unsustainable in this context, despite their use in other locations. And in a small evaluation of the pilot program, the life skills training—not typically seen as "economic" strengthening—was identified as an integral part of the program, with potential cross-over influence into HIV risk behavior territory. Having specific goals and feeling confident and empowered through use of a budget and a developing business plan could help women better negotiate condom use or decline sex with a particular partner altogether.

Though small, this study provided essential information on what type of economic strengthening programming to incorporate into HIV prevention efforts for this population of women. And, importantly, it recognized that FSWs are more than vectors for disease—they are women making critical decisions in an environment of constrained choices. Qualitative research facilitates understanding of the complex linkages between socio-economic realities and health behaviors by asking the populations affected to explain the 'hows' and 'whys' of those connections. Programs based on these types of grounded knowledge are more likely to address the perceived needs of those at risk, and therefore, have greater potential for success. As one FSW expressed, "... This project is an opportunity for us. This is the first time they did not come to talk about AIDS with us, but to help us manage our money. Thank you very much."

Example 2: IMRAD Format

Research Brief: Communicating Partial Protection of Voluntary Medical Male Circumcision

This brief was disseminated to implementers of voluntary medical male circumcision (VMMC) in Kenya via electronic mailing lists and in print format. It was also featured in an issue of the *Clearinghouse on Male Circumcision* newsletter. In addition, a link to the brief was provided on the FHI 360 website.

Communicating Male Circumcision's Partial Protection from HIV

Male circumcision reduces men's risk of acquiring HIV infection through vaginal intercourse, but it does not provide complete protection against the virus. Circumcised men and their partners are advised to take additional steps to protect themselves from HIV infection, such as using condoms consistently and having fewer partners.

But do men and women understand these messages about partial protection? And do they act on the messages to protect themselves from HIV after male circumcision?

Kelly L'Engle and colleagues from FHI 360 conducted a study, with support from the Male Circumcision Consortium, to examine understanding of partial protection among men and women in Kenya's Nyanza Province and identify the best ways to convey to men and women the need for safe sex after voluntary medical male circumcision (VMMC).

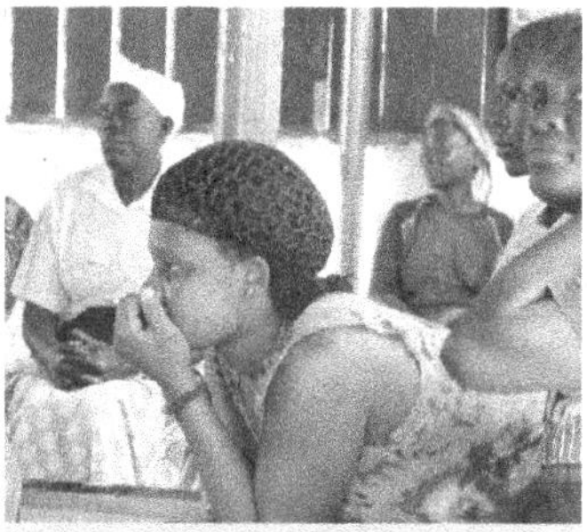

PHOTO: SILAS ACHAR/FHI 360

- **Men and women in Nyanza understand the concept of partial protection from HIV.**
- **Counseling is a critical and effective part of voluntary medical male circumcision.**
- **Women should be involved in VMMC promotion, counseling and follow-up support.**

Study Design

Participants in the Communicating Partial Protection Study were recruited through community mobilizers and health clinic staff in urban Kisumu East and the more rural Siaya District. The study consisted of:

In-depth interviews with 44 men and 22 women ages 18 to 35 conducted in April-May 2010. Half the men had been circumcised in the past six months; half planned to get circumcised soon. Women were evenly divided between those with circumcised and uncircumcised partners.

Focus group discussions conducted in March-April 2011: eight involving a total of 89 men who had been circumcised within the past six months and reported changing their behavior after VMMC to further reduce the risk of HIV infection, and four involving 44 women whose partners had recently been circumcised.

A content analysis of 48 communications on VMMC: 23 print materials and audiotapes of 10 radio broadcasts, eight health education sessions and seven counseling sessions.

MALE CIRCUMCISION CONSORTIUM

The Male Circumcision Consortium worked with the Government of Kenya and other partners — including the US President's Emergency Plan for AIDS Relief (PEPFAR), which supports service delivery — to prevent HIV and save lives by expanding access to safe and voluntary male circumcision services. FHI 360 received a grant from the Bill & Melinda Gates Foundation to collaborate on the consortium with EngenderHealth and the University of Illinois at Chicago, working with the Nyanza Reproductive Health Society.

Source: The Male Circumcision Consortium.

Results

Both men and women demonstrated a high level of awareness of partial HIV protection. Participants described partial protection in different ways, including the need to continue using other HIV-protective measures after VMMC and with numbers, such as "not 100 percent" protection.

Circumcised men were better able to explain partial protection, compared to women and uncircumcised men. They attributed their knowledge to the counseling they had received as part of VMMC.

Women held no misconceptions about partial protection, but some were unable to elaborate on its meaning. When women in the focus groups were given more information about partial protection, they understood it well.

The ways men and women explained partial protection mirrored how partial protection was presented in the communication materials, suggesting that the messages are reaching and resonating with target audiences.

Most of the materials mentioned that VMMC provides partial protection from HIV, and two-thirds included other ways to protect against HIV infection following VMMC. One-third of the materials addressed partner communication.

There was little evidence that men were engaging in riskier sexual behavior after VMMC. A number of men said they had actually increased their HIV-protective behaviours after circumcision. Only a few uncircumcised men planned to take fewer precautions against HIV after VMMC. Some men reported that being circumcised made it easier to use condoms.

The main reasons reported for positive behavior changes were VMMC counseling and getting tested for HIV prior to being circumcised.

Male participants' decisions about circumcision were strongly influenced by men who had recently been circumcised and by their own female partners. Men and women said partners often discuss the decision to get circumcised. They also talk about partial protection and the six weeks of abstinence required during wound healing.

RECOMMENDATIONS

- The program's emphasis on VMMC counseling — which appears to be effectively communicating the concept of partial protection — should be maintained and strengthened.
- Messages about male circumcision should reiterate that VMMC provides only partial HIV protection, specify additional ways to reduce HIV risk, and emphasize that VMMC services are based on scientific evidence.
- Couples' counseling should be encouraged to increase women's understanding of partial protection and foster discussion between partners about HIV prevention following VMMC.
- The VMMC program should redouble its efforts to engage women in promotion, counseling and follow-up support. VMMC communications should be more effectively targeted to reach women, particularly in venues recommended by the women in interviews such as markets, women's group meetings and maternal-child health clinics.
- The program should consider having recently circumcised men provide "testimonials" and serve as role models for VMMC adoption.

References

Lanham M, L'Engle KL, Loolpapit M, Oguma IO. Women's roles in voluntary medical male circumcision in Nyanza Province, Kenya. 2012; PLoS One 7(9):e4482. doi:10.1371/journjal.pone.0044825.

L'Engle KL, Lanham M, Loolpapit M, Oguma IO. Understanding partial protection and HIV risk and behavior following voluntary medical male circumcision rollout in Kenya. Health Education Research 2014; 29(1): 22-30. doi:10.1093/her/cyt103.

L'Engle KL, Lanham M, Oguma IO, Loolpapit M. Communicating Partial Protection: Results from In-depth Interviews and Focus Group Discussions with Men and Women, and Content Analysis of Voluntary Medical Male Circumcision Messages in Nyanza Province, Kenya. Final Report. FHI 360: Durham, NC, USA, 2011.

AUGUST 2014

MCC MALE CIRCUMCISION CONSORTIUM · fhi360 THE SCIENCE OF IMPROVING LIVES · UIC UNIVERSITY OF ILLINOIS AT CHICAGO

EMAIL: mccinfo@fhi360.org
WEBSITE: http://www.fhi360.org/projects/male-circumcision-consortium-mcc

Source: The Male Circumcision Consortium.

Example 3: Newsletter

This newsletter shares developments undertaken by a research team preparing for baseline assessments of the Mphatlalatsane project in northeastern Lesotho, an integrated intervention to improve early child development and nutrition outcomes and increase HIV testing and treatment support for young children in Lesotho. A randomized controlled trial will evaluate the outcomes of the project, which is funded by the U.S. Agency for International Development through Management Sciences for Health's Building Local Capacity for Delivery of HIV Services in Southern Africa Project, in collaboration with the local civil society organization GROW and research partner Stellenbosch University. It is reprinted with permission from Marguerite Marlow and the Mphatlalatsane study team.

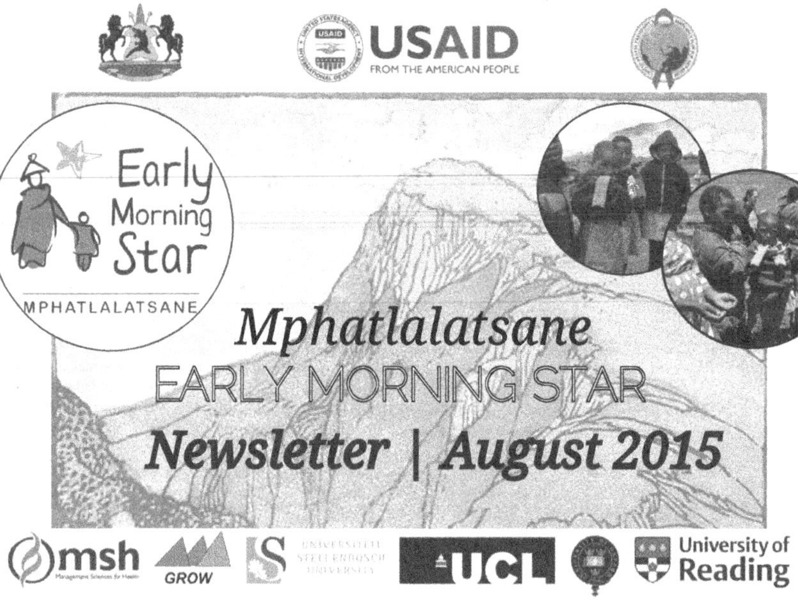

MPHATLALATSANE | EARLY MORNING STAR | LESOTHO

The Mphatlalatsane project, meaning "early morning star" in Sesotho, aims to improve early child development and nutrition outcomes and increase HIV testing and treatment support for young children in Lesotho. A randomized controlled trial will be used to evaluate the outcomes of this integrated intervention. The research study will take place in 32 villages in the Mokhotlong district of north-eastern Lesotho.

This project is funded by USAID through Management Sciences for Health Building Local Capacity for Delivery of HIV Services in Southern Africa Project, in collaboration with local civil society organisation GROW and research partners Stellenbosch University, University College London, the University of Oxford and the University of Reading.

This newsletter looks at the latest developments undertaken by the Mphatlalatsane research team as they train and prepare for baseline assessments.

Early Morning Star

MPHATLALATSANE

Mokhotlong Lesotho: A Challenging Terrain

Conducting research in the remote mountains of Mokhotlong presents some unique logistical challenges to the research team. Some villages are only accessible by horse or donkey, which means the only way for teams to access these areas is to saddle up! Steep ascents and descents make the journey even more of a challenge, especially during the winter months. During recruitment, several villages were inaccessible by roads after heavy snowfall. Footpaths which connect different villages in the district were also affected due to the sub-zero temperatures. The main roads which connect Mokhotlong with Underberg (South Africa) were also at times impassable due to snow. This created some delays in delivery of supplies and logistical challenges for those travelling from Stellenbosch University, Although the teams encountered many logistical obstacles during recruitment, they remain in good spirits and look forward to their next adventure in the field.

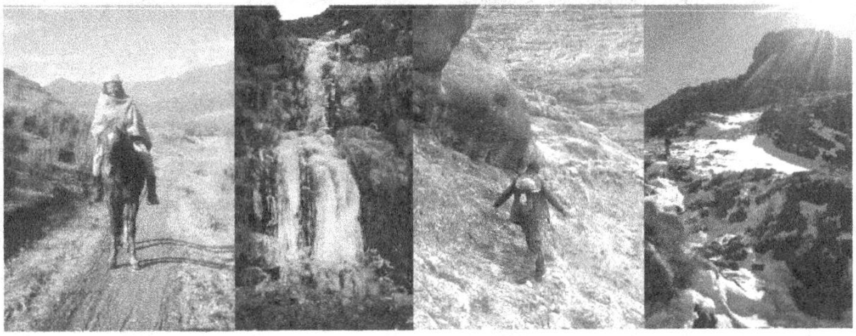

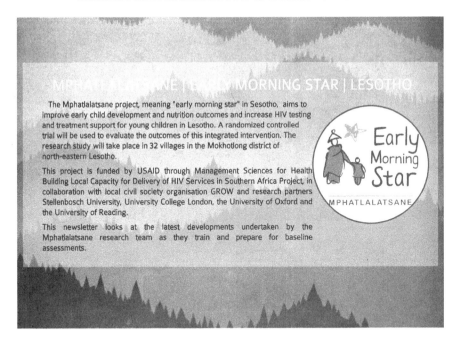

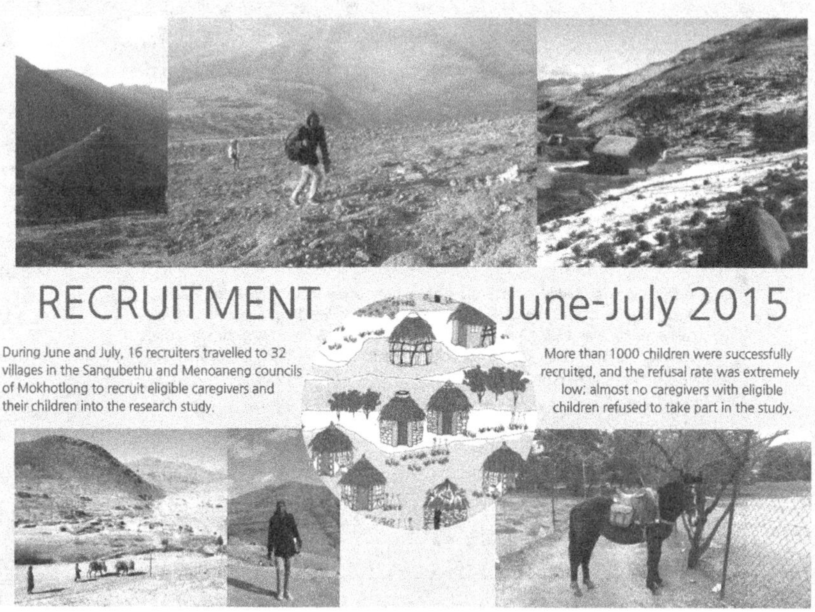
RECRUITMENT
June-July 2015
During June and July, 16 recruiters travelled to 32 villages in the Sanqubethu and Menoaneng councils of Mokhotlong to recruit eligible caregivers and their children into the research study.
More than 1000 children were successfully recruited, and the refusal rate was extremely low; almost no caregivers with eligible children refused to take part in the study.

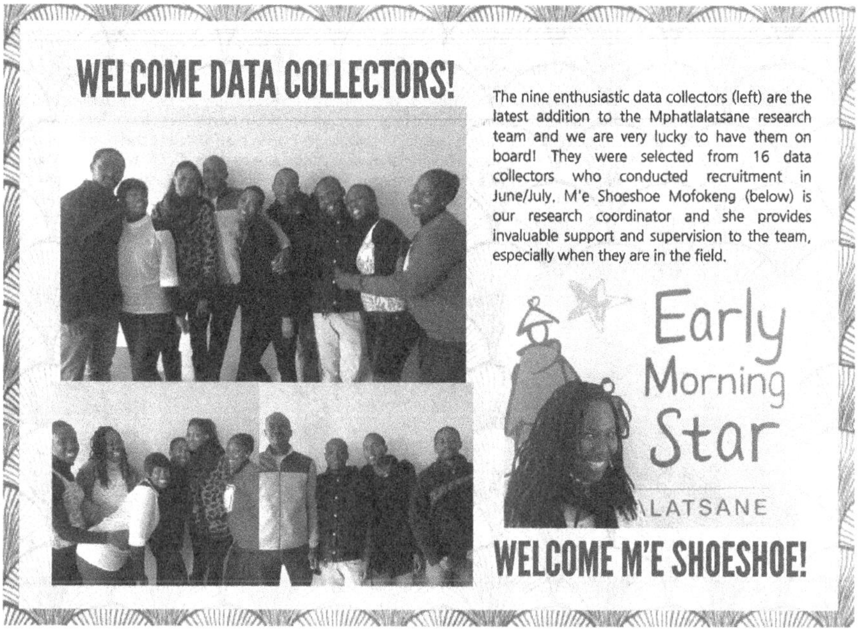
WELCOME DATA COLLECTORS!
The nine enthusiastic data collectors (left) are the latest addition to the Mphatlalatsane research team and we are very lucky to have them on board! They were selected from 16 data collectors who conducted recruitment in June/July. M'e Shoeshoe Mofokeng (below) is our research coordinator and she provides invaluable support and supervision to the team, especially when they are in the field.
Early Morning Star
LATSANE
WELCOME M'E SHOESHOE!

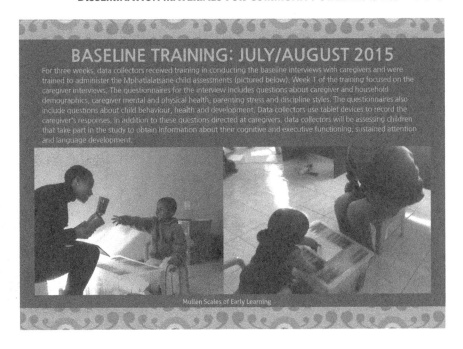

BASELINE TRAINING: JULY/AUGUST 2015

For three weeks, data collectors received training in conducting the baseline interviews with caregivers and were trained to administer the Mphatlalatsane child assessments (pictured below). Week 1 of the training focused on the caregiver interviews. The questionnaires for the interview includes questions about caregiver and household demographics, caregiver mental and physical health, parenting stress and discipline styles. The questionnaires also include questions about child behaviour, health and development. Data collectors use tablet devices to record the caregiver's responses. In addition to these questions directed at caregivers, data collectors will be assessing children that take part in the study to obtain information about their cognitive and executive functioning, sustained attention and language development.

Mullen Scales of Early Learning

Peabody Picture Vocabulary Test

Early Childhood Vigilance Task

CHILD ASSESSMENTS TRAINING

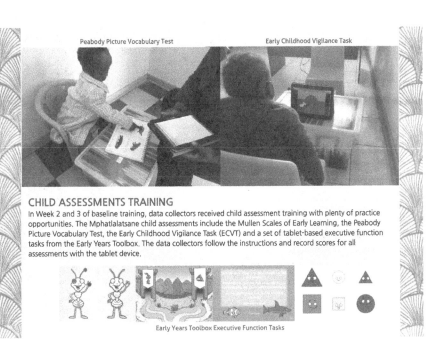

In Week 2 and 3 of baseline training, data collectors received child assessment training with plenty of practice opportunities. The Mphatlalatsane child assessments include the Mullen Scales of Early Learning, the Peabody Picture Vocabulary Test, the Early Childhood Vigilance Task (ECVT) and a set of tablet-based executive function tasks from the Early Years Toolbox. The data collectors follow the instructions and record scores for all assessments with the tablet device.

Early Years Toolbox Executive Function Tasks

COMMUNITY ADVISORY BOARD MEETING: JULY 2015

In July, the first community advisory board meeting was held at MSH Offices in Mokhotlong. The purpose of the advisory board is to provide input on particular issues arising during implementation of the research protocol of the Mphatlalatsane Project. Representatives from the Ministry of Social Development, Ministry of Education and Training, Ministry of Health and the Food and Nutrition Coordinating Office make up the advisory board. Chief Seeiso of Thabang also joined the meeting to provide advice on governance related issues that may arise in the communities to ensure smooth run of the project. The next meeting will be held in October of this year. We are very grateful for their expert advice and guidance.

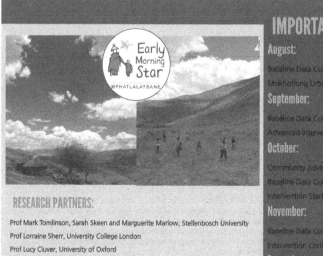

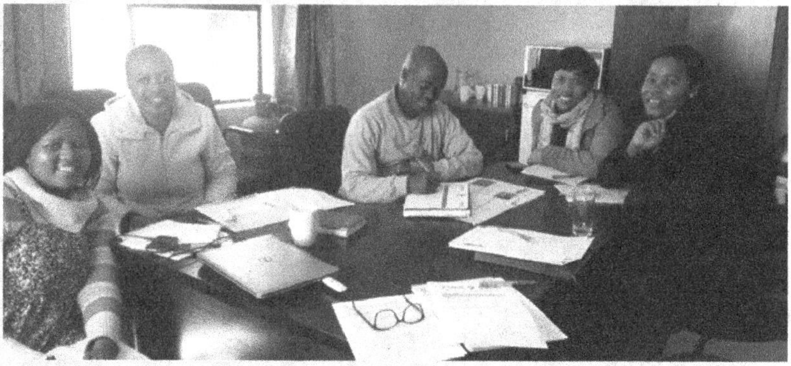

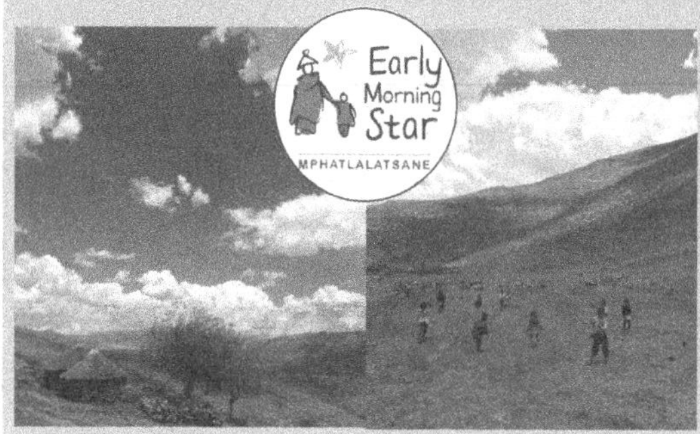

RESEARCH PARTNERS:

Prof Mark Tomlinson, Sarah Skeen and Marguerite Marlow, Stellenbosch University

Prof Lorraine Sherr, University College London

Prof Lucy Cluver, University of Oxford

Prof Lynne Murray and Prof Peter Cooper, University of Reading

This project is funded by USAID through Management Sciences for Health Building Local Capacity for Delivery of HIV Services in Southern Africa Project

IMPORTANT DATES

August:

Baseline Data Collection Starts

Mokhotlong Urban Intervention

September:

Baseline Data Collection Continues

Advanced Intervention Training

October:

Community Advisory Board Meeting

Baseline Data Collection Continues

Intervention Starts

November:

Baseline Data Collection Continues

Intervention Continues

December:

3 Month Follow Up Data Collection Begins

SAMPLE BRIEFS TO SHARE QUALITATIVE STUDY FINDINGS WITH POLICY AUDIENCES

Example 1

This brochure was developed by Susan Settergren and the staff of the POLICY Project to share findings with members of the communities in Zimbabwe where a qualitative study on unsafe abortion and postabortion care was conducted. It is reprinted with permission from the POLICY Project, an international effort funded by the U.S. Agency for International Development and undertaken by the Futures Group International, Research Triangle Institute, and the Centre for Development and Population Activities in 1999. For more information, see:

http://www.policyproject.com/pubs/policymatters/pm-01.pdf.

POLICY *Matters*
www.policyproject.com No. 1, January 2000

Unsafe Abortion and Postabortion Care in Zimbabwe: Community Perspectives

Based on the report "Community Perspectives on Unsafe Abortion and Postabortion Care in Zimbabwe" by Susan Settergren, Cont Mhlanga, Joyce Mpofu, Dennis Ncube, and Cynthia Woodsong, April 1999. Emily Pierce and Susan Settergren prepared this brief.

Background

Abortion complications pose a serious health risk to women and account for 13 percent of maternal deaths worldwide.[1] Effective and safe postabortion care would save women's lives by reducing maternal mortality rates by as much as one-fifth in many low-income countries.[2] Complications of unsafe abortion cost health care systems a tremendous amount in terms of hospital space, providers' time, antibiotics, blood, and supplies. Experts note that "It is not uncommon for the majority of beds in emergency gynecology wards to be occupied by women suffering abortion complications ... Treating a patient with abortion complications can cost upward of five times the annual per capita health budget."[3] Given the magnitude of the health burden and costs associated with abortion complications, it is vital for countries to extend postabortion care services to women. To do so, it is important to understand the roles communities can play in reducing abortion and promoting good quality postabortion care.

In East and Southern Africa, USAID has implemented a regional initiative to reduce the number and consequences of unsafe abortions by promoting postabortion care (PAC). PAC is a widely accepted public health strategy to reduce maternal mortality and morbidity from unsafe abortion and provide links between postabortion emergency treatment services and comprehensive family planning/reproductive health services. Most PAC program efforts focus on service delivery, emphasizing operations research, training of service providers, and service delivery strategies. However, community perspectives, such as knowledge and attitudes about unsafe abortion and health-seeking behavior among those who experience complications of abortion, also need to be considered in program design. This research is intended to enhance understanding of the role of communities in the prevention of unsafe abortion and provision of client-oriented PAC services.

Methodology

Collecting information about community perspectives on abortion is difficult. Traditional methods of data collection, such as surveys, have proved inadequate in gathering valid data on this sensitive topic. Restrictions on abortion and the social stigma attached to it often make people reluctant to discuss the issue openly with researchers.[4]

The POLICY Project and Amakhosi Theatre Group are using an innovative approach to overcome these research challenges. They are using methods of social theater to promote community dialogue and document community perspectives

[1] Starrs, A. 1998. *The Safe Motherhood Action Agenda: Priorities for the Next Decade—Report on the Safe Motherhood Technical Consultation 18-23 October 1997, Colombo, Sri Lanka.* New York: Family Care International in collaboration with the Interagency Group for Safe Motherhood.

[2] Maine, D. 1997. *Safe Motherhood Programs: Options and Issues.* New York: Center for Population and Family Health, Columbia University.

[3] REDSO. n.d. Postabortion Care Initiative Brochure. Kenya: USAID/REDSO.

[4] Abortion is heavily restricted in most African countries. In Zimbabwe, abortion is permitted only in cases of threat to the life or permanent physical impairment of the pregnant woman, grave physical or mental defects to the child, or conception by unlawful intercourse (i.e., rape, incest, or intercourse with a mentally handicapped woman).

Source: The POLICY Project.

on unsafe abortion and PAC. Amakhosi Theatre Group, a leading professional theatre company in Zimbabwe, produced a play on adolescent pregnancy, unsafe abortion, and postabortion care, entitled *Don't—Ungaqali.*[5] The play uses drama, music, and comedy to tell the story of a teenage girl who has an unsafe abortion and suffers complications. (See *Don't—Ungaqali!* box for plot summary.)

Performances were held in nine rural and urban locations in Hwange and Bulawayo Districts in Matebeleland North Province of Zimbabwe. Following each performance, the audience was invited to stay for a discussion of the issues raised by the play. The author of the play and a public health nurse led discussions, while two researchers documented what was said.

Altogether, approximately 2,500 people attended the performances. Post-performance discussions ranged in size from 18 to 100 participants. Participants included elected city officials, traditional chiefs, health care professionals, traditional healers, teachers and education administrators, clergy and religious leaders, police, court magistrates, business leaders, military officials, representatives of national- and community-level NGOs, and community members-at-large. Researchers also conducted over 60 key informant interviews with selected community members before and after the performances.

[5] The University of Zimbabwe Medical Library commissioned Cont Mhlanga, Artistic Director of Amakhosi Theatre Group, to write and produce the play with support from the USAID-funded Support to Analysis and Research in Africa (SARA) Project. The play is based on Amakhosi's community research on unsafe abortion and the policy guidelines published by the Commonwealth Regional Health Community Secretariat.

Don't—Ungaqali!

In an all-too-common scenario, a teenage couple in Zimbabwe succumbs to peer pressure, and they have sex. The girl becomes pregnant. When her boyfriend learns of her condition, he abandons her. Both are thrown out of their homes by their parents. Faced with few alternatives, the boy runs away to South Africa; the girl takes up residence with a professional sex worker who arranges for her to have an abortion. The abortion is performed by a *nyanga* (a traditional healer) who provides the girl with *muti* (herbal medicine), but the girl suffers serious complications. When her parents learn of the situation, her mother arranges to take her to the hospital, while her father, in his anger, focuses on the arrest of the nyanga. The girl survives but will never be able to bear children. At the end of the play, the mother warns the audience about the dangers of unsafe abortion and advises that if a woman experiences complications from an abortion, she should receive immediate medical attention and family planning counseling.

Findings

Community members of all ages engaged in lively discussions following the performances. Community perspectives from these discussions and the key informant interviews are highlighted below.

Community Knowledge about Abortion

Although most abortions are done secretly, the majority of community members recognize that unsafe abortion is a serious problem. Sources of information about the magnitude of the problem include rumors, personal observation in health care and social services settings, and the media.

"The problem of abortions is a well-known fact in the communities, even if they're done in secrecy."
—Residents' association member

POLICY Matters presents the findings and implications of POLICY-supported research. The POLICY Project is funded by the U.S. Agency for International Development (USAID) under Contract No. CCP-C-00-95-00023-04 and is implemented by The Futures Group International in collaboration with Research Triangle Institute (RTI) and The Centre for Development and Population Activities (CEDPA). The views expressed in this series do not necessarily reflect those of USAID.

For more information, please contact:

The POLICY Project
1050 17th Street, NW, Suite 1000
Washington, DC 20036

Tel: (202) 775-9680
Fax: (202) 775-9694
E-mail: policyinfo@tfgi.com
Internet: www.policyproject.com

The POLICY Project

The common assumption is that young, unmarried girls are most affected by unwanted pregnancy and unsafe abortion. However, older, married women also are acknowledged to experience these problems. Causes of unwanted pregnancy cited by the respondents include the following:

- Economic hardship that leads to sex for income;
- Poor parenting;
- Ignorance about sex and reproductive health, early physical maturity and experimentation with sex;
- Promiscuity;
- Unprotected sex and inaccessibility of contraceptives;
- Breakdown of traditional family and societal values;
- Women's lack of control of their sexuality;
- Boys and men "cheating" girls into having sex by promising marriage; and
- Lack of respect between a man and a woman.

The most frequently cited reasons for inducing an abortion are denial of responsibility for the pregnancy by the boy or man and fear of parents discovering the pregnancy.

Abortion Sources and Methods

Traditional healers, certain community members (often female elders), and medical doctors are reported to induce abortions. Abortions also are self-induced with assistance from friends and other community members. Most abortionists are unskilled, although some are more qualified than others. Abortion methods used outside the formal health care system include oral administration of traditional medicine or herbs, overdoses of malaria tablets or contraceptive pills, and insertion of knitting needles or roots into the vagina.

Health-seeking Behavior for Abortion Complications and PAC Services

Girls and women who experience complications of induced abortion often delay or do not seek medical treatment. Fear of being reported to the police by clinic or hospital staff, fear of harsh treatment and exposure by nurses, and fear of parents' reactions are the primary reasons for avoiding medical attention. The law requires health care facilities to report abortion cases to the police. However, the practice of reporting appears to vary among service delivery sites and individuals. Parents and community members also report cases to authorities. Frequently, they file these reports because they are concerned with arresting the abortionist. Other reasons for delaying treatment include financial constraints, difficulty with transport, and "mild" symptoms.

"When they find they can no longer hide the pregnancy, they decide to abort and still keep on hiding and hope that things will be all right. As a result, they come late for help when they can no longer cope."

—Private medical doctor

Nurses' attitudes and behavior toward postabortion clients have an impact on clients' decisions to seek care. In particular, community members are concerned about nurses' gossip to family members and neighbors, harsh treatment, and unfriendliness to youth. At the same time, nurses express frustration with the client's failure to explain the reason for her condition and delay in seeking treatment until complications are severe.

Recommended Community Actions

Respondents acknowledged that abortion and unwanted pregnancy have far-reaching effects on the community and assumed ownership of the problem. They recommended specific actions for communities to take to address the issue.

Many community members stated that better parenting would reduce the problems of unwanted pregnancy and unsafe abortion. They also encouraged schools to work with parents to teach sex education.

"There is no point blaming this and that. Abortion is a community problem."

—Woman at a performance discussion

Community members acknowledged that family planning helps prevent unwanted pregnancy, but voiced several concerns. In particular, opinions regarding provision of contraceptives to young, unmarried teens greatly diverged. Some respondents also expressed fear of contraceptive side effects. Others complained of financial constraints. Many people can no longer afford to purchase

Source: The POLICY Project.

contraceptives since the government raised prices in early 1999.

In general, respondents encouraged better community dialogue and mobilization. Specific recommendations include the following:

- Sensitize and educate on the dangers of unsafe abortion, the need for prompt medical attention for complications, and PAC;
- Broadcast information on the radio and in newspapers, host drama performances and workshops;
- Encourage church attendance and dialogue at church on unsafe abortion;
- Establish and support programs for youth;
- Facilitate networking among community organizations;
- Engage elected officials and politicians;
- Continue dialogue on sensitive policy issues, such as legalization of abortion and family planning services for youth; and
- Expand and improve PAC services by offering clients confidentiality, counseling, and support.

Policy Implications

The health community must recognize the important role of the broader community in solving the problems of unwanted pregnancy and unsafe abortion and in strengthening PAC services. These research findings suggest three key strategies:

- Listen to the community. Community members have information that health care managers and providers need in order to design and provide services that will better meet client needs. Incorporating client perspectives is critical because many clients in need are not seeking services. Community members are eager to provide their perspectives if they feel they are being listened to and respected.
- Educate the community. Education should be a cornerstone of PAC service delivery. Many people, particularly young people, do not understand the seriousness of abortion complications. More broadly, knowledge about sex and reproductive health is seriously lacking. The health community must reach out to the larger community to provide this education.
- Partner with the community. Unwanted pregnancy and unsafe abortion are multidimensional problems deeply embedded in societal and cultural norms and practices. The health community cannot, and should not, operate alone. As PAC programs are established and improved, opportunities to create linkages and synergies with other community services and organizations must be explored.

The first phase of this social theatre project aimed to sensitize communities to the problems of unsafe abortion and motivate community action, while gathering data on community perspectives in the process. The second phase will focus on measuring the impact of the social theatre intervention to mobilize community action.

Acknowledgments The editorial, production, and design team for this issue of *POLICY Matters* includes Nancy McGirr, Karen Hardee, Charles Wilkinson, and Jen Marenberg of The Futures Group International. Barbara Crane and Elizabeth Schoenecker of USAID also reviewed various drafts and provided helpful comments. Graphic design by CGS, Inc. Printed on recycled paper.

Source: The POLICY Project.

Example 2

Lessons From a Female Condom Community Intervention Trial in Rural Kenya

What impact will a general distribution of the female condom have on sexually transmitted infection (STI) rates in a rural area? To address this question, FHI conducted a community intervention trial and follow-up service delivery assessment in rural Kenya, collaborating with the University of Nairobi, Department of Medical Microbiology, and the Family Planning Association of Kenya. The researchers concluded:

- The availability of the female condom did not reduce STI rates, relative to the reductions achieved by distribution of the male condom alone.
- Female condom users generally liked the device, recognized its dual protection properties and appreciated its advantages over the male condom.
- Provider preconceptions may have limited opportunities for women to use the device.

The community intervention trial was conducted in six matched pairs of tea, coffee and flower plantations, each served by at least one primary health care clinic. Each matched pair comprised an intervention and a control site. In the intervention areas, providers and outreach workers received training in providing male and female condoms, STI risk reduction and treatment, and were supplied with free male and female condoms. The control areas received training, supplies and training only on the male condom. A thorough educational campaign reached residents throughout all sites with activities in control sites covering only the male condom.

The study followed about 1,600 women, testing and treating them at baseline, six months and 12 months for three infections—gonorrhea, chlamydia, and trichomoniasis. At both control and intervention plantations, about 24 percent of the women tested and treated had one or more of the three STIs at the beginning of the study. After 12 months, STI rates had declined to about 18 percent at both the intervention and control sites.[1]

These results indicate that adding the female condom to the male condom distribution system did not contribute to any additional reductions in disease prevalence. At the same time, the intensive promotional campaign in the male-condom-only distribution system was not sufficient to have an important impact on disease rates either.

Reported female condom use was not sufficiently frequent to make a substantial difference in the overall number of protected sex acts in the intervention sites. Also, providing female condoms did not result in more overall condoms distributed in intervention sites. At the end of the study, 58 percent of study participants in intervention sites reported that they had not used the female condom at all in the previous six months.[2]

Service Delivery Impact

To assess why so few women used the female condom, researchers visited 16 of the 23 sites participating in the community trial, including a balance of high- and low-performing intervention and control sites. At each site, surveys were conducted with all available clinicians, outreach workers, recent family planning clients, and community key informants. Also, researchers observed all family planning service delivery encounters in the clinic on the day of the visit.[3]

A gap existed between clinicians' reported condom promotion activities and their observed behaviors. In 42 observed family planning visits, the woman in every case chose a hormonal method, but only once did a provider suggest a condom as a supplemental method for STI protection. Moreover, 91 percent of providers interviewed said they had a major influence on whether clients used condoms. Many clinicians viewed the female condom as a feasible method only for single women and sex workers, not for women in stable unions. This provider opinion regarding appropriate female condom users may have contributed to inadequate interest on the part of clients. Only one of 10 intervention site clinics distributed female condoms all 12 months of the trial as called for by the protocol.

Despite the provider behaviors, outreach workers reported that the female condom was viewed by clients as an acceptable method, credited for being warmer, roomier, and stronger than the male condom. Some women felt safer with the female condom because it was perceived as being less prone than the male condom to break. Further, women appreciated being able to insert the female condom themselves, avoiding the risk of men tampering with the device, as was suspected with the male condom.

At the same time, social norms and personal preferences appeared to limit true acceptability of the female condom and impede its introduction into sexual relationships. Community members expressed concern that the female condom may allow women too much freedom, enabling them to "move around" on their husbands. Some feared that intensified distribution of condoms might lead to increased prostitution.

With limited understanding of female anatomy, some users expressed fears that it could "slip into the stomach," get "lost inside the womb," or get "stuck in the vagina." Others rumored it was laced with HIV or that the lubricant could cause infertility or produce infections. Some men worried that a woman can take semen captured in the female condom to a witch doctor and put a hex on the partner.

When considering the introduction of the female condom in rural areas, program planners need to take into consideration the local culture and address the negative influence that traditional gender roles can have on female condom use.

Notes

1. Feldblum PJ, Kuyoh MA, Bwayo JJ, et al. Female condom introduction and sexually transmitted infection prevalence: results of a community intervention trial in Kenya. AIDS 2001 May 25;15(8):1037–1044.
2. Welsh MJ, Feldblum PJ, Kuyoh MA, et al. Condom use during a community intervention trial in Kenya. Int J AIDS STDs 2001 July;12(7):469–474.
3. Toroitich-Ruto C. Assessment of the Intervention: Was It Implemented as Intended? Presented at Conference on Female Condom and STDs: A Community Intervention Trial, May 9, 2000, Nairobi, Kenya.

APPENDIX 12

SAMPLE DISSEMINATION STRATEGY FOR ADVOCACY

This pocket card was developed by Sonke Gender Justice and FHI 360 in partnership with the South Africa National AIDS Commission (SANAC). It was used as an advocacy tool to promote support for microbicides among SANAC members and other government bodies. It presents findings from a gender analysis conducted in South Africa and is an excellent example of a dissemination strategy tailored for advocacy.

For more information:

email: info@genderjustice.org.za

www.genderjustice.org.za

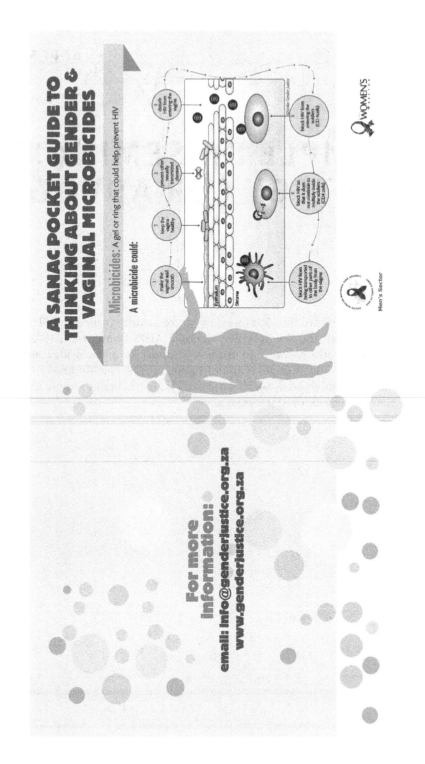

A SANAC POCKET GUIDE TO THINKING ABOUT GENDER & VAGINAL MICROBICIDES

Microbicides: A gel or ring that could help prevent HIV

A microbicide could:

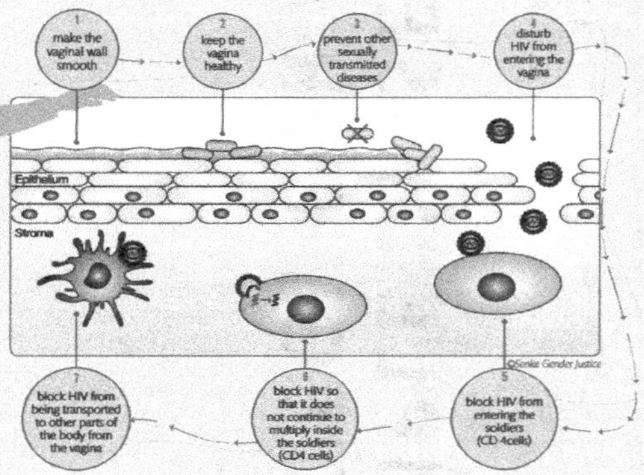

1 make the vaginal wall smooth
2 keep the vagina healthy
3 prevent other sexually transmitted diseases
4 disturb HIV from entering the vagina
5 block HIV from entering the soldiers (CD 4cells)
6 block HIV so that it does not continue to multiply inside the soldiers (CD4 cells)
7 block HIV from being transported to other parts of the body from the vagina
Epithelium
Stroma
©Sonke Gender Justice

Men's Sector

WOMEN'S SECTOR

MICROBICIDES

are substances being tested in clinical trials that could be used in the vagina and/or rectum to reduce the risk of HIV transmission during sex. If proven effective, they will offer women an important and fundamentally different HIV prevention option – one that could possibly be used without their partners' knowledge, if desired. Sonke Gender Justice & FHI 360, with funding from the United States Agency for International Development (USAID), conducted a gender analysis to make recommendations for an effective and rights-based microbicides roll out in South Africa. In addition to access to microbicides reaffirming every woman's right to health and to live free from HIV, the analysis found:

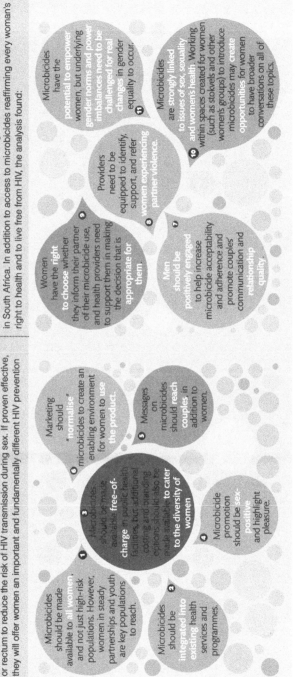

1. Microbicides should be made available to **all women**, and not just high-risk populations. However, women in steady partnerships and youth are key populations to reach.
2. Microbicides should be **integrated into existing** health services and programmes.
3. Microbicides should be made available **free-of-charge** in public health facilities, but additional costing and branding options should also be made available **to cater to the diversity of women**
4. Microbicide promotion should be **sex-positive** and highlight pleasure.
5. Messages on microbicides should **reach couples** in addition to women.
6. Marketing should **"normalise"** microbicides to create an enabling environment for women to **use the product.**
7. **Men should be positively engaged** to help increase microbicide acceptability and adherence and promote couples' communication and **relationship quality**.
8. Providers need to be equipped to identify, support, and refer **women experiencing partner violence.**
9. Women have the **right to choose** whether they inform their partner of their microbicide use, and health providers need to support them in making the decision that is **appropriate for them**.
10. Microbicides are **strongly linked to issues of sex, sexuality and women's health**. Working within spaces created for women (such as stokvels and other women's groups) to introduce microbicides may **create opportunities** for women to have broader conversations on all of these topics.
11. Microbicides have the **potential to empower** women, but underlying **gender norms and power imbalances need to be challenged for real changes** in gender equality to occur.

APPENDIX 13

WHERE TO PUBLISH

Many scientific journals that cover public health issues accept articles that report on qualitative studies or studies using mixed methods. The journals and presses listed here represent a selection of publishing venues for qualitative researchers to consider.

Journals

African Journal of Reproductive Health

Editor: Friday Okonofua

Women's Health and Action Research Centre

4 Alofoje Avenue, Off Uwasota Street

P.O. Box 10231, Ugbowo

Benin City, Edo State

Nigeria

Tel: 234.52.602334/600151

Fax: 234.52.602091

Email: wharc@hyperia.com, wharc@warri.rcl.nig.com

Website: http://www.wharc.freehosting.net

AIDS

Editor-in-Chief: J.A. Levy (San Francisco)

Editorial Coordinator, Chris Mowat

250 Waterloo Road

London SE1 8RD UK

Tel: 44 20 7981 0672

Fax: 44 20 7981 0556

Email: Christopher.Mowat@wolterskluwer.com

Website: http://www.aidsonline.com

AIDS and Behavior

Editor: Seth C. Kalichman, PhD

Center for HIV Prevention & Intervention

2006 Hillside Road, Unit 1248

University of Connecticut

Storrs, CT 06269

Email: aidsandbehavior@yahoo.com

Submit online: http://www.editorialmanager.com/aibe/

Website: http://www.springer.com/public+health/journal/10461

AIDS Education and Prevention

Editor: Francisco S. Sy, MD, DrPH

NCMHD, National Institutes of Health

6707 Democracy Blvd., Suite 800

Bethesda, MD 20892-5465

Tel: 301-496-7074

Fax: 301-480-4049

E-mail: syf@ncmhd.nih.gov

Website: http://www.atypon-link.com/GPI/loi/aeap?cookieSet=1

American Anthropologist

Editor-in-Chief: Michael Chibnik

Department of Anthropology

University of Iowa

Iowa City, IA 52242

Email: amanthro@uiowa.edu

Website: http://mc.manuscriptcentral.com/aman

American Ethnologist Journal

Editor-in-Chief: Angelique Haugerud

P.O. Box 1185

Davis, CA 95617

E-mail: haugerud@rci.rutgers.edu

Website: http://americanethnologist.org/for-contributors/guidelines-for-articles/

American Journal of Public Health

Executive Editor, Nancy J. Johnson, MA

APHA

800 I Street NW

Washington, DC 20001

Tel: 202-777-2465

Email: ajph.submissions@apha.org

Website: http://www.ajph.org/

American Journal of Sociology

Editor: Andrew Abbott

5835 S. Kimbark Avenue

Chicago, IL 60637-1684

Tel: 773-702-8580

Fax: 773-702-6207

Email: ajs@press.uchicago.edu

Website: http://www.journals.uchicago.edu/AJS/home.html

***Cross Cultural Research* (formerly *Behavior Science Research*)**

Editor: Melvin Ember

Human Relations Area Files

755 Prospect Street

New Haven, CT 06511

Email: Melvin.ember@yale.edu

Website: http://ccr.sagepub.com/

Culture, Health and Sexuality

Editor: Peter Aggleton

Thomas Coram Research Unit

Institute of Education, University of London

27-28 Woburn Square

London WC1H 0AA UK

Submit online: http://mc.manuscriptcentral.com/tchs

Website: http://www.informaworld.com/smpp/title~content=t713693164

Field Methods

Dr. H. Russell Bernard

Department of Anthropology

University of Florida

1112 Turlington Hall

Gainesville, FL 32606

E-mail: ufruss@ufl.edu

Website: http://www.sagepub.com/journals/Journal200810/manuscript Submission

Health Affairs

Editor-in-Chief: Andrew Weil

Email: aweil@projecthope.org

Website: https://mc.manuscriptcentral.com/ha

Health Education and Behavior

Editor: Marc A. Zimmerman, PhD

Department of Health Behavior and Health Education

School of Public Health

University of Michigan

1420 Washington Heights

Ann Arbor, MI 48109

Email: marcz@umich.edu

Online submission: https://www.editorialmanager.com/heb/

Website: http://heb.sagepub.com/

Human Organization

Editor: Sarah Lyon

Department of Anthropology

University of Kentucky

202 Lafferty Hall

Lexington, KY 40506-0024

Tel: 859-257-5038

Email: humanorg@uky.edu

Website: http://www.sfaa.net/publications/human-organization/authors/

International Journal of Health Economics and Management

Editors-in-Chief: P. P. Barros, L. Dafny, G. David, D. Dranove, M. Pauly, R. Town

Website: http://www.springer.com/public+health/journal/10754

International Journal of STD and AIDS

Editor-in-Chief: W.W. Dinsmore

Royal Society of Medicine Press Ltd.

1 Wimpole Street

London W1G 0AE UK

Tel: 44 (0)20 7290 2921

Fax: 44 (0)20 7290 2929

Email: publishing@rsm.ac.uk

Submit online: http://mc.manuscriptcentral.com/ijsa

Website: http://www.rsmpress.co.uk/std.htm

International Perspectives on Sexual and Reproductive Health

Editor: Fran Althaus

Guttmacher Institute

New York, NY

Email: falthaus@guttmacher.org

Website: http://www.guttmacher.org/guidelines/guidelines_ipsrh.html

International Quarterly of Community Health Education

Editor: Dr. George P. Cernada

PO Box 3585

Amherst, MA 01004

Email: gcernada@schoolph.umass.edu

Website: http://www.baywood.com/journals/PreviewJournals.asp?Id=0272-684x

Journal of Acquired Immune Deficiency Syndrome (JAIDS)

William A. Blattner, MD

Email: lbarrett@ihv.umaryland.edu

Epidemiology

Online submission: http://www.editorialmanager.com/jaids-epidemiology/

Website: www.jaids.com

Journal of Contemporary Ethnography

Editor: Charles Edgley

Department of Anthropology

University of Arkansas

405 Stabler Hall

2801 S. University Avenue

Little Rock, AR 72204

Tel: 501-569-3173

Website: http://www.sagepub.com/journals/Journal200975/manuscript Submission

Journal of Family Practice

Editor-in-Chief: John Hickner, MD, MSc

Managing Editor: Jeff Bauer

Email: jfp.eic@gmail.com

Website: http://www.jfponline.com/corporate-links/journal-info/author-guidelines.html

Journal of Immigrant and Minority Health

Editor: Sana Loue

Case Western Reserve University School of Medicine

Cleveland, OH

Website: http://link.springer.com/journal/10903

Journal of Interpersonal Violence

Editor: Jon R. Conte

School of Social Work JH-30

University of Washington

4101 15th Avenue, N.E.

Seattle, WA 98195

Website: http://www.sagepub.com/journals/Journal200855/manuscript Submission

Journal of Social Issues

Editor: Rick Hoyle

Department of Psychology and Neuroscience

Box 90086, 9 Flowers Drive

Duke University

Durham, NC 27708-0086

Tel: 919-660-5791

Fax: 919-660-5728

Email: rhoyle@duke.edu

Journal of Women's Health

Editor-in-Chief: Susan G. Kornstein, MD

Virginia Commonwealth University School of Medicine

Journal of Women's Health

3805 Cutshaw Ave., Suite 504

Richmond, VA 23230

Tel: 802-457-3635

Fax: 802-457-3649

Email: jwh@vcu.edu

Submit online: http://mc.manuscriptcentral.com/womenshealth

Website: http://www.liebertpub.com/publication.aspx?pub_id=42

***Lancet* (England)**

32 Jamestown Road

London NW1 7BY UK

Tel: 44 (0) 20 7424 4910

Fax: 44 (0) 20 7424 4911

Email (inquiries only): editorial@lancet.com

Website: http://ees.elsevier.com/thelancet/

Lancet Global Health

Editor: Zoë Mullan

Email: globalhealth@lancet.com

Website: http://www.thelancet.com/langlo/information-for-authors

Medical Anthropology

Steve Ferzacca

University of Lethbridge

Department of Anthropology

4401 University Drive

Lethbridge, AB T1K 3M4, Canada

Tel: 403-329-2489

Fax: 403-329-5109

Email: medanth@uleth.ca

Submit online: http://www.uleth.ca/medanth/index.php?journal=medanth

Website: http://www.tandf.co.uk/journals/titles/01459740.asp

Medical Anthropology Quarterly

Editor: Clarence C. Gravlee, PhD

Department of Anthropology

University of Florida

Email: cgravlee@ufl.edu

Website: https://mc.manuscriptcentral.com/maq

PLoS Medicine

Editor: Virginia Barbour

Email: plosmedicine@plos.org

Submit online: http://medicine.plosjms.org/cgi-bin/main.plex

Website: http://medicine.plosjournals.org

Population Research and Policy Review

Editor: David A. Swanson

Submit online: http://www.editorialmanager.com/popu/

Website: http://www.springer.com/social+sciences/demography/journal/11113

Psychology & Health

Paul Norman, Editor

Department of Psychology

University of Sheffield

Sheffield, UK S10 2TP

Tel: (44-114) 2226505

Fax: (44-114) 2766515

Email: P. Norman@sheffield.ac.uk

Website: https://mc.manuscriptcentral.com/ehps-journal

Qualitative Health Research

Editor: Janice M. Morse, PhD

International Institute for Qualitative Methodology

6-10 University Extension Center

Edmonton, Alberta T6G 2T4 Canada

Submit online: http://mc.manuscriptcentral.com/qhr

Website: http://qhr.sagepub.com/

Qualitative Inquiry

Editors: Norman K. Denzin and Yvonna Lincoln

Department of Sociology

University of Illinois

810 South Wright Street, 228 Gregory Hall

Urbana, IL 61801

Tel: 217-333-1950

Fax: 217-333-5225

Email: n-denzin@uiuc.edu

Website: http://qix.sagepub.com/

Qualitative Sociology

Editor: Javier Auyero

Qualitative Sociology

Sociology Department

SUNY at Stony Brook

Stony Brook, NY 11794-4356

Tel: 631-632-4884

Fax: 631-632-8203

Email: Qualitative_Sociology@notes.cc.sunysb.edu

Website: http://www.springer.com/social+sciences/sociology/journal/11133

Reproductive Health Matters

Editor: Shirin Heidar, PhD

444 Highgate Studios

53-79 Highgate Road

London NW5 1 TL UK

Tel: 44 20 7267 6567

Fax: 44 20 7267 2551

Email: SHeidari@rhmjournal.org.uk

Website: http://www.rhmjournal.org.uk/

Sexual Health

Editors: Christopher Fairly and Roy Chan

Sexual Health

CSIRO Publishing

PO Box 1139 (150 Oxford Street)

Collingwood, Vic. 3066 Australia

Email: publishing.sh@csiro.au

Website: http://www.publish.csiro.au/nid/164.htm

Sexually Transmitted Diseases

Editor: Julius Schachter, PhD

Managing Editor: Jeanne Moncada

Tel: (415) 824-5115

Fax: (415) 821-8945

Email: std@itsa.ucsf.edu

Submit online: http://www.editorialmanager.com/std/

Website: www.stdjournal.com

Sexually Transmitted Infections

Editors: Dr. Helen Ward and Professor Rob Miller

BMA House

Tavistock Square

London WC1H 9JR UK

Tel: 44 (0) 20 7383 6204

Fax: 44 (0) 20 7383 6668

Email: sti@bmjgroup.com

Submit online: http://sextrans.bmj.com/ifora/

Website: http://sti.bmj.com/

Social Science and Medicine

Editor-in-Chief: E. Annandale

Submit online: http://www.ees.elsevier.com/ssm/

Sociological Quarterly

Editors: Betty A. Dobratz and Lisa K. Waldner

Managing Editor: Leslie B. Kawaler

Iowa State University

Email: tsq@iastate.edu

Website: https://mc.manuscriptcentral.com/socq

Studies in Family Planning

Managing Editor: Gary Bologh

Studies in Family Planning

Population Council

One Dag Hammarskjold Plaza

New York, NY, 10017

Email: sfp@popcouncil.org

Website: http://www.popcouncil.org/publications/sfp/default.htm

Symbolic Interaction

Editor-in-Chief: Robert Dingwall

Managing Editor: Patricia Hulme

Nottingham Trent University

Nottingham NG1 4BU UK

Web: https://mc.manuscriptcentral.com/si

Tropical Medicine and International Health

Managing Editor: Susanne Groener

London School of Hygiene and Tropical Medicine

Keppel Street

London WC1E 7HT UK

Tel: 44 20 7927 2433

Fax: 44 20 7637 4314

Email: susanne.groener@lshtm.ac.uk

Submit online: http://www.editorialmanager.com/tmih/

Website: http://www.blackwellpublishing.com/journal.asp?ref=1360-2276

World Health and Population

Editor-in-Chief: John E. Paul, PhD

260 Adelaide Street East, No. 8

Toronto ON M5A 1N1 Canada

Tel: 416-864-9667

Fax: 416-368-4443

Email: DKent@longwoods.com

Website: http://www.longwoods.com/home.php?cat=381

APPENDIX 14

WHO IS AN AUTHOR?

In qualitative research, the data collection and analysis phases tend to be less temporally distinct than in quantitative research, and team members who collect study data are called on to conduct iterative analysis as they go. Such active participation by all study team members in refining questions, coding data, and generating insights has implications for authorship roles on study papers. Although different journals have different rules for authorship, this one, by the International Committee of Medical Journal Editors (2003), is most widely accepted:

- Authorship credit should be based on (1) substantial contributions to conception and design, or acquisition of data, or analysis and interpretation of data; (2) drafting the article or revising it critically for important intellectual content; and (3) final approval of the version to be published. Authors should meet conditions 1, 2, and 3.
- When a large, multicenter group has conducted the work, the group should identify the individuals who accept direct responsibility for the manuscript. These individuals should fully meet the criteria for authorship defined previously, and editors will ask these individuals to complete journal-specific author and conflict of interest disclosure forms. When submitting a group authored manuscript, the corresponding author should clearly indicate the preferred citation and should clearly identify all individual authors as well as the group name. Journals will generally list other members of the group in the acknowledgments. The National Library of Medicine indexes the group name and the names of individuals the group has identified as being directly responsible for the manuscript.
- Acquisition of funding, collection of data, or general supervision of the research group, alone, does not justify authorship.

- All persons designated as authors should qualify for authorship, and all those who qualify should be listed.
- Each author should have participated sufficiently in the work to take public responsibility for appropriate portions of the content.
- Some journals now also request that one or more authors, referred to as "guarantors," be identified as the persons who take responsibility for the integrity of the work as a whole, from inception to published article, and publish that information.
- Increasingly, authorship of multicenter trials is attributed to a group. All members of the group who are named as authors should fully meet the previous criteria for authorship.
- The order of authorship on the byline should be a joint decision of the co-authors. Authors should be prepared to explain the order in which authors are listed.

International Committee of Medical Journal Editors. (2003). Uniform requirements for manuscripts submitted to biomedical journals. Available at http://www.icmje.org.

INDEX

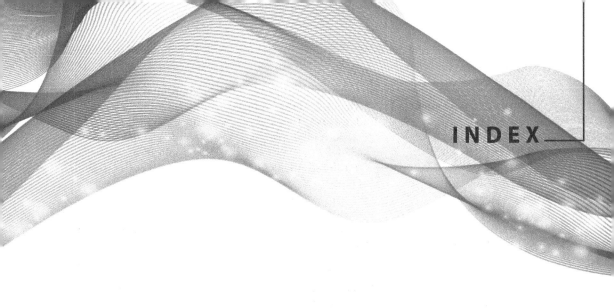

Q

S